Introduction to Breast Care

by

CAROL BIRD

RGN, DNCERT, Diploma in Community Health, OND

District Nursing Sister
Morecambe Health Centre, Morecambe

W

WHURR PUBLISHERS
LONDON AND PHILADELPHIA

© 2003 Whurr Publishers Ltd
First published 2003
by Whurr Publishers Ltd
19b Compton Terrace
London N1 2UN England and
325 Chestnut Street, Philadelphia PA 19106 USA

Reprinted 2004

British Library Cataloguing in Publication Data

A catalogue record for this book
is available from the British Library.

ISBN 1 86156 357 4

Typeset by Adrian McLaughlin, a@microguides.net
Printed and bound in the UK by Athenæum Press Ltd, Gateshead, Tyne & Wear.

Contents

Preface

As a former breast care nurse and now as a community nurse, I have seen first-hand what a devastating effect a breast cancer diagnosis has on a woman and her family. One in nine women in the UK will be diagnosed with this disease and some will die from it despite advances in research and technology. It is vital that the patient receives holistic, sensitive care from diagnosis through to outcome from a committed multidisciplinary team. The breast care nurse is a vital part of this team as often she is the health care professional with whom the patient will have the most contact. She is the person to whom the patient turns for support and information. The breast care nurse is often privy to confidences and private thoughts.

This book is intended to help student and qualified nurses, and newly appointed breast care nurses to care for patients with breast cancer from screening and diagnosis through to outcome. A chapter on benign breast disease is included as these patients too require sensitive, holistic care.

The impact of a breast cancer diagnosis affects all patients and their families differently. This book will endeavour to give straightforward, evidence-based factual information. Recent studies have been included so that information is as up to date as possible.

The book commences with the anatomy and physiology of the breast, risk factors for breast cancer and genetics. The chapters move in a logical order through diagnosis and surgical treatments, adjuvant therapies and psychological care. National government strategies relating to breast cancer are discussed. The Breast Screening Programme and the importance of breast awareness are also covered. Chapters relating to lymphoedema, prosthetics and complementary therapies are included as are chapters on fungating wounds and advanced breast cancer. However, palliative care is a vast, specialized subject in its own right and it is beyond the scope of this book to include much detail. Chapter 15 concentrates on areas relevant to advanced breast cancer, but symptom control, hospice care and loss and grief can be found in texts devoted to palliative care.

In breast cancer, as in other fields in medicine and nursing, there are constant developments and advances in research and treatments. Therefore although every effort has been made to keep the text as up to date as possible, it is impossible to include all new developments especially those in areas such as chemotherapy and endocrine therapies.

The role of the nurse is emphasised throughout. It is also, however, beyond the scope of this book to discuss in depth financial aspects and employment and benefit issues but, where applicable, the appropriate agency or professional through which information can be accessed is suggested.

This book is intended to be useful to all nurses who meet and care for patients with breast problems. I hope that it will broaden the reader's knowledge about breast cancer and ability to help the patients and families to cope with this disease.

I also hope that this book will encourage the reader's interest and enthusiasm for breast care nursing, which although challenging is extremely rewarding. If the reader wishes to learn more about breast care in the future it will have achieved its goal. I feel very privileged to have been given the chance to care for women with breast cancer and for their families.

Acknowledgements

I am extremely grateful to all the people who have helped with my research, especially all those at the North Lancs and South Cumbria Breast Care Unit, but also to other friends and colleagues who have been so helpful and supportive. Thanks also to the staff of the Rosemere Cancer Centre at the Royal Preston Hospital for the time spent in the radiotherapy unit. In no particular order I would like to thank the following: Jose Bates, Noelle Bennett, Deborah Booth, Heather Cruickshank, Clare Fox, Dr Janet Lavelle, Dorothy Loxam, Chris McCann, Marie Rodden, Moya Ruddick, Lizzie Watson, Sheila Whittaker and Helen Williams.

Special thanks to Barbara Moss who, as a breast care nurse, was an inspiration to both patients and practitioners.

Thank you to my hugely supportive and long-suffering husband, daughters, friends and my colleagues and friends at Morecambe Health Centre.

Lastly, thank you to the women I have cared for with breast problems. They are all, without exception, very special.

CHAPTER ONE

Physiology of the breast

Anatomy and physiology

The two normal female adult breasts contain mammary glands which are modified sweat glands that produce milk. The breasts lie over the pectoralis major and serratus anterior muscles. They are attached to these by a layer of fascia (irregular, dense connective tissue) called the ligaments of Cooper. The size of the breast is determined by the amount of fat around the glandular or milk-secreting tissue rather than by the amount of glandular tissue itself. The mammary glands are structurally related to the skin but functionally related to the reproductive system as they produce milk to nourish offspring.

The breast is composed of two separate functional parts. The first part is the epithelial component and is concerned with production, secretion and ejection of breast milk. These functions are known as lactation and are associated with pregnancy and childbirth. The second part consists of all the other tissues making up and supporting the breast. These tissues include fat, fascia and muscles. In non-pregnant women and men the mammary glands are relatively underdeveloped. The Cooper's ligaments supporting the breast become looser with age or with stress caused by long-term vigorous exercise.

In each breast are 15–20 divisions of glandular tissue called lobes, which are arranged radially. Each lobe is separated by adipose tissue and is further divided into lobules that are separated and supported by fibrous tissue. Each lobule contains small, sac-like alveoli that produce and hold breast milk. The alveoli are embedded in connective tissue and are surrounded by spindle-shaped cells called myoepithelial cells, which are muscular and contract to propel milk towards the nipple during lactation. Milk collects in small ducts called terminal ducts, which then lead to the mammary ducts. These drain the alveoli and open onto the surface of the nipple, converging towards the nipple like the spokes of a wheel. There are

1

about 20 of these mammary ducts. Each duct drains milk from a different lobe of the breast. Close to the nipple the mammary ducts expand and form lactiferous sinuses. Some milk may be stored here before draining into a lactiferous duct, which then carries milk to the exterior.

It is important that this arrangement is understood when exploring cancer development. Most breast cancers form in the ducts of the breast. When the disease is confined to the ducts it is non-invasive and does not spread initially. This is known as ductal carcinoma *in situ* and is often classed as a pre-cancerous condition. It is always treated to reduce the chance of invasive cancer developing. The upper outer quadrant of the breast has the most ducts and therefore this is where most breast cancers occur. When the cancer cells break out of the duct it is known as invasive or infiltrating ductal carcinoma. This is the most common type of breast cancer.

The coloured area around the nipple is known as the areola. In lactation, there is a lactiferous sinus just below the areola where milk accumulates.

Blood supply

The breast receives its blood supply from two main sources. The internal mammary artery runs down on either side behind the sternum. The artery gives off perforating branches to the breast that enter under its surface between the ribs. The lateral thoracic artery is a branch of the axillary artery. This reaches the breast from under the arm up in the armpit. The acromiothoracic and intercostal arteries supply further blood to the breast.

When trying to understand breast cancer and how it spreads, knowledge of the blood supply is very important. The most common method of cancer spread in the case of the breast is by direct invasion and via the lymphatics (see 'Lymphatic drainage' section later in this chapter). Lymph vessels draining an organ run alongside the arteries which supply that organ with blood. The lymph drainage from the breast will be along the lymph vessels running with the internal mammary and lateral thoracic arteries. However, spread via blood vessels (haematogenous spread) also occurs. Breast cancer can spread to other organs by this route including brain, liver, lungs and ovaries.

Blood drains from the breast via the veins that run with the arteries mentioned above. This is important in the case of the intercostals veins as these connect with the azygos veins deep in the chest and therefore allow cancer to spread to the spinal column – a site to which breast cancer can spread.

The spread of breast cancer is dependent also on establishment of a blood supply to the tumour. This is accomplished by the extension of existing blood vessels into the tumour mass by the growth of the cells that line the intruding blood vessels. Highly vascular tumours are large and more likely to spread to other organs.

Development and function

Oestrogens produced in the ovary and circulated by follicular cells are important as they promote development and maintenance of female reproductive structures including the breasts (Tortora and Grabowski 1996). These oestrogens cause the breast to develop rapidly at puberty. During a woman's life the breast is constantly under the influence of hormonal stimulation and does not enter a resting phase until after the menopause. Then oestrogen output virtually ceases and the size of the breasts may reduce.

The discrepancy between glandular and adipose tissue in the breast allows the lobes to be felt on breast palpation. The difference in density is the basis for mammographic imaging. The ducts of the breast are not usually palpable unless they contain tumour or are inflamed or engorged with milk.

Young women's breasts are mostly composed of glandular tissue and are firm. As women age the lobes involute (shrivel) due to loss of density and are replaced by fat. Therefore they become softer and easier to examine and image with mammography.

Glandular tissue is very sensitive and many changes take place in the breast during the menstrual cycle. These changes are most evident prior to menstruation when oestrogen and progesterone are peaking. The breast glandular tissue may enlarge and become tender and painful in some women. After the menopause hormone levels are low and the breast becomes less tender and is easier to examine.

Considerable changes are also undergone during lactation. Milk formation after pregnancy is under hormonal control. In pregnancy high oestrogen and progesterone levels prepare the alveolar glands for the production of milk. The synthesis of milk after pregnancy is caused by prolactin from the anterior pituitary gland. Prolactin is a principal hormone in promoting lactation. It is released in response to prolactin releasing hormone, which is secreted by the hypothalamus. During pregnancy the high progesterone levels inhibits prolactin so no milk is secreted. After delivery the oestrogen and progesterone levels in the blood reduce and the inhibition is removed.

The sucking action initiates nerve impulses to the posterior pituitary gland via the hypothalamus. These stimulate oxytocin release, which causes the myoepithelial cells around the walls of the alveoli to contract therefore ejecting milk. Milk moves from the alveoli of the mammary glands into the ducts where it can be suckled from the nipple.

Congenital problems and variations on normal are often seen. Up to five per cent of the population present with aberrant breast tissue and super-numerary and accessory nipples. Breast asymmetry and hypoplasia are often caused by defects in the pectoral muscles. Unilateral enlargement of the breast or general uncontrolled overgrowth of breast tissue in adoles-cent girls can cause concern especially if pain and discomfort are also present.

Uncontrolled overgrowth of the breast tissue can be seen in adolescent girls who have a normal hormonal profile and can be severe enough to require breast reduction surgery for cosmetic and social reasons (Leinster et al. 2000).

Lymphatic drainage

A knowledge of the lymphatic drainage of the breast is necessary because cancerous cells from tumours often spread to other parts of the body via the lymphatic system.

The circulatory system brings many substances to cells and then removes waste products accumulated as a result of metabolism. Many addi-tional substances including excess fluid and protein molecules are returned to the blood as lymph. This is a specialized fluid formed in the tis-sue spaces that is transported via specialized lymphatic vessels to re-enter the circulatory system. The lymphatic system also includes lymph nodes and lymphatic organs such as the spleen and thymus.

Lymph nodes are located in clusters along the pathway of lymphatic ves-sels. Some are the size of a pinhead; others are larger. Lymph nodes perform biological filtration of bacteria and other abnormal cells. Knowledge of lymph node location is vital when surgery for breast cancer is being performed. Lymph passes through the node and is filtered so that cancer cells are removed and prevented from entering the blood. Axillary nodes are removed during breast cancer surgery as they may contain can-cer cells filtered out of the lymph drained from the breast.

Unfortunately cancer cells from a single breast tumour can often spread to other areas of the body via the lymph system. Swollen but pain-free lymph nodes can be a result of cancer spreading via the lymph system and infiltrating the nodes (Hubbard and Mechan 1997). Knowledge of the loca-tion of nodes and flow of lymph is important when diagnosing metastatic spread. Secondary tumour sites are predictable by the direction of lymph flow from the organ primarily involved (Tortora and Grabowski 1996).

Following lymph node removal a patient may suffer from lymphoedema (swelling of the arm), which will be discussed in Chapter 12.

Pathology of breast tumours

How a tumour develops

A cancerous tumour is an expanding mass of disorganized tissue produced by the multiplication of abnormal cells. A tumour may develop when exposed to a carcinogen (Richardson 1995). External agents such as a chemical or virus, or further genetic alterations can promote tumour development by causing irreversible changes to the DNA. These agents do not change the structure of DNA but stimulate normal growth-controlling genes (proto-oncogenes) into abnormal expression as oncogenes (tumour causing genes). The resulting changes may progress to malignancy first as a pre-invasive lesion then as invasive cancer. The malignant tumour will invade adjacent tissue, destroying it and metastasizing via the lymph and blood (Mera 1997). A tumour can also develop a blood supply of its own and will sometimes outgrow it causing necrosis in the middle.

Most malignant breast tumours originate in epithelial cells in the undifferentiated terminal structures of the mammary gland, an area called Lob 1, and are classified as carcinomas. Lob 1 is particularly sensitive to carcinogens. Pregnancy and breastfeeding reduce the amount of Lob 1 in the breast (Brashers 1998).

The tumour cells infiltrating the tissue are surrounded by dense connective tissue, which is produced by the body in response to the tumour. This dense tissue pulls on the adjacent tissue causing skin puckering and nipple retraction, which are typical signs of a malignant lesion. The tumour feels firm on palpation and does not have sharp margins as it infiltrates into surrounding tissue (Damjanov 1996).

Malignant breast tumours can be divided into *in situ* and invasive cancers.

In situ carcinomas

There are three types of *in situ* carcinomas – ductal carcinoma *in situ* (DCIS), lobular carcinoma *in situ* (LCIS) and Paget's disease. Although generally classed as pre-invasive, each has the potential to progress to invasive carcinoma.

DCIS (Ductal carcinoma in situ or intraduct carcinoma)

In pure DCIS malignant cells are confined to the ducts of the lobules and there is no invasion of surrounding tissue. The tumour cells cannot metastasize to other areas of the body as the ducts do not contain blood or lymphatic vessels. Up to 20 per cent of screening cancers are pure DCIS but sometimes it may present as a palpable mass, Paget's disease or nipple discharge. There is a proliferation of cells with cytological features of malignancy within the ducts. Several patterns can frequently be seen in the same lesion, so whereas previously DCIS was classified according to the architectural pattern (for example comedo, cribriform, solid) now more emphasis is placed on nuclear grade. Currently DCIS is divided into three grades: high, intermediate and low based on size and pleomorphism of the nuclei.

DCIS can progress to invasive carcinoma if not completely excised. It is not clear how long it takes to progress or how many cancers do become invasive, although some studies suggest 30–40 per cent. Low grade DCIS is less likely to progress than high and intermediate. If excision is inadequate DCIS or invasive carcinoma may recur.

LCIS (Lobular carcinoma in situ)

In LCIS the lobules at the end of the mammary ducts are filled with a uniform population of regular tumour cells which may spread along adjacent ducts. These cells distort the ducts and may often undergo necrosis (Kumar et al. 1997).

As LCIS usually does not produce a mass and is not usually found on a mammogram, it is generally an incidental finding. There may be a slight association with adjacent calcification. It tends to be multifocal and bilateral, complicating the approach to treatment. It is generally regarded as a risk indication for the development of carcinoma – about 10 times that of the general population and carrying a 20 per cent risk of developing cancer in 10–15 years time.

Paget's disease

This is a manifestation of high-grade comedo DCIS in which the malignant cells (Paget cells) extend from the subareolar ducts to the epidermis of the nipple. Here they can be seen lying either singly or in groups between the squamous cells. Between a third and a half of cases have an associated invasive cancer. Women affected are usually in a slightly older age group than those who experience the usual invasive ductal carcinoma (Kumar et al. 1997). There may be a palpable mass in the breast. Involved areolar skin tends to be fissured and ulcerated.

Invasive carcinomas

It is important that pathologists recognize that there are a number of differing types of invasive breast carcinoma, based on the cell morphology and histological pattern. They may have different prognoses and therefore choice of treatment will be affected.

Invasive ductal carcinoma

This is the commonest type, accounting for 50–70 per cent of invasive cancers. They usually have an irregular stellate outline, are firm to palpate and are gritty when cut. They often accompany DCIS.

Invasive lobular carcinoma

This accounts for 10–15 per cent of invasive cancers. These cancers may be bilateral or multifocal. They consist of small regular tumour cells, which infiltrate in a diffuse manner. Contralateral disease is more common in patients with infiltrating lobular carcinoma. Patients who have had treatment for breast cancer should have regular follow-ups to detect cancer in the second breast (Orel et al. 1992). Development of contralateral disease is associated with the risk of distant recurrence (Heron et al. 2000).

Tubular carcinoma

This accounts for two per cent of symptomatic cancers but up to 15 per cent of screen detected. Tubular structures form a well-differentiated carcinoma. Little cell activity is displayed and the prognosis is good.

Mucinous carcinoma

This is commoner in older women and will form two per cent of invasive cancers. Nests of tumour cells compose well-differentiated gelatinous masses. The prognosis is better than the usual invasive cancers (Kumar et al. 1997).

Medullary carcinoma

This represents one per cent of invasive cancers. It is usually found in postmenopausal women. Again, the prognosis is good.

Inflammatory breast cancer

This is a rare form of breast cancer which affects a small number of women. The cancer cells block the lymph vessels in the skin of the breast giving the breast an acutely inflamed appearance. The lymph nodes may be swollen. Inflammatory breast cancer grows rapidly and often spreads to other sites. It can be mistaken for an infection so treatment may be delayed. Systemic treatment and then surgery are usually necessary. The prognosis is poor but as treatment methods improve the prognosis improves slightly.

Staging

Staging is used to determine the extent of the disease beyond the primary site, therefore the need for adjuvant treatment can be determined. The stage may determine whether or not the patient will undergo surgery. It is also important to determine the prognosis. A small, early, localized tumour is likely to carry a good prognosis whereas an advanced tumour with metastases will have a poor prognosis.

Tumour differentiation

Prognostic information can be gained by grading the degree of differentiation of the tumour. The degree of tubule formation, nuclear pleomorphism and frequency of cell division are graded from one to three (Sainsbury et al. 2000). These are added and the tumour is given a final grade of 1, 2 or 3. A grade 3 tumour will show no glandular formation and its cells will have large pleomorphic nuclei and show frequent mitoses. A grade 1 tumour will show many glands and will be composed of small tumour cells with few mitoses. Therefore, a grade 3 tumour will show an aggressive nature and suggest a poorer prognosis. This histological grade is an important predictor of disease free and overall survival.

Other features in a tumour are of value in predicting local recurrence and prognosis.

Vascular or lymphatic invasion

Any cancer cells in the lymphatic or blood vessels are an indicator of more aggressive disease. The number of lymph nodes involved and the level of axillary involvement is important. A patient with this feature is at risk from local and systemic recurrence (Sainsbury et al. 2000). Ten-year survival drops to 25–30 per cent for patients with positive nodes from 70 per cent for patients with negative nodes.

Extensive *in situ* component

If more than 25 per cent of the main tumour consists of non-invasive disease and there is *in situ* cancer in the surrounding tissue, the cancer is classified as having an extensive *in situ* component. Local recurrence is more likely following breast conservation surgery (Sainsbury et al. 2000).

Staging of invasive breast cancers

On diagnosis of a breast cancer the extent of disease is assessed and the tumour staged in order for the most appropriate treatment to be established. This is performed on the basis of the gross appearance of the tumour and how it has spread to lymph nodes and distant organs. There appear to be three major classification systems.

The 4 stage system

Stage 1 – early disease – the tumour less than 2.5cm and confined to the breast; 5-year survival rate is 80 per cent.

Stage 2 – early disease – the tumour is 2–5cm; there is some spread to the axillary lymph nodes; 5-year survival rate is 65 per cent.

Stage 3 – locally advanced disease – the tumour is more than 5cm; it has spread to chest wall; there is involvement of supraclavicular or internal mammary nodes; 5-year survival rate is 40 per cent.

Stage 4 – advanced disease – the tumour is any size; metastases are present at distant sites, for example bone, brain, liver, lungs; 5-year survival rate is 10 per cent (Damjanov 1996).

Stages 1 and 2 are potentially curable with surgery and chemotherapy and/or radiotherapy and anti-hormone drugs. Stages 3 and 4 are advanced where symptom control is a priority.

This system may also be known as the Manchester Staging System (Denton 1996).

The TNM system

The International Union against Cancer details this system (Tumour, Node, Metastasis) as given below:

T – Tumour stage
Tx – Cannot be assessed
T0 – No evidence of primary tumour
Tis – Carcinoma *in situ*
T1 – Tumour 2cm or less in its greatest dimension
T2 – Tumour greater than 2cm but less than 5cm
T3 – Tumour greater than 5cm
T4 – Tumour of any size with direct extension to chest wall or skin

N – Lymph node stage
Nx – Cannot be assessed
N0 – No nodal metastases detected
N1 – Metastasis to mobile nodes on same side
N2 – Metastasis to nodes on the same side that are fixed to each other or another structure
N3 – Metastasis to internal mammary nodes on the same side

M – Metastasis stage

Mx – Cannot be assessed

M0 – No distant metastasis present

M1 – Distant metastasis present (Sobin and Wittekind 1997).

The Nottingham prognostic index (NPI)

This is often used as a prognostic tool. It gives an accurate prediction of survival for women with breast cancer and aids the decision regarding adjuvant therapy. An equation is used:

The size of the tumour (cm) by 0.2 + the grade (1–3) + the nodal status (1–3).

1 = no nodes involved.

2 = 1–3 nodes involved.

3 = > 3 nodes involved.

The higher the final figure the worse the prognosis.

A NPI of < 3 = 90 per cent 15-year survival rate and no adjuvant therapy.

A NPI of 3.01–3.4 = 80 per cent 15-year survival rate and no adjuvant therapy.

A NPI of 3.41-4.4 = 50 per cent 15-year survival rate. If the patient is ER+ = endocrine therapy. If ER- = chemotherapy.

A NPI of 4.41–5.3 = 30 per cent 15-year survival rate. Adjuvant therapy as above.

A NPI of >5.4 = 8 per cent 15-year survival rate. Adjuvant therapy as above but administer chemotherapy only if the patient is fit enough (Galea et al. 1992).

Hormone receptors

Oestrogen receptors are proteins present on the cell surface of breast cells and on breast tumours. Oestrogen binds to these receptors and stimulates growth factor production. This results in uncontrolled cell proliferation in malignant cells. Oestrogen and progesterone status can be assessed where labelled antibodies against the receptors are applied to tissue sections. Sixty per cent of tumours are considered ER positive. These tend to have a better prognosis. Many tumours also have progesterone receptors (PR). These also carry a better prognosis. Receptor status provides information as to the likely response to adjuvant therapies (Brashers 1998). More information on oestrogen receptors can be found in Chapter 9.

Other prognostic markers

Other markers of prognosis are constantly being sought. These include angiogenesis (a high density of new vessels indicates a worse prognosis), peptide growth factors and receptors such as epidermal growth factor (EGF) and its receptor (EGFR – this is associated with a poor prognosis), proliferation markers, for example Ki 67 or PCNA, c-erbB-2 and oncogenes and tumour suppressor genes.

Epidemiology

Breast cancer is the most common female cancer in westernized countries, responsible for 20 per cent of all female cancers. In the UK one in five cancers in women are breast cancers and it is estimated that one in nine women will develop breast cancer at some point in their life (Cancer Research Campaign 2001). Mortality from breast cancer in this country is among the highest in the world (Evans et al. 1998). Each year there are 14,000 deaths and 38,000 new cases. The incidence appears to be higher in the upper socio-economic groups. Breast cancer is also the commonest cancer in minority ethnic groups in the UK (Cancer Research Campaign 1996).

There is a regional variation in England and Wales – more cases occur in the south in post-menopausal women. However, post-menopausal women account anyway for 80 per cent of breast cancers. Breast cancer does occur in men but is rare, accounting for about 300 cases per year.

Risk factors

Age is the strongest risk factor – the older woman is at greater risk. Although 80 per cent of cases are post-menopausal, nearly 7000 cases per year are pre-menopausal. In addition, one in five cases in women of child bearing age occur when the woman is pregnant or lactating, or in the first year following the birth. Over 1000 women per year are diagnosed in the age group 35–39 years. The rate of increase prior to the menopause suggests that hormonal status is a link (Cancer Research Campaign 1996).

Reproductive factors play a part. The greater the exposure to oestrogen the higher the risk. In countries such as Japan, China, Arabia and Africa where women have an average age of 17 years at menarche, the risk is low. An early age at menarche appears to increase the risk – in the USA the average age is 12.8 years and one in nine women will face breast cancer in their life (Tortora and Grabowski 1996). A late menopause (after 55 years) approximately doubles the risk compared to undergoing the menopause before 45 years. Having a child after the age of 30 years and nulliparity doubles the risk in comparison to the risk of a woman who had a child before the age of 20 years.

A woman who has had benign breast disease proven on biopsy, especially atypical hyperplasia will have an increased risk of malignancy occurring. However, this will only account for 10 per cent of benign biopsy specimens. If a woman has already had cancer in the other breast her risk will be quadrupled.

Ionizing radiation in large quantities is a risk factor but is unlikely to occur under modern clinical conditions (Cancer Research Campaign 1996). Research suggests that young girls who have had thoracic radiotherapy for Hodgkin's disease in the past may be at increased risk of breast cancer. The breast at puberty is very sensitive and it has been suggested that girls under 21 years who have undergone this treatment should be identified and screened. Radiation doses are now lower and radiotherapists try to exclude breast tissue from the radiation field.

The risk of breast cancer occurring due to taking the oral contraceptive and HRT has been studied. There is a small increase in risk of contracting breast cancer during use of the combined oral contraceptive and for 10 years afterwards, but the excess disappears 10 years after the cessation of use (Collaborative Group on Hormonal Factors in Breast Cancer 1996).

Combined HRT (oestrogen and progesterone) is now more common. At present the health benefits of HRT outweigh the disadvantages, but some studies show an increase in risk after more than 10 years of use of unopposed oestrogen. Other evidence suggests that there is an increased risk of about 50 per cent for use of HRT for more than five years (Colditz et al. 1995). However, most studies show that shorter term use is not associated with increased risk. HRT reduces CHD and osteoporosis, which possibly gives an advantage in terms of years of life (Mera 1997). Due to the possibility that oestrogens stimulate the production of growth factors by cancer cells, women who have had breast cancer or who have a family history may be advised to avoid HRT. HRT is discussed in more detail in Chapter 9.

Dietary factors may play a part but this is still unclear. A high fat diet may be a risk but this appears to be inconclusive. Fat intake in an individual's early years may be more significant than during middle age (Hunter and Willett 1996). However, obesity may be a risk factor in postmenopausal women. This may be because oestrogen is stored in adipose tissue and may be released over a longer period than in non-obese women. High alcohol consumption has also been implicated possibly because high alcohol levels can lead to obesity and raise oestrogen levels. Migrants who move from low incidence areas (for example Japan) to high incidence areas (such as the USA) are at greater risk of breast cancer than women who do not migrate. Incidence and mortality is five times higher in the USA than in Japan (Kumar et al. 1997). This difference would appear to be environmental and involve diet and reproductive patterns. The migrants tend to adopt the habits of the host country and vice versa.

Some factors may protect against breast cancer, for example high levels of exercise, breastfeeding and a high-fibre diet rich in fruit and vegetables

(Cancer Research Campaign 1996). Cigarette smoking has been implicated in the past but a recent study has shown that teenage girls who smoke have a 70 per cent greater risk of developing breast cancer in later life. The results showed that the effects of smoking were especially harmful during adolescence when breast tissue is most sensitive to environmental carcinogens. The study also showed that childless women who smoked 20 cigarettes a day for 20 years were also at similar risk (Breast Cancer Care 2002). These results suggest that there is a role for breast care nurses to undertake health promotion in schools to raise the awareness of young girls about the risks of smoking and breast cancer.

Although 11,340 women died of breast cancer in England and Wales in 2000, breast cancer survival rates continue to improve. Earlier diagnosis through breast screening and improved treatments contribute to this (National Institute for Clinical Excellence 2002). Survival rates have increased in recent years. Survival figures at the moment mean staying alive five years after diagnosis. As improvements in screening programmes and treatment are recent, 10-year survival rates are not yet available. If breast cancer is detected at its earliest stage there is a 92 per cent survival rate.

However, research undertaken nearly 10 years ago states that the 10-year survival rate for patients with non-palpable invasive breast cancer of 10mm or less in diameter is over 85 per cent, a better rate by 15–40 per cent than for patients with a palpable breast cancer (Rosen et al. 1993).

The survival rate for patients diagnosed between 1993 and 1995 was 93 per cent at one year and 76 per cent after five years. Five-year survival rates are highest among people aged 50–59 years at diagnosis. Younger and older have a lower survival rate. Survival rates vary with the characteristics of the tumour and the stage at which it was detected. About 50 per cent have early disease at initial diagnosis and have an excellent prognosis. Fewer than five per cent have metastatic disease at diagnosis although the likelihood of an initial advanced cancer diagnosis increases with age (National Institute for Clinical Excellence 2002).

Genetics

The genetic link to breast cancer is widely believed to be common. In actual fact only 5–10 per cent of women are at increased risk due to an inherited form of breast cancer occurring in women in their 30s and 40s. In some families, the high incidence of breast cancer is accompanied by clusters of ovarian cancer (Mera 1997).

Most cases of breast cancer are sporadic in which genetic changes occur only within the cancer cells. However, in a few cases a genetic change will have been inherited. This means that it is present in every cell and can be passed down through the family in each generation. Carriers have a 50 per cent chance of passing the gene down to each of their children but although the risk is increased it does not mean that cancer will definitely develop (Eeles 1996).

BRCA1 and BRCA2

A number of different genes are involved. Since 1990 two highly penetrant autosomal dominant genes have been localized and cloned. (Penetrance is the likelihood of getting the disease.) These are BRCA1 and BRCA2. These account for five per cent of breast cancers showing a clear inherited pattern due to autosomal dominant inheritance (Miki et al. 1994).

BRCA1 is an inherited susceptibility gene present on the long arm of chromosome 17. BRCA1 is a tumour suppressor gene, which plays a part in regulating cell growth and repairing DNA. However, when one copy of BRCA1 is inherited in a defective or mutant form the woman is predisposed to breast or ovarian cancer. More than 100 different types of mutation have been found in BRCA1. Many of these are confined to a very small number of families. It is a large gene and screening for mutations is difficult. Screening is undertaken on samples from affected family members. The test is very difficult technically and takes many months. If a faulty gene is not found it is not possible for subsequent relatives to be tested. If the patient is tested and does not carry a faulty gene the chance of developing breast cancer is the same as the general population.

If the number of breast/ovarian cancer cases within a family increases the probability of detecting a BRCA1 mutation also increases. The lifetime risk of breast cancer if mutations in BRCA1 are detected is 85 per cent and ovarian cancer 30–50 per cent. There is also an increased risk of prostate cancer 8 per cent and bowel cancer 10 per cent (Evans et al. unpublished notes). BRCA1 is associated with medullary cancers in some cases. A high proportion of BRCA1 cancers is grade 3 with a high mitotic frequency and lymphocytic infiltration. They also tend to be oestrogen/progesterone receptor negative and the prognosis may be worse than that of patients who do not have the gene.

BRCA2 is found on the long arm of chromosome 13. Mutations in this area can account for as many inherited breast cancer cases as BRCA1 but probably not as many ovarian cancers. The lifetime risk of breast cancer is 85 per cent and ovarian cancer 20 per cent. This gene is also associated with an increase in male breast cancer and also prostate and bowel cancer (Wooster et al. 1995).

A pattern of malignancies within a pedigree determines which gene is most likely to have a mutation present. Specific mutations occur with increasing frequency. Three mutations – two in BRCA1 and one in BRCA2 – occur frequently in Ashkenazi Jewish women. An estimated 20 per cent of these women affected by breast cancer before the age of 40 years will show a mutation (Eeles 1996). Breast cancers caused by BRCA1 and BRCA2 are generally of early onset (before 40 years). Both breasts may be affected and another woman within the family may also be affected.

Other genetic alterations in breast cancer involve a mutation in oncogenes. When this occurs, the control of cell growth is lost.

P53

P53 is the most common tumour suppressor gene that is mutated in breast cancer. Tumour suppressor genes are part of the normal mechanism that controls the cell cycle. Normal p53 is activated when abnormalities occur in DNA transcription. The cell cycle is arrested and the cell undergoes programmed cell death, therefore the abnormal DNA is prevented from replicating. When mutant p53 replaces the normal, the DNA continues to replicate giving rise to cancer tumours. A tumour containing p53 will have a worse prognosis than one that does not (Leinster et al. 2000).

Li-Fraumeni syndrome is due to an autosomal dominant germline mutation in p53. This is a rare syndrome causing brain tumours, soft tissue and bone sarcomas, adrenocortical carcinomas and early onset breast cancer. Most of these occur early, breast cancer presents before the age of 40 years. Early mammography is recommended.

ErbB, c-erbB-2, and erbB-3

Amplification of erbB, c-erbB-2 and erbB-3 oncogenes is seen in approximately two-thirds of breast cancer patients. Over expression of erbB-2 appears to be linked with a poor prognosis. The c-erbB-2 gene product has been found in post-menopausal patients with a family history of breast cancer, whereas the BRCA1 mutation is generally found in younger women (Leinster et al. 2000).

Cowden's disease

PTEN is the gene involved in Cowden's disease, a rare syndrome of multiple hamartomas of the skin, thyroid, mucous membranes and breast. There is an increased risk of breast cancer associated with the syndrome, possibly occurring in 50 per cent of affected females; 33 per cent are bilateral. The onset can be very young but the average age is 38 years (Hodgson and Maher 1999).

Risk assessment and genetic counselling

Genetic counselling is increasingly in demand to determine risk and measures to reduce it among women with a family history of breast cancer.
Counselling requires an initial assessment of the lifetime risk of developing
breast cancer on the basis of data obtained by taking a thorough family history. This would include information about types of cancer in the family,
ages at onset, bilateral breast diseases and multiple cases. This includes all
first- and second-degree relatives and as many distant relatives as possible
(Hodgson and Maher 1999).

Currently regional genetics services are able to offer genetic testing and
counselling to a small number of these women at the Family History
Clinics. Also some local breast units are able to offer risk assessment to low
and moderate risk women. Some breast care nurses have undergone training and are running clinics for these women.

Women with a family history of breast cancer are advised to visit their
GP who will advise on increased risk or will refer to a cancer genetics clinic or cancer specialist. Information and counselling will be provided and
the patient informed whether they are at low, medium or increased risk.
If there is a strong family history and the woman is at moderate risk she
may be asked to take part in a study which is looking at ways to monitor
people at moderate risk, and will include regular screening (Cancer Bacup
2001).

Risk calculation

Where four first-degree relatives have early onset or bilateral breast cancer
the risk of inheriting a gene is nearly 50 per cent (Evans et al. 1994). About
80 per cent of gene carriers will develop breast cancer in their lifetime.
Therefore, the maximum risk counselled is 40–45 per cent unless there is
significant family history on both sides. A dominant history on a father's
side of the family would give at least a 20–25 per cent lifetime risk to daughters as breast cancer genes can be inherited through the father.

The daughter of a breast cancer gene carrier has a prior risk of 50 per
cent of inheriting the susceptibility so her lifetime risk of developing breast
cancer is about 40 per cent. However, if she remains unaffected after the
age of 50 years her risk will fall because she has lived through a large
amount of her risk period. Most hereditary breast cancers occur at a
younger age (Evans et al. 1994). If she remains healthy the older she
becomes it is less likely that she has inherited the susceptibility. The risk
gradually equalizes to normal after the age of 60 years in those with a family history of breast cancer.

Women who have an identical twin sister with breast cancer are also at least three times more likely to develop breast cancer. Identical twins may gain their increased risk by inheriting the same set of genes. Non-identical twins are at much smaller risk.

If a family history shows an increased risk the woman could be offered a predictive test to ascertain if she carries a BRCA1 or BRCA2 mutation. Permission is requested to offer other at risk family members predictive testing and counselling (Hodgson and Maher 1999).

Criteria for referral to the Family History Clinic

The following criteria are suggested:

1 First-degree relative with breast cancer under 40 years.
2 First-degree relative or one first- and one second-degree relative with breast cancer under 60 years.
3 Three or more cases of breast/ovarian cancer, any age on the same side of the family.
4 One case of breast cancer at less than 50 years and one ovarian cancer on the same side of the family where one is the first-degree relative of the referred patient.
5 Double primary cancer involving breast and ovary, sarcoma or colon when the first occurred at less than 50 years.
6 Breast cancer in father or brother – any age.
7 History of related cancer in mother/father – any age.
8 BRCA1, BRCA2 or Cowden's disease confirmed.
9 Ashkenazi Jewish with breast cancer at less than 60 years or ovarian cancer any age in a close relative.

Women at moderate risk fit the following criteria:

1 First-degree relative with a breast cancer diagnosis at less than 40 years old.
2 First/second-degree relatives with breast cancer diagnosis under 60 years or ovarian cancer at any age.
3 First/second-degree relatives with breast/ovarian cancer at any age.
4 First-degree relative with bilateral breast cancer under 60 years.
5 First-degree male relative with breast cancer at any age.

The relative risk in this group is at least three times that of the general population. Below 30 years no mammogram would be carried out, the patient would be advised on breast awareness. At age 35–49 years annual mammography would be carried out. Screening may be done from five years prior to the age at diagnosis of the relative if this age is greater than 39 years. After 50 years mammograms would be carried out every 18 months (in between screening via the National Breast Screening Programme).

The difference between familial and non-familial breast cancer would be discussed with women at low risk and they would be reassured that their risk is not significantly raised. They would be encouraged to be breast aware and are entered into the screening programme at the appropriate age (British Association of Surgical Oncologists 1998).

Reducing the risk

For a young woman with a significantly increased risk the options are limited. She could be advised to plan her family early, avoid the oral contraceptive pill and HRT, stop smoking and maintain a good diet. She will also be advised to become breast aware and self-examine.

A study published recently suggests that the longer women breastfeed the more they are protected against breast cancer. The study found that the relative risk of breast cancer decreased by 4.3 per cent for every 12 months of breastfeeding in addition to a seven per cent decrease already for each birth. This may explain why breast cancer is less prevalent in countries where having large families and breastfeeding for longer is common (Collaborative Group on Hormonal Factors in Breast Cancer 2002).

Annual screening may identify over 60 per cent of cancers in younger women but the young breast is difficult to interpret as tissue is dense (Tabar et al. 1987). Women are eligible for annual screening from 35 years if at a lifetime risk of one in six (twice the national average) or greater. If breast cancer in a first-degree relative has occurred when the relative was less than 40 years, screening of the patient begins at five years before the age the relative was at diagnosis (for example, if the first-degree relative was 39 years at diagnosis, the patient will be screened from age 34 years). After 50 years mammograms are undertaken every 18 months.

Mammography can detect lesions in the 35–49 year age group especially. Although there is a small theoretical risk of repeated scans inducing a breast cancer, it is generally considered that the benefits of early detection outweigh any possible hazards (Law 1997).

The potential use of MRI (magnetic resonance imaging) for screening women aged 35–50 years at high risk is currently being evaluated. This uses IV contrast and therefore is a more invasive test than mammography but it gives more information on any tumour present. It is the most sensitive practical technique, although it will not detect a proportion of DCIS. Ideally it would be undertaken yearly in high-risk women, but MRI is also extremely expensive.

For some women at very high risk of breast cancer bilateral prophylactic mastectomy may be carried out. These women need to be made aware of the residual risk of cancer following mastectomy leaving the nipple – total mastectomy may be preferable (Hodgson and Maher 1999). Also patients having unilateral mastectomy have to live with the risk of still having breast tissue – contralateral breast cancer is much more likely in gene carriers. A recent report suggests that prophylactic bilateral mastectomy reduces the risk of breast cancer by 90 per cent in those with a BRCA1 mutation (Kennedy et al. 2002). Bilateral breast reconstruction will also be discussed with the patient. Some women may be psychologically unprepared for preventive surgery and may be unhappy with the final result. It is necessary to offer these women extensive counselling.

Prophylactic oopherectomy can reduce the risk of ovarian cancer but cancer can still occur in the abdominal cavity lining (Struewing et al. 1995). Some centres may recommend hysterectomy. These procedures can have a major impact on the patient's sexuality, family planning issues and career as many are young, working women. Extensive support from the multidisciplinary breast team and genetic centre is required.

Tamoxifen is a drug that has been shown to reduce contralateral breast cancer in treated patients by 30–40 per cent. This has been the subject of an international collaborative trial (Powles et al. 1990). Tamoxifen is also well tolerated. However, it does have side effects such as hot flushes, vaginal dryness, altered libido, weight gain and menstrual disturbance. There is also an increased risk of endometrial cancer and uterine sarcoma with long-term Tamoxifen therapy (3–5 years). In post-menopausal women taking Tamoxifen as a preventive measure the potential side effects need to be carefully considered. Many will not develop breast cancer even if they are high risk and will have been given a drug that could cause endometrial disease needlessly (Mera 1997). Tamoxifen may be given as a preventive measure in women of child-bearing age if they are at high risk but they are advised not to become pregnant as Tamoxifen may cause foetal harm. Research and clinical trials into Tamoxifen as a preventive measure are ongoing.

In women who have been treated for DCIS, treatment with Tamoxifen reduces the rate of breast cancer recurrence from 13.4 per cent to 8.2 per cent over five years. However, when the risk of recurrence is low, the absolute benefit is small and the adverse effects such as the increased risk of endometrial cancer should be considered (NICE 2002). (Tamoxifen is discussed more fully in Chapter 9.)

Genetic testing

In the main part research laboratories will test those with a probability of a BRCA1, BRCA2 or p53 mutation. About 60 per cent of women take up the option (Watson et al. 1995). A blood sample from a living affected patient has to be screened prior to testing being offered to at risk family members. Full informed consent is obtained for these tests (Hodgson and Maher 1999).

The highest risk families and Ashkenazi Jews with breast/ovarian cancer in the family are given priority as mutation screening is lengthy. Screening for BRCA1 takes many months although screening for the Ashkenazi mutation takes 4–6 weeks.

Counselling

At the North West Regional Genetic Service each new family is assigned a genetic co-worker. A home visit may be carried out. A detailed family history is taken and concerns and anxieties are addressed. Hospital records, death certificates and cancer registries are consulted to confirm cancer diagnoses and details of the patients. A clinic consultation following this includes discussion of the family history, assessment of risk and discussion of options.

If a genetic screen is decided on the counsellor will provide emotional support and offer counselling/predictive testing to other family members. Individuals eligible for predictive testing once a mutation has been identified will have three counselling sessions prior to blood being taken. The first is an information session, the second explains the test and the third takes place a month later when the individual has had time to reflect.

Counselling involves helping the individual comprehend the way heredity contributes to the disorder, providing information as required, discussing options to manage risk and helping the individual understand the implications of the risk. Support is offered regardless of the decision or outcome of the test.

Patients may have many issues to address, possibly having had to cope with the loss of affected family members. Unresolved grief, anxiety about their own health, concerns about children and fears of testing may be among these.

Individuals at a higher than one in four lifetime risk are given the option to discuss preventive surgery; that is, prophylactic mastectomy. The unknown residual risks are discussed and psychological evaluation is carried out. The possible psychological and family dynamic consequences are discussed. A surgical referral is then made.

A recent report from Professor Peter Harper and commissioned by the Department of Health recommended a three-tier system for screening women with a family history of breast cancer. Those at no significant increased risk should be reassured in primary care. Those at moderate risk should be seen at their local Calman breast unit and those at high risk should be seen by the local Regional Genetics Centre.

At St Mary's Hospital in Manchester an integrated education programme for specialist nurses is in progress to allow low and moderate risk counselling at unit level. This centre also runs the only MSc course in Europe on genetic counselling.

References

Brashers VL (1998) Clinical Applications of Pathophysiology – Assessment, Diagnostic Reasoning and Management. St Louis, MI: Mosby.

Breast Cancer Care (2002) Breast cancer risk up to 70% in teenagers who smoke. www.breastcancercare.org.uk (accessed October 2002).

British Association of Surgical Oncologists (BASO) (1998 Revision) Guidelines for surgeons in the management of symptomatic breast disease in the United Kingdom. The BASO Breast Specialty Group. BASO: London. www.baso.org/breast.html (accessed October 2002).

Cancer Bacup (2001) Genetics in bowel, breast and ovarian cancer. www.cancerbacup.org.uk (accessed August 2002).

Cancer Research Campaign (1996) Breast Cancer. UK Factsheet 6.1. London: CRC.

Cancer Research Campaign (2001) Now Cancer Research UK. http://cancerresearch.org.uk

Colditz GA, Hankinson SE, Hunter DJ, et al. (1995) The Nurses Health study. New England Journal of Medicine 332: 1589–93.

Collaborative Group on Hormonal Factors in Breast Cancer (1996) Breast cancer and hormonal contraceptives: collaborative reanalysis of individual data on 53,297 women with breast cancer and 100,239 women without breast cancer from 54 epidemiological studies. Lancet 347 (9017): 1713–27.

Collaborative Group on Hormonal Factors in Breast Cancer (2002) Breast cancer and breast feeding: collaborative reanalysis of individual data from 47 epidemiological studies in 30 countries including 50,302 women with breast cancer and 96,973 women without the disease. Lancet 360 (9328): 187.

Damjanov I (1996) Pathology for the Health Related Professions. Philadelphia, PA: WB Saunders.

Denton S (1996) (Ed.) Breast Cancer Nursing. London: Chapman and Hall.

Eeles R (1996) Testing for the breast cancer disposition gene BRCA1. British Medical Journal 313: 572–3.

Evans AJ, Wilson ARM, Blamey RW, et al. (1998) Atlas of Breast Disease Management. 50 Illustrative Cases. London: WB Saunders.

Evans DGR, Fentiman IS, McPherson K, Asbury D, Ponder BAJ, Howell A (1994) Familial breast cancer. British Medical Journal 308: 183–7.

Galea MH, Blamey RW, Elston CW, Ellis IO (1992) The Nottingham Prognostic Index in primary breast cancer. Breast Cancer Research and Treatment 22: 207–19.

Heron DE, Komarnicky LT, Hyslop T, et al. (2000) Bilateral breast carcinoma: Risk factors and outcomes for patients with synchronous and metachronus disease. Cancer 88(12): 2739–50.

Hodgson S, Maher E (1999) A practical guide to human cancer genetics. Cambridge: Cambridge University Press.

Hubbard J, Mechan D (1997) The Physiology of Health and Illness with Related Anatomy. Cheltenham: Stanley Thornes.

Hunter DJ, Willett WC (1996) Nutrition and breast cancer. Cancer Causes and Control 7: 56–68.

Kennedy RD, Quinn JE, Johnston PG, Harkin DP (2002) BRCA1: mechanisms of inactivation and implications for management of patients. Lancet 360(9338): 1007–14.

Kumar V, Cotran SC, Robbins SL (1997) Basic Pathology. 6th edn. Philadelphia, PA: WB Saunders.

Law J (1997) Cancers detected and induced in mammographic screening: new screening schedules and younger women with a family history. British Journal of Radiology 70(829): 62–9.

Leinster SJ, Gibbs TJ, Downey H (2000) Shared Care for Breast Disease. Oxford: Isis Medical Media.

Mera S (1997) Pathology and Understanding Disease Prevention. Cheltenham: Stanley Thornes.

Miki Y, Swensen J, Shattuck-Eidens D, et al. (1994) A strong candidate for the breast and ovarian susceptibility gene BRCA1. Science 266: 66–71.

National Institute for Clinical Excellence (NICE) (2002) Guidance on Cancer Services. Improving Outcomes in Breast Cancer. Manual Update. London: NICE.

Orel SG, Troupin RH, Patterson EA, et al. (1992) Breast cancer recurrence after lumpectomy and irradiation: role of mammography in detection. Radiology 183(1): 201–6.

Powles TJ, Tillyer CR, Jones AL, et al. (1990) Prevention of breast cancer with tamoxifen: an update on the Royal Marsden Hospital pilot programme. European Journal of Cancer 26: 680–4.

Richardson P (1995) What is Cancer? In David J (Ed.) CancerCare: Prevention, Treatment and Palliation. London: Chapman and Hall.

Rosen PP, Groshen S, Kinne DW, Norton L (1993) Factors influencing prognosis in node-negative breast carcinoma: analysis of 767 T1N0M0/T2N0M0 patients with long-term follow up. Journal of Clinical Oncology 11: 2090–100.

Sainsbury JRC, Anderson TJ, Morgan DAL (2000) ABC of breast diseases: breast cancer. British Medical Journal 321: 745–9.

Sobin LH, Wittekind CH (eds) (1997) UICC – TNM – Classification of Malignant Tumours. 5th edn. New York: Wiley-Liss.

Struewing JP, Watson P, Easton DF, et al. (1995). Prophylactic oopherectomy in inherited breast/ovarian cancer families. Journal of the National Cancer Institute Monograph 17: 33–5.

Tabar L, Faberberg G, Day N, Holmberg L (1987) What is the optimum screening interval between mammographic screening examinations? An analysis based on the Swedish two county breast cancer screening trial. British Journal of Cancer 56: 547–51.

Tortora GJ, Grabowski SR (1996) Principles of Anatomy and Physiology. 8th edn. New York: Harper Collins College.

Watson M, Murday V, Lloyd S et al. (1995) Genetic testing in breast/ovarian cancer (BRCA1) families. Lancet 346: 583.

Wooster R, Ford D, Mangion J, et al. (1995) Identification of the breast cancer susceptibility gene BRCA2. Nature 378: 789–92.

CHAPTER TWO

Breast awareness and the breast screening programme

National strategies

The prevention of cancer was selected as a key area in the government report 'The Health of the Nation' (Department of Health 1992) because of the part cancers play in ill-health and death. Cancer was also targeted as some can be prevented and cured as a result of screening and early detection.

One of the main targets was to reduce the death rate for breast cancer in the population invited for screening by at least 25 per cent by the year 2000.

The UK was the first country in the European Community to launch a nationwide breast cancer screening programme, using a computerized call and recall system. Women aged 50–64 years are invited three yearly to be screened and older women can be screened three yearly on request. Women under 50 years are not offered screening. There appears to be insufficient evidence to show that screening women under 50 is effective in reducing mortality from breast cancer. Pre-menopausal women have dense breast tissue and it is difficult to detect problem areas on the mammogram. Also, the incidence of breast cancer is lower in younger women. As women go past the menopause the breast tissue is increasingly made up of fat and is clearer on a mammogram.

Symptomatic women under 50 years who have a suspicious breast lump or breast changes seemingly inconsistent with benign changes are referred by their GP to a breast unit for investigations.

A study (the Age Trial) is at present underway to consider if there is any benefit in screening women under 50 years. Approximately 65,000 women aged 40–49 are being screened annually for seven years. After this they are automatically put back into the NHS Breast Screening Programme. The incidence of breast cancer in these women and in a control group of 130,000 who do not receive annual screening is being monitored. The trial started in 1991 and is running for 15 years. It is funded by the United Kingdom Committee on Cancer Research and is being co-ordinated by the

Cancer Screening Evaluation Unit of the Institute of Cancer Research. An analysis of interim outcome measures is being conducted and published in 2003. This will include a study of the prognostic indicators of all diagnosed breast cancers. This will in turn be used to predict the outcome in terms of breast cancer mortality. A full mortality analysis will be done in 2005.

In 1993 the Government funded a pilot programme that included the aim to improve uptake of screening invitations by women, especially those from black and ethnic minority groups. 'Targeting Practice: The Contribution of Nurses, Midwives and Health Visitors' (Department of Health 1993) was drawn up by nurses and midwives describing key areas in which they are involved. It describes how nurses lead screening services, develop information services, improve access to services, work in 'centres of excellence' as part of a multidisciplinary team, develop initiatives in nurse education and evaluate outcomes.

The most important contribution of nurses in preventing breast cancer is to encourage women to be breast aware and to attend screening clinics. Other contributions by nurses include participating in research, teaching breast awareness, developing literature encouraging self-awareness and targeting ethnic minority groups.

'The New NHS: Modern, Dependable' (Department of Health 1999a), a Government White Paper, led to 'Saving Lives: Our Healthier Nation' (Department of Health 1999b), an action plan to tackle ill-health. This committed the health service to ensuring that all women with suspected breast cancer are referred to a specialist by their GP and seen within two weeks. The latest monitoring data show that 96.1 per cent of women referred urgently were seen within two weeks (Department of Health 1999b). The new NHS Plan (including the National Cancer Plan) has now superseded all other White Papers.

The Cancer Services Collaborative (CSC) is a national NHS programme designed to improve the way that cancer services are provided. It offers practical approaches to delivering the targets set by the NHS Cancer Plan. Its goal is to improve the experience and outcomes for patients who have suspected or diagnosed cancer by optimizing care delivery systems. Since April 2001 the cancer networks in England have been taking part in the programme. This encourages local clinical teams to look at their services and supports them in making improvements to the way care is delivered. Targets include reducing the number of days from referral to treatment, increasing the percentage of patients with a booked appointment time/admission, reducing unnecessary delays, improving patient and carer experience. Breast is one of the main tumour areas in which changes will be implemented. The CSC has set up work to improve services relating to cancers in such areas as screening, primary care, radiotherapy, chemotherapy and palliative care (NHS Modernisation Agency 2002).

Pilot studies have been undertaken as to the feasibility of screening women aged 65–69 years. In September 2000 a report from the Institute of Cancer Research showed that the Breast Screening Programme saves lives due to the high quality of the programme, increased uptake, the increasing experience of radiologists and awareness of the disease as well as improved treatments and drugs. The National Cancer Plan (Department of Health 2000) announced a major expansion in equipment for breast screening in order to include women aged 65–70 years. This should be in place by 2004. This plan also promises that from 2002 no patient with breast cancer should wait longer than eight weeks from an urgent GP referral to treatment. Cancer units are trying to achieve the recommendation at the moment that no patient with breast cancer waits longer than four weeks from being diagnosed with cancer to treatment. There are vast variations in waiting times from referral to first hospital visit across the UK.

This major expansion of the programme will lead to a re-organization of staffing in screening units to increase the programme's capacity. A new skill mix is being tested with a new grade of assistant practitioner included. This involves radiographers undergoing extra training to be able to read mammograms, undertake fine needle aspiration, core biopsy and ultrasound and do assessment clinics. This will lead to a 40 per cent increase in workload. Four sites in the UK are piloting this. These are Warwickshire, Solihull and Coventry Breast Screening Unit, South Derbyshire Breast Screening Unit, Bolton, Bury and Rochdale Breast Screening Unit and Norfolk and Norwich Breast Screening Unit (Department of Health 2000). This of course has a huge training and cost implication. Bids from screening units are being considered for equipment, clinic space, etc.

Figures from the Department of Health (2000) show an increase in uptake for screening by 1–2%; 76 per cent of those invited were screened and 8215 cancers were found.

The Calman-Hine Report

This report by the Expert Advisory Group on Cancer (Department of Health 1995) set out a framework for cancer services. Several recommendations were made including:

- All patients should have access to a uniformly high quality of care wherever they live.
- Public/professional education regarding early recognition of cancer symptoms and availability of national screening programmes are vital.
- Patients, carers and families should receive clear information and assistance.

- Cancer services should be patient centred and take into account patients', families' and carers' views.
- Good communication is vital.
- The primary health care team is a central element in cancer care from prevention, screening and diagnosis to follow-up and death.
- The impact of screening, diagnosis and treatment of cancer on patients, carers and families should be recognized.

There are three levels of care:

1 Primary care – seen as the focus of care. Detailed discussion between primary care, cancer units and cancer centres is necessary.
2 Designated Cancer Units – in many district hospitals. These should have the expertise and facilities to manage the commoner cancers.
3 Designated Cancer Centres – expert in management of all cancers. Provide specialist diagnostic and therapeutic techniques, for example radiotherapy.

In a Cancer Unit nursing care must be planned and led by nurses who have had post-registration education in oncology. Access to specialist nurses, such as breast care nurses, must be ensured.

Supportive care must include counselling, prosthetics, complementary therapies, access to self-help groups, physiotherapy and dietetics.

Cancer Centres must provide a high degree of specialization and Clinical Nurse Specialists including breast care. The Centre should also provide advanced cancer nursing education.

Breast awareness

Being breast aware includes the woman being familiar with the appearance and feel of her breasts and also being informed about breast diseases. Many women practise breast self-examination but there does not appear to be any evidence that this is effective. It should not be used solely as a diagnostic test. Breast self-examination tends to increase awareness of lumps but does not give information on other signs and symptoms. It can also lead to feelings of guilt whatever the decision – either for not carrying it out at all or not carrying it out properly. Plus the reward is poor – if examination is successful the outcome is the discovery of disease.

A large number of women present to their GP with symptoms having practised self-examination. It would seem obvious that if women carry out self-examination regularly, cancers will be detected earlier. However, studies show that populations who have been taught this procedure do not show any improvement in the stage at which breast cancer presents (Leinster et al. 2000).

This may be because of poor compliance. Younger women tend to practise breast self-examination and the risk of cancer is low anyway. The at risk age group tends not to practise it. Therefore younger women tend to present with an increased number of benign lumps leading to investigations and increased anxiety in the women. So in the UK women are encouraged to practise breast awareness rather that breast self-examination.

Breast Cancer Care (2001) advocate a five-point code for breast awareness:

1 Know what is normal for you.
2 Know what changes to look and feel for.
3 Look and feel.
4 Report any changes to a GP immediately.
5 Attend for routine breast screening if aged 50 or over.

Changes to look out for include:

• change in outline/shape/size of the breast
• dimpling/puckering of the skin
• new/discrete lumps
• persistent asymmetrical nodularity present early in the menstrual cycle
• unusual pain/discomfort, different from normal, persistent, localized
• nipple discharge, new, serous, bloody
• persistent single duct discharge
• a swelling under the armpit or around the collarbone.

Women can check their breasts from time to time to become aware of how breast tissue changes at different times of the month. A woman who has gone through the menopause can choose the same time each month. The woman can then get used to the look and feel of her breasts. She may use a mirror to check from different angles. Raising the arms above the head with elbows bent allows any change in shape or skin changes to be noted. Leaning forward with the hands on the hips also allows these changes to be seen. Feeling the breasts and armpits is probably easier to do in the bath or shower with a soapy hand.

The letter from the Chief Medical and Nursing Officers (1998) regarding clinical examination of the breast emphasizes the importance of teaching breast awareness to women. Women should be aware of what is normal for them, and be aware of their breasts in activities of living such as showering, bathing and dressing. The breast awareness concept is now widely accepted.

The role of the primary care nurse in breast awareness

Nurses work at all levels in breast care providing a continuous service, starting with health promotion and promoting breast awareness, and continuing through to the specialist work of the breast care nurse in the breast unit.

People are very anxious about breast cancer, this leads to increased pressure on GPs, practice and community nurses – often the first point of contact for anxious patients. This anxiety can be reduced by primary care nurses through well-women services. Education about what is a normal breast and what to look for can be given. Further information can then be supplied if required (Royal College of Nursing 1999).

Nurses are discouraged from examining women's breasts, a joint letter from the Chief Medical and Nursing Officers (1998) discourages this practice as lesions may be missed and false reassurance given (Leinster et al. 2000). The Royal College of Nursing Breast Care Nursing Forum has produced guidelines for breast palpation and breast awareness (Royal College of Nursing 2002). It is recognized that pressure is placed on nurses to relieve the anxieties of women with breast problems both in the primary care setting and in hospital. Breast palpation alone is not a valid screening tool, it should be carried out as part of the clinical assessment at specialist units (Department of Health 1996). The only exception would be specialist breast care nurses who undertake breast palpation as a part of their role (Royal College of Nursing 2002). It is acknowledged that some breast care nurses will include breast palpation as part of their role but it must be within the breast unit and with full professional support from the rest of the breast care team.

The primary care nurse's role is one of education and giving support and education to women (Royal College of Nursing 2002).

The primary care nurse will be aware of how to manage breast problems and about specialist referral within the National Health Service Breast Screening Programme guidelines so that any woman who has been referred with a breast problem can be supported. Breast care in the primary care setting involves a knowledge of normal breast development and any changes associated with age, cyclical changes, use of HRT and oral contraceptives. It also involves a realistic perception of the risk factors for breast cancer such as family history and increased age (Cancer Research Campaign 1997). Practice and screening nurses need to be trained to a uniformly high standard to support the patient and provide written and verbal information.

Practice and community nurses also need to be aware of how they can facilitate breast awareness for women who have a problem examining their breasts. Some physical problems, for example rheumatoid arthritis or blindness make self-examination impossible. A patient may have a learning difficulty and decreased self-awareness. The nurse may need to educate those caring for women with handicapping conditions to be increasingly aware of what to look for.

Primary care nurses can provide information on the normal breast and normal changes. As well as teaching breast awareness, primary care nurses can encourage women to accept the invitation to breast screening mammography and to attend regularly once over the age of 65. The screening programme can be discussed and support and advice can be provided throughout the screening procedure (Royal College of Nursing 1999). Specialist breast care nurses are ideally placed to offer training and support to primary care nurses. Although the breast care nurse has a large part to play in health promotion, the primary care and community nurses can disseminate information to larger numbers in the community.

Women may seek referral to the specialist unit as breast palpation is not carried out in primary care. This means that the system is becoming overloaded and delaying women who may have serious breast problems. The national Guidelines for Referral of Patients with Breast Problems (Austoker and Mansel 1999) provides support for the primary care team. Nurses in primary care increase women's self-awareness, provide advice and management once cancer has been excluded and provide ongoing support and care for women who have undergone acute treatments (Royal College of Nursing 1999).

The breast screening programme

Reductions in mortality can be achieved by earlier detection and treatment. This is recognized in the Health of the Nation (Department of Health 1992) targets, which refer only to reducing mortality from breast cancer by screening.

In screening, healthy individuals are tested to see if they have disease at an early stage. A screening test must meet several criteria:

- It must be specific and only detect the disease it is looking for.
- It must be sensitive – must detect the disease if present to avoid a false negative.
- The disease must be common – socially and economically there is no point screening for a rare disease.
- The disease's natural history must be known. If a disease is incurable even when detected early the screen is of no value. A patient would be aware of a terminal illness years before the disease shows.

- Treatment must be available.
- The test must be acceptable to patients – a painful, embarrassing test would not be accepted by healthy people as routine.
- It should be cost-effective.

Screening for breast cancer using X-ray mammography fulfils many of the above criteria (The Breast Clinic online 2001). The Forrest Report (Department of Health 1986) examined the evidence from a number of countries and concluded that for women aged 50 and above screening can reduce mortality from breast cancer by up to a third. The National Health Service Breast Screening Programme (NHSBSP) commenced in 1987 and was nationwide by 1994. It is responsible for the assessment and diagnosis of mammographically detected abnormalities. Its aim is to reduce mortality from breast cancer by regularly screening women aged 50–64 in order to identify asymptomatic breast cancer (Comptroller and Auditor General 1992).

Many deaths in the 1990s were of women diagnosed before invitation to screening in the 1980s and early 1990s. Evidence from the programme indicates that the prevalent round was not completed until 1995. However, the latest survival figures for England and Wales show an average of 75 per cent of women with breast cancer in 1992–94 were alive five years later. The British Association of Surgical Oncologists carried out an audit of screen-detected breast cancers between 1992 and 1996 and found that the five-year survival rate was 93 per cent (BASO 2002). By 1998 both screening and other factors including improvements in treatment had resulted in substantial reductions in mortality from breast cancer. Research published in 2000 demonstrated that the programme has lowered mortality rates in the 55–69 age group (Blanks et al. 2000). It is estimated that the programme will save 1250 lives by the year 2010. A Swedish study showed that screening reduces deaths from breast cancer by nearly two-thirds (Mayor 2001). The World Health Organisation Inter-Agency for Research on Cancer (2002) concluded that screening reduces mortality. A working group concluded that there is a 35 per cent reduction in mortality among women who are screened in the 50–64 age group.

As most deaths (89 per cent in the UK) from breast cancer are women over 50, the screening programme targets this age group. Exceptions would be women previously described who carry the BRCA1/BRCA2 breast cancer genes. At the moment the programme stops screening women after age 64 as the Forrest Report suggested that screening would be ineffective in older women due to low compliance. However, in a study by Hobbs et al. (1990) 61 per cent of women over 64 in Manchester responded to an invitation to screening. Women over 64 can request an appointment to be screened.

A national co-ordinating body with a national co-ordinator was established at the beginning of the programme. The role includes quality assurance, training and information systems. A Department of Health Advisory Committee supplies policy and professional advice. In 1995 the purchase of screening services became the responsibility of purchasing authorities. Local purchasers and providers are required to offer a three-yearly screening programme and attain national quality standards (Dey et al. 1997).

The Royal College of Surgeons is responsible for advising on training, audit and working practices in relation to surgery in the breast screening programme. The British Association of Surgical Oncology (BASO) has established a group of surgeons working in breast cancer screening to represent surgeons in the screening programme. This group advises on surgical aspects of breast screening and reports to the College. The screening programme is only successful if followed by appropriate and timely surgical management. Women must be diagnosed quickly and accurately and not be over- or under-treated (NHS Breast Screening Programme 1996).

Breast screening and assessment of screen-detected abnormalities are undertaken in specifically dedicated centres. A core team of radiologists, radiographers, surgeons, pathologists, administrative and technical support staff are involved. Breast care nurses, the primary health care team, the FHSA, and health promotion officers all contribute towards the uptake of screening. The women are identified from GP registers and invited to a fixed site or mobile unit.

The Forrest Report recommended that each of these specialist centres should include an appropriately trained registered nurse to support women undergoing screening. The NHSBSP guidelines for quality assurance in breast cancer nursing (NHS Breast Screening Programme 1998) sets out standards for Clinical Nurse Specialists in Breast Care (Screening). These guidelines also contain an assessment tool for the audit of the breast care nursing role within the screening assessment unit. The National Coordination Group for Nurses in Breast Cancer Screening co-ordinates quality assurance issues at national level.

All women attending for breast screening should have access to a breast care nurse and know how to contact her. The breast care nurse is an important part of the multidisciplinary team and has a commitment to ensure that women receive appropriate care and information throughout the screening process.

Initially the service used single view mammography (oblique view). All screening centres now provide two-view mammography in the prevalent round. This allows accurate determination of the position of any abnormality discovered. It also reduces the chance of false positives – normal breast tissue may appear as a dense region on just one view but be seen as normal on the second (The Breast Clinic online 2001). By 2003 all women will have two views of the breast taken at every screening – a craniocaudal and an oblique view. Also being introduced is digital mammography – instead of conventional mammograms, which are on film and viewed in a light box, images will be viewed and reported from the computer monitor. This technology allows the digital image of the breast to be manipulated on screen enabling it to be seen more clearly. This may be more effective in detecting cancer in dense breasts. Digital mammography is not widely used at the moment.

At the screening unit, the procedure takes about half an hour. The radiographer takes details of previous breast disease and explains the procedure. It is important that radiographers have good communication skills. She also answers any questions the woman might have and reinforces the need to be breast aware. The radiographer then positions the woman so that the whole breast is included on the X-ray. Each breast will be placed on turn on the X-ray machine and gently but firmly compressed with a clear plate. This can be slightly uncomfortable and a small number of women report short-lived pain. The result is usually received within two weeks (NHSBSP online 2001).

If anything unusual is discovered the woman is asked to attend an assessment clinic. About eight per cent of women will be recalled generally to clarify an area seen on the first two X-rays. One per cent of these will require a biopsy. At this point, because of careful investigation, most biopsies will reveal a breast cancer (Mera 1997). Often at this stage a cancerous abnormality is DCIS (cancer in its pre-invasive form) and can be treated long before it progresses to ductal cancer. Pre-cancerous changes cannot be detected by mammography – DCIS is the earliest and comprises 15–20 per cent of screen-detected cancers. Some tumours can be detected as microcalcifications of only 2–3mm. This can be compared with tumours found on self-examination and palpation of 1–2cm.

In 1999/2000 8.1 per cent attending for a first screen and 4.3 per cent attending for a subsequent screen were asked to attend an assessment clinic for technical reasons or because an abnormality was found (Department of Health 2001). A total of 8215 cancers were discovered by screening in 1999/2000 (invasive and *in situ*).

The optimum screening interval remains uncertain. A report by Woodman et al. (1995) reveals that the rate of interval cancers in the third year after screening approaches that which would be expected if screening had not been carried out. This suggests that the screening interval may be too long. More frequently than three yearly may reduce compliance due to discomfort and the possible fear of frequent X-rays. However, for women willing to attend annual or biennial screening the incidence of interval cancers is lower (Mera 1997).

From its inception the NHSBSP has recognized that screening can never be a perfect test and interval cancers will occur (Department of Health 1986). All film readers are expected to audit interval cancers as part of their continued professional development. These cancers are retrospectively reviewed to see if they could have been diagnosed earlier, therefore helping to improve performance (NHSBSP 1997). Brown and co-workers (2001) have developed a database to collect and audit interval cancers. This allows systematic recording of radiological and pathological information regarding breast cancers. The geographic distribution of interval cancers can also be recorded. Statistical differences in the distribution of screen-detected and false negative cancers have been demonstrated. The position of the cancer is plotted on a stylized diagram, which reinforces the importance of the conventional review areas. Although no 'blind spots' have been found, it still provides film readers with an audit tool.

Interval cancers are divided into two types. False negatives are cancers present but unidentified on a previous screening and true intervals are cancers appearing since the last screen. The sensitivity of the test can be improved by optimizing the optical density of the mammographic film (Young et al. 1994), by involving two-view mammography (Van Dijck et al. 1992) and by two radiologists reading the mammogram independently (Anderson et al. 1994).

However, it must be taken into account that a screening programme will potentially have negative effects on a healthy population. The possibility of psychological problems has been of concern since the beginning of the screening programme. Disadvantages include anxiety generated by a screening invitation, especially a recall, discomfort during the procedure, possible over-diagnosis and over-treatment, maintaining quality assurance and false reassurance for those with a false negative result (Cancer Research Campaign 1997).

There is also the danger that the widespread notion that the smaller the cancer is at the time of detection, the earlier the stage of the disease and the greater the likelihood of cure ignores the disease's capacity for dissemination even in the sub-clinical stage (Baum 1994). However, screening is beneficial but this must be balanced financially and in terms of physical or psychological morbidity. The anxiety of false alarms, the costs both financially and psychologically of unnecessary biopsies and the problems of women diagnosed as having DCIS fearing cancer when in theory it may not actually progress, must all be taken into account.

False positive results occur in a broad group of women who are eventually given an all-clear after further investigations. Psychiatric morbidity increases among women who have had a mammogram and are recalled for further investigation (Olsson et al. 1999). An initial false positive result can cause anxiety as it challenges the belief that the individual is healthy.

Further investigations can include physical examinations, ultrasound scans, fine needle aspiration, core biopsy and surgical biopsy as well as mammograms. Brett et al. (1998) found that women who were found to be clear after further investigations still suffered adverse psychological consequences five months after their final appointment. Olsson et al. (1999) also found that six months after the all-clear 15 per cent of women were still significantly more anxious than those who had been screened and not recalled. The women who did not cope well tended to be of low educational level so possibly this was due to the inability to assimilate the relevant information. Others who showed high levels of distress lived in densely populated urban areas so they had less social contact and more anonymity.

Despite these findings the evidence is clear that the breast screening programme is saving lives. Every effort is made to minimize anxiety. Invitations to breast screening and recall letters are carefully worded and contain contact numbers so women can phone the unit and have their questions answered. Less than 10 per cent of women screened for the first time and less than seven per cent screened for a subsequent time should be recalled. Standards are in place to minimize the number recalled (NHSBSP online 2001).

However, some women still do not attend. There could be many reasons for this – possibly they do not receive their invitation, forget the appointment, are away on holiday, are busy or ill, or simply choose not to attend. Other reasons can include:

- fear of the test/fear of cancer
- embarrassment
- dislike of clinics/hospitals
- previous bad experience
- do not wish to know.

Practical factors may be:

- other people's experiences
- the style of the invitation
- the convenience of the appointment
- the image of the local Screening Unit and the environment where screening is offered
- unclear, inadequate information
- impersonal, uncaring treatment
- pain or discomfort caused by the procedure and not properly managed by the staff.

Women may also be influenced by the information available regarding the procedure, the effectiveness, the seriousness of the disease and general health issues (Austoker 1992). A woman's right to make her own decisions should be respected and women who do not attend should not be made to feel guilty.

To achieve high attendance rates:

- administration – having correct addresses and providing accurate information
- publicizing the programme
- encouraging positive attitudes towards breast screening
- if a woman cannot attend, encourage her to change the appointment or make another if one is missed – and make the process of changing appointments easy to do
- encourage primary care nurses to give information and advice on all aspects of the screening programme (Austoker 1992).

From 2001 all invitations to breast screening will contain a leaflet explaining the benefits and limitations of screening so that the patient can make an informed decision. This is part of the National Cancer Plan (Department of Health 2000).

References

Anderson EDC, Muir BB, Walsh JS, et al. (1994) The efficacy of double reading mammograms in breast screening for breast cancer: a review. Clinical Radiology 49: 248–51.

Austoker J (1992) NHS Breast Screening Programme. Breast Cancer Screening: Practical Guide for Primary Care Teams. London: Meditext.

Austoker J, Mansel R (1999). Guidelines for Referral of Patients with Breast Problems. Revised 2nd edn. Sheffield: NHSBSP.

Baum M (1994) Cost benefit analysis of screening for breast cancer in the UK and US. In Wise L, Johnson H junior (eds) Breast Cancer – Controversies in Management. New York: Futura Publishing.

Blanks RG, Moss SM, McGahan CE, et al. (2000) Effect of the NHS breast screening programme on mortality from breast cancer in England and Wales 1990–98: comparison of observed with predicted mortality. British Medical Journal 321: 665–9.

Breast Cancer Care online (2001) Breast Health. www.breastcancercare.org.uk/Breasthealth (accessed May 2001).

Brett J, Austoker J, Ong G (1998) Do women who undergo further investigation for breast screening suffer adverse psychological consequences? A multi-centre follow-up study comparing different breast screening result groups five months after their last breast screening appointment. Journal of Public Health Medicine 20(4): 396–403.

British Association of Surgical Oncologists (BASO) (2002) An Audit of Screen Detected Cancers for the Year of Screening April 2000–March 2001. Sheffield: BASO and NHSBSP. Available at www.cancerscreening.nhs.uk/breastscreen

Brown M, Eccles C, Wallis MG (2001) Geographical distribution of breast cancers on the mammogram: an interval cancer database. British Journal of Radiology 74: 317–22.

Cancer Research Campaign (1997) Factsheet 7.1 Breast Cancer Screening. London: Cancer Research Campaign.

Chief Medical Officer and Chief Nursing Officer (1998) Clinical Examination of the Breast. Advisory Letter. London: Department of Health.

Comptroller and Auditor General (1992) Cervical and Breast Screening in England. Report by the Comptroller and Auditor General. London: National Audit Office/HMSO (House of Commons papers 1991–2, 236).

Department of Health (1986) Breast Cancer Screening – Report to the Health Ministers of England, Wales, Scotland and N. Ireland. Working Group chaired by Sir Patrick Forrest. London: HMSO.

Department of Health (1992) The Health of the Nation. A Strategy for Health in England. London: HMSO.

Department of Health (1993) The Health of the Nation. Targeting Practice: The Contribution of Nurses, Midwives and Health Visitors. London: HMSO.

Department of Health (1995) A Policy Framework for Commisioning Cancer Services. A Report by the Expert Advisory Group on Cancer to the Chief Medical Officers of England and Wales. London: Department of Health.

Department of Health (1996) Cancer Guidance Sub-group of the Clinical Outcomes Group. Improving outcomes in breast cancer. London: The Stationery Office.

Department of Health (1999a) The New NHS: Modern, Dependable. London: HMSO.

Department of Health (1999b) Saving Lives: Our Healthier Nation. London: HMSO.

Department of Health (2000) NHS National Cancer Plan. A plan for investment, a plan for reform. London: Department of Health.

Department of Health (2001) Breast Screening Programme, England, 1999–2000. (Bulletin) www.doh.gov.uk/pdfs/sbo110.pdf (accessed June 2001).

Dey P, Twelves E, Woodman CBJ (1997) Breast Cancer: Health Care Needs Assessment. Oxford: Radcliffe Medical Press.

Hobbs P, Kay C, Friedmore E (1990) Response by women aged 65–79 to an invitation for screening for breast cancer by mammography; a pilot study. British Medical Journal 301: 1314–16.

Leinster SJ, Gibbs TJ, Downey H (2000) Shared Care for Breast Disease. Oxford: Isis Medical.

Mayor S (2001) Study confirms that screening reduces deaths from breast cancer. News. British Medical Journal 332: 1140.

Mera S (1997) Pathology and Understanding Disease Prevention. Cheltenham: Stanley Thomas.

NHS Breast Screening Programme (1996) Quality Assurance Guidelines for Surgeons in Breast Cancer Screening. Publication no. 20. Sheffield: NHSBSP.

NHS Breast Screening Programme (1997) Quality assurance guidelines for radiologists. Publication no. 15. Sheffield: NHSBSP.

NHS Breast Screening Programme (1998) Quality Assurance Guidelines for Nurses in Breast Cancer Screening. National Coordination Group for Nurses in Breast Cancer Screening. Publication no. 29. Sheffield: NHSBSP.

NHSBSP online (2001) www.cancerscreening.nhs.uk/breastscreen (accessed May 2001).

NHS Modernisation Agency (2002) Cancer Services Collaborative, www.modern.nhs.uk (accessed October 2002).

Olsson P, Armelius K, Nordahl G, et al. (1999) Women with false positive screening mammograms: how do they cope? Journal of Medical Screening 6: 89–93.

Royal College of Nursing (1999) Developing Roles: Nurses Working in Breast Care. London: Royal College of Nursing.

Royal College of Nursing (2002) Breast Palpation and Breast Awareness. The Role of the Nurse. London: Royal College of Nursing.

The Breast Clinic online (2001) www.thebreastclinic.com/screening.htm (accessed May 2001).

van Dijck JAAM, Verbeek ALM, Hendriks JHCL (1992) One view vs two view mammography in baseline screening for breast cancer: a review. British Journal of Radiology 65: 971–6.

Woodman CBJ, Threlfall AJ, Boggis CMR, et al. (1995) Is the three year breast screening interval too long? Occurrence of interval cancers in the NHS Breast Screening Programmes' NWR. British Medical Journal 319: 224–6.

World Health Organisation Inter-Agency for Research on Cancer (2002) 7th Handbook on Cancer Prevention. Lyons: IARC.

Young KC, Wallis MG, Ramsdale ML (1994) Mammographic film density and detection of small breast cancers. Clinical Radiology 49: 461–5.

CHAPTER THREE

Benign breast disease

Introduction

Most breast complaints are benign, with only 1 in 15 referrals being diagnosed with malignancy (Henderson 1998). Despite this, however, most women fear the worst. The 14 out of 15 diagnosed with benign conditions may be due to raised public awareness of breast cancer and frequent coverage in the media prompting women to seek a medical opinion for breast problems. To help allay these women's fears an understanding of benign breast disorders is necessary.

The breast is identical in both sexes until puberty. At around 10 years growth begins and may be asymmetrical initially. A breast lump in a girl of 9–10 years is usually a developing breast and biopsy should not be done as it can damage the breast bud. Most benign conditions as well as breast cancer arise within the terminal duct lobules of the breast.

Pregnancy doubles the weight of the breast at term and the breast involutes after the pregnancy. Most benign changes in pregnancy are due to swollen milk glands, however, women should not assume that any lumpiness is due to this. Although breast cancer is uncommon in pregnancy, any problem should be checked.

Breast involution begins at around 30 years of age in nulliparous women. During involution the breast becomes less radiodense as the stroma is replaced by fat. It also becomes softer and ptotic. Most benign breast conditions are so common they are regarded as aberrations rather than disease (Dixon and Mansel 1994). Therefore, the term often used for benign conditions in general is Anomalies of Development and Involution or ANDI. Benign conditions are most often diagnosed in 30–40 year olds.

There are many types of benign problems but in general they can be classified according to symptom: lumps, pain, nipple problems and infections. There can be many causes of these. Most benign disorders are physiological extremes but still normal. Support, reassurance and explanation are often the only treatment required. A true abnormality may require treatment but is still not life threatening.

In a few specific benign conditions there is a risk of breast cancer but not in the majority of cases. However, a study in 1999 showed that pre-menopausal women with fibrocystic breast disease have an almost six-fold higher risk of future breast cancer (Dixon et al. 1999). It is important that these women are taught to continue to be breast aware.

Investigation follows the same principles as investigations for breast cancer although young women may not require every test (Breast Clinic 2001). The high levels of anxiety in women with breast problems tend to lead to over-investigation (Leinster et al. 2000).

Guidelines for the referral of breast problems

Guidelines have been produced to reduce the number of unnecessary referrals to breast clinics, increasing the pressure already on clinics following the introduction of the two-week rule. The two-week rule was introduced in April 1999 and originated from the White Paper *The New NHS* (Department of Health 1997). It states that every person with suspected cancer will be seen by a specialist within two weeks of their GP deciding that they need to be seen as an urgent case. The increased rate of referrals has led to over-crowded breast clinics. This is partly due to large numbers of women who contact GPs as a result of raised awareness of a genetic link to breast cancer. Women who are at low risk are another source of unnecessary referrals. Conditions such as moderate breast pain and bilateral symmetrical nodularity can be safely managed in the primary health care setting.

The guidelines give specific advice on which patients should be referred as 'urgent'. They should allow GPs to reassure patients and categorize them confidently as urgent or non-urgent, confining the urgent group to those at risk of cancer (Austoker and Mansel 1999). If GPs are trained to incorporate the guidelines the number of unnecessary referrals should drop (Henderson 1998). The guidelines also allow GPs to reassure women at low risk of breast cancer connected to family history and to refer those at high risk to a genetic clinic. If guidelines are adhered to specialist breast clinics can see patients more quickly and can observe the two-week rule. Patients with cancer should then receive earlier diagnosis and treatment.

If the GP suspects that the patient has breast cancer an urgent referral should be made to the breast clinic on the same day. The classification of 'urgent' should be applied only to those whose symptoms suggest breast cancer:

- a discrete lump in those over 30 years
- definite signs of cancer such as skin distortion, skin nodule or ulceration.

Conditions requiring a referral to a breast surgeon include:

- any new discrete lump
- any asymmetrical nodularity that persists after menstruation
- a new lump in pre-existing nodularity
- abscess
- cyst
- pain associated with a lump
- intractable pain
- unilateral persistent pain in post-menopausal women
- nipple discharge, nipple distortion or eczema
- change in skin contour
- women with a strong family history (Austoker and Mansell 1999).

Benign breast conditions

Fibrocystic change

This is a general term referring to a group of anomalies, conditions and symptoms forming part of the spectrum of breast pathology. The term is still used clinically although often conditions such as mastitis, fibroadenosis and fibrocystic disease are known as benign breast change. Benign breast disease is also given the general blanket term of ANDI as previously mentioned. This condition causes the tenderness and lumpiness that occurs in many women mid-menstrual cycle as this is the time of maximum hormonal stimulation.

D'Amelio et al. (2001) found an association between polycystic ovary and fibrocystic breast disease or benign breast change. This raises the question of whether some form of screening should be encouraged for women with polycystic ovary.

Mastalgia

Breast pain is known as mastalgia and is very common. It is often the main and only symptom. It indicates some underlying process or disease within the breast, which is in most cases benign. Pain is associated rarely with breast cancer. Breast pain can be cyclical or non-cyclical depending on the relationship to the patient's menstrual cycle. Before each monthly period the breast may store about 15–30cc of fluid causing enlargement and tenderness (Avillion 1998).

Cyclical is the most common type. It often occurs in the week prior to menstruation. Some women can experience quite severe pain which can result in problems with work, leisure and relationships. The pain tends to be greatest in the upper outer quadrant of the breast, or may be a dull, heavy, aching sensation. The cause is thought to be hormonal. An abnormality in the secretion of prolactin has been suggested. Other causes could be too much caffeine or a deficiency of essential fatty acids. Patients are usually aged 30–40 years. A few will experience pain for the whole month with relief at the onset of menstruation, others will experience pain for a few days prior to menstruation. Mastalgia can occur unilaterally or in both breasts along with lumpiness and being able to feel nodules (Breast Clinic 2001).

Treatment involves the reassurance that cancer is not present and that the mastalgia will probably settle in a few months. On examination of the breasts there is usually tenderness with nodularity. The breast tissue tends to be glandular and dense with no abnormality of the nipple. A fine needle aspiration gives a benign result.

The patient is often asked to record a breast pain chart. Pain is scored on a daily basis from severe to moderate to none. The chart is recorded for a few months. With the onset of menstruation it can be seen if the pain is cyclical.

The use of Evening Primrose Oil to replace essential fatty acids is usually recommended. This should be prescribed as Efamast 40mg (gamolenic acid) concentrated capsules to achieve the recommended dose of 240–320mg daily. This should be taken for at least three months, ideally six months, and will take 2–4 weeks to have any effect. Fifty per cent of patients will respond to this.

Cyclical mastalgia may be caused by the abnormal secretion of prolactin and therefore drugs that inhibit prolactin secretion can be tried. Danazol 200–400mg daily may be prescribed; this inhibits the follicle stimulating hormone and lutenizing hormone in the pituitary gland. This will be effective in 70 per cent of patients but 25 per cent will have side effects. These include hirsutism, acne, a deep voice (possibly permanent), weight gain and amennorhoea. The patient should be advised to change to a different form of contraception if on the oral contraceptive pill, as Danazol interferes with the effectiveness of this (Dixon, Breast Care Campaign online 2001).

If Danazol is ineffective bromocriptine can be tried. This lowers the levels of prolactin. The dose needs gradually building up to try to reduce side effects:

- 1.25mg for three days.
- 1.25mg twice daily for four days.
- 1.25mg morning and 2.5mg afternoon for four days.
- 2.5mg twice daily (Leinster et al. 2000).

Side effects can include dizziness, nausea and headaches. Bromocriptine will be effective in 50 per cent of patients but is not used very often due to the side effects.

Other measures which can be tried are wearing a well-fitting bra day and night and reducing caffeine intake. Removing caffeine from the diet can reduce breast cyst formation and eliminate pain (Minton et al. 1981). A study by two British surgeons has also shown that pre-menopausal women can reduce breast pain by going without a bra, wearing a camisole if they wish. The study concluded that the majority of pre-menopausal women found that their breast pain decreased during a three-month period of not wearing a bra. Some women claim to be now pain-free (Cawthorne and Mansel 2000). This study was undertaken in conjunction with Channel 4 UK and a documentary was shown in November 2000.

Women should be informed of the options and can then make an informed decision.

Gregory et al. (1999) found that applied kinesiology was effective for mastalgia in a study of 88 women. This is a hands-on technique involving rubbing a series of lymphatic reflex points while touching painful areas of the breasts. Self-rated pain scores showed immediately that there was a reduction in pain in 60 per cent of patients and complete resolution in 21 per cent. After two months there was a reduction in pain in 50 per cent of the group. This may be an effective treatment.

Non-cyclical breast pain tends to occur in a number of conditions. Breast cancer must be excluded. True non-cyclical breast pain (not emanating from the chest wall or referred pain) can be difficult to treat. Once investigations reveal a benign diagnosis it may be found that the problem is inflammatory. The inflammatory process may be aggravated by smoking so smokers are strongly advised to cease. Oral non-steroidal anti-inflammatories are tried first. If pain still persists the medication used for cyclical pain can be prescribed. Around 40 per cent of women will obtain a response. Gamolenic acid should be tried first due to low side effects (Dixon, Breast Care Campaign online 2001).

Some medications may cause non-cyclical breast pain, for example drugs for hormonal problems, blood pressure, gastrointestinal problems and antidepressants. Some herbal remedies such as ginseng and dong quai may cause some pain.

An injection of local anaesthetic and a corticosteroid may help some women who have pain localized to one tender area (Leinster et al. 2000).

Sclerosis

This is the development of localized areas of excessive fibrosis. It may be sclerosis (over-proliferation of the terminal duct lobules can impinge on adjacent nerve endings and cause pain), radial scar or a complex sclerosing lesion. This can present as a painful lump or a stellate, calcified mass on mammography. As this can be confused with breast cancer surgical excision is usually carried out.

Tietz's Syndrome

Inflammation of the costochondrial junctions and costal cartilages causes pain on the anterior chest wall and can be mistaken for breast pain. Anti-inflammatories and a small steroid injection generally help.

Mastitis

Mastitis is inflammation or infection of the breast. The infective organism gains entry to the breast tissue via the nipple and ducts or from trauma. Infection or inflammation affecting the nipple and drainage of major ducts is known as periductal mastitis. A superficial infection can lead to cellulitis, a deeper infection can lead to abscesses. If an abscess lasts long enough it can lead to the development of a mammary fistula, therefore establishing a chronic infection. The abscess cavity drains onto the breast surface leaving a connection from the skin to the breast tissue, draining pus.

A wound infection can cause a breast infection following surgery or trauma. Breast surgery can result in cavities forming where tissue has been removed. These can fill with blood and inflammatory fluid and an abscess can result (Breast Clinic 2001).

Breast infections caused by *Mycobacterium tuberculosis* can be the cause of a breast lump presenting clinically and radiologically as a breast cancer. This tends to be in older patients with a history of TB and is rare in Western countries. Treatment includes anti-TB drugs (O'Reilly et al. 2000).

Breast abscess

Breast abscesses are common during breastfeeding. The mode of entry for the causative organism (*Staphylococcus aureus*) is through a cracked nipple or damaged skin. Signs and symptoms include pain, erythema, hardening of the breast tissue and signs of fever including nausea, sweating and tachycardia. Treatment consists of antibiotics and possible drainage of pus by needle aspiration. Surgical drainage may be carried out if all else fails.

Non-lactating abscesses can occur in association with periductal mastitis in women over 30 years. The abscess tends to occur close to the areola. Treatment includes antibiotics, aspiration and surgical drainage, if recommended. Abnormal ducts need to be excised to prevent a mammary fistula developing (Breast Clinic 2001). Should a fistula develop, it can be treated by excision of the fistula tract and affected duct.

Fibroadenoma

This is very common in young women aged 15–25 years. It consists of a proliferation of tissue around the breast lobule and has a rubbery texture on
palpation. A fibroadenoma is usually smooth but can be lobulated and feel
like several lumps in one. The size is typically 1–3cm. Highly mobile on
examination, it has earned the term 'breast mouse' or 'breast mice'. Totally
benign but cancer must always be excluded.

Full investigations are usually carried out (triple assessment). As these
occur in young women with very dense breast tissue, an ultrasound is usually done instead of a mammogram. A fine needle aspiration will reveal a
benign diagnosis.

Treatment will depend on size, position, pain/discomfort and the anxiety of the patient. A large fibroadenoma can be confused with a phyllodes
tumour, which can be malignant. If there is any risk that this is the case an
excision biopsy is performed. Any growth of 4–5cm would be surgically
excised. A large fibroadenoma in a small breast would also be removed for
cosmetic reasons as it will look unsightly. Removal may also be undertaken
if it is growing rapidly (Breast Clinic 2001). Generally a fibroadenoma will
be excised if it is over 2cm or the patient is over 40 years.

The level of anxiety of the patient must be taken into account, the
patient may request removal even if the fibroadenoma is small. If left alone
a fibroadenoma may resolve over time, it may stay the same or enlarge,
necessitating removal.

A very new procedure is being undertaken at two selected UK centres.
This involves the use of a laser inserted into the lesion to provide thermal
heat and can treat a lesion of up to 3cm. This is a minimally invasive procedure and gradually decreases the size of the fibroadenoma over 12
months. A MRI scan is done to check shrinkage.

Cysts

Cysts are common in pre-menopausal women and women taking HRT.
They present as fluid filled cavities within the breast tissue, and can be
painful prior to the menstrual period. These take the form of a lump, causing anxiety as the patient assumes that it is breast cancer and indeed
recurrent cysts may slightly increase the chance of cancer. As breast cancer
can present as a cyst, confusion may often arise. Cysts tend to be recurrent
and bilateral and feel smooth on examination. The fluid can vary from a
clear or turbid colour to black. Treatment is generally ultrasound and aspiration (2–10mls may be obtained). If the fluid appears blood stained a
sample will be sent to the laboratory. Ordinary cyst fluid will not usually be

blood stained. Danazol 100mg twice daily for six months can stop cysts developing but side effects need to be taken into account (see above) (Leinster et al. 2000).

Nipple disorders

Common symptoms are inversion and discharge. Inversion can be present from birth. Nipple discharge is usually caused by infection or benign breast conditions. A sample may be sent for examination and antibiotics will clear an infection. Blood stained discharge should always be sent for microscopic examination. Discharge is not uncommon and not always a sign of disease, healthy women may experience a discharge from the nipple.

Periductal mastitis/duct ectasia

Periductal mastitis, as previously mentioned, is a form of infection. The major ducts draining into the nipple distend (ectasia) and become infected and inflamed. Discharge from the nipple may be bloody and chronic infection can form scar tissue pulling the nipple in. This is often seen in older women, a 'transverse slit' appearance is often seen. Investigations must be carried out to exclude breast cancer when there is a history of recent nipple inversion in an older woman.

The condition can be bilateral. Pain and a lump beneath the nipple is not uncommon. An abscess and a fistula may form.

Duct ectasia is often associated with smokers. On mammography it can be seen to cause microcalcification and dilated ducts. Surgical removal of the milk ducts is often required and can be quite mutilating. The nipple will be left numb.

Microdochectomy (removal of one duct) is carried out to establish a diagnosis when the nipple discharge is serous or blood stained and coming from a single duct. This is to exclude intraduct carcinoma (Leinster et al. 2000).

Duct papilloma

Duct papilloma is a benign wart-like tumour of a single major duct near the nipple. One in 60 may be cancerous therefore excision is carried out especially if there is a blood stained nipple discharge. The patient may experience numbness in the nipple/areola area following excision. Multiple papillomas can occur in young women and should always be removed.

Galactorrhoea

This is the term for the discharge of milk outside pregnancy. It can be due to a number of causes including some drugs and certain types of cancer such as a pituitary tumour. However, it is often normal and occurs in relation to the menarche and menopause.

Phyllodes tumour

Phyllodes tumours are rare and around two-thirds are usually benign. However, they can exist in a malignant form accounting for less than two per cent of breast cancers. They are most common in women of 40–50 years and can be enormous. Phyllodes tumours require treatment by wide excision or they tend to recur.

Breast trauma

Trauma to the breast can produce an oil cyst, fat necrosis or a haematoma. An oil cyst can present as a breast mass. There may be calcification present on the wall of an oil cyst, which may mimic cancer on mammography. An oil cyst can be aspirated and a core biopsy will establish the diagnosis. Fat necrosis is seen as painless round firm lumps formed by damaged and disintegrating fatty tissue. Radiological features also mimic cancer. A diagnosis of haematoma should be considered where there is a history of trauma with bruising. Radiological and ultrasound features can be extremely varied. Again core biopsy can confirm diagnosis (Evans et al. 1998).

Sclerosing adenoma

These are excessive growth of lobule tissues and are painful and impalpable. The lesion is detected on mammography and core biopsy confirms the diagnosis.

Granulomatous mastitis

Multiple granulomata form in the terminal ducts and lobules. The condition is uncommon but well recognized. It can appear as a locally advanced breast cancer but TB, sarcoid and toxoplasmosis brucellosis should also be excluded. Surgery can lead to a discharging sinus so the problem is difficult to treat and there does not appear to be any consensus as to treatment.

Screen-detected benign calcification

This is usually confirmed by a stereotactically guided core biopsy to exclude DCIS or malignancy. A core biopsy avoids an unnecessary surgical biopsy and reassures the patient. Calcification tends to be the most common cause of a benign biopsy of a lesion detected during screening (Evans et al. 1998).

Extra nipples and breasts

Between one per cent and five per cent of people have supernumerary or accessory nipples, or less frequently, supernumerary or accessory breasts. Nipples usually develop below the breast and extra breast tissue develops in the lower axilla. These rarely require treatment but they are subject to the same diseases as breasts and nipples.

Hypoplasia

The absence of one breast usually associated with defects in the pectoral muscle. Treatment is usually augmentation, reduction or a combination.

Juvenile hypertrophy

Juvenile hypertrophy is the term for pre-pubertal breast enlargement. Uncontrolled growth can occur in adolescent girls. Reduction mammoplasty cures social embarrassment, discomfort, pain and the inability to carry out daily tasks.

Epithelial hyperplasia

This is the increase in the number of cells lining the terminal duct lobule. It is also known as proliferative breast disease. If the hyperplastic cells also show cellular atypia the condition is known as atypical hyperplasia. The absolute risk of breast cancer developing in a patient with atypical hyperplasia who does not have a first-degree relative with breast cancer is eight per cent at 10 years. For a woman with a first-degree relative with cancer the risk is 20–25 per cent at 15 years. Closer clinical follow-up than the rest of the population may be advised.

Gynaecomastia

Gynaecomastia is the growth of breast tissue in males. Benign and reversible, it can be seen in 30–60 per cent of boys, aged 10–16 years.

Eighty per cent resolve spontaneously. If there is further enlargement or embarrassment surgery can be performed. Causes include puberty, testicular tumours, some drugs, malnutrition and hypothroidism.

In men aged 50–80 years the condition is known as senescent gynaecomastia and is not associated with endocrine abnormalities.

Body builders taking anabolic steroids can develop gynaecomastia. Danazol produces some improvement in the older man (Dixon and Mansel 1994).

Core biopsy and mammotome

Core biopsy is carried out as part of the assessment process. When an abnormality is palpable as a discrete lump a fine needle aspiration is often done but core biopsy provides histological detail. Core biopsy is performed using a spring-loaded gun with a 14-gauge needle. Local anaesthetic is administered prior to the procedure.

For screen-detected, impalpable lesions, such as microcalcification, X-ray guided (stereotactic) core biopsy is required. Five separate cores are taken and the specimens X-rayed to confirm that representative tissue has been obtained (Evans et al. 1998). Core biopsy will be discussed further in Chapter 4.

The mammotome has recently been approved by the US Food and Drug Administration but is available around the world. The mammotome is a minimally invasive alternative to a surgical biopsy but removes more tissue than a core biopsy. It is also known as a vacuum-assisted biopsy. Suction is used to draw tissue into an opening in the side of a cylinder inserted into the breast tissue. A rotating knife then cuts the tissue samples from the rest of the breast. A local anaesthetic is administered and the procedure takes about an hour (American Cancer Society online 2001).

Benign breast disease and women's anxieties

It has been found that women with benign breast disease and those with breast cancer can suffer similar levels of psychological distress and anxiety in the period from being aware of a problem to diagnosis. Post diagnosis the anxiety levels in the patients with a benign condition fall more quickly. Women who have had several benign episodes worry more about breast cancer and see themselves at greater risk. Therefore it would seem that women require more support pre-diagnosis (Woodward and Webb 2001). Breast care nurses tend to see the women diagnosed with cancer. However, all women need their anxieties addressing in the lead up to diagnosis. The most important information need appears to be knowing when the diagnosis will be received. Other important anxieties are the risk of developing cancer and information about other diagnostic tests and follow-up (Deane and Degner 1998).

The British Surgeons Group of the British Association of Surgical Oncology recommend that specialist nurses should be available to all breast patients and recognize that women with a benign diagnosis may still have questions (BASO 1998). BASO also recommends that breast cancer patients should bring a relative or friend to consultations, and that possibly the same should apply to women with benign diseases to reduce distress. Much of the work of a Breast Unit outpatient clinic is the reassurance of the 'worried well'.

Immediate reporting of results of investigations can benefit patients with benign disorders (Ubhi et al. 1996). In a study at Frenchay Hospital, Bristol, one-stop clinics were found to ease anxiety as the investigations, results and counselling are all undertaken in one day. Women receive advocacy from a nurse counsellor, who meets them before the tests and acts as advocate when the results are given. Women feel more in control, less anxious and better informed. However, there still may not be enough time allowed for questions (Cawthorne 1999).

Nurse-led clinics

At some centres nurses run breast pain clinics, aspirate cysts, lead the assessment process and undertake counselling. Garvican et al. (1998) found that technical expertise in fine needle aspiration was better when performed by nurses than by other health care professionals. Benefits also include helping to cope with the workload of breast units and increasing the quality of patient care. However, these nurse-led clinics are only part of the solution to overcrowded clinics. Training and accrediting nurses to fulfil Calman Hine requirements is a major problem as nurses are undertaking medical tasks and responsibilities usually associated with doctors (Thomson 1999). Further research is required to assess where nurses are most valuable. Nurse-led clinics must not compromise the conventional role of the breast care nurse.

References

American Cancer Society online (2001) How is Breast Cancer Diagnosed? Cancer Reference Information: Breast Cancer. http://www.cancer.org (accessed June 2001).

Austoker J, Mansel R (1999) Guidelines for Referral of Patients with Breast Problems. 2nd edn. Sheffield: NHSBSP.

Avillion A (1998) Evaluating breast pain. Pennsylvania Nurse 53(2): 8–11.

Breast Clinic (2001) www.thebreastclinic.com/thebreast.htm (accessed June 2001).

British Association of Surgical Oncologists (BASO) (1998) Guidelines for Surgeons in the Management of Symptomatic Breast Disease in the United Kingdom. The BASO Breast Specialty Group. London: BASO. Also available online at http://www.baso.org/breast.html (accessed June 2001).

Cawthorne S (1999) Prompt diagnosis allays fears in women with benign breast disease. International Symposium on Benign Breast Disease abstract: Breast Care Campaign website. www.breastcare.co.uk (accessed June 2001).

Cawthorne S, Mansel R (2000) Study in conjunction with Dispatches – 'Bras The Bare Facts'. Documentary shown November 2000, Channel 4 Television UK.

D'Amelio R, Farris M, Grande S, et al. (2001) Association between polycystic ovary and fibrocystic breast disease. Gynaecological and Obstetric Investigation 51(2): 134–7.

Deane KA, Degner LF (1998) Information needs, uncertainty and anxiety in women who had a breast biopsy with benign outcome. Cancer Nursing 21(2): 117–26.

Department of Health (1997) The New NHS, Modern, Dependable. London: HMSO.

Dixon JM, Breast Care Campaign online (2001) Managing Breast Pain www.breastcare.co.uk (accessed June 2001).

Dixon JM, Mansel RE (1994) ABC of breast diseases: Congenital problems and aberrations of normal breast development and involution. British Medical Journal 309: 797–800.

Dixon JM, McDonald C, Elton RA, Miller WR (1999) Risk of breast cancer in women with palpable breast cysts: a prospective study. The Lancet 353(9166): 1742–5.

Evans AJ, Wilson ARM, Blamey RW, Robertson JFR, et al. (1998) Atlas of Breast Disease Management. 50 Illustrative Cases. London: WB Saunders.

Garvican L, Grimsey E, Littlejohns P, et al. (1998) Satisfaction with the Clinical Nurse Specialist in a breast care clinic questionairre survey. British Medical Journal 316: 976–7.

Gregory WM, Mills SP, Hamed HH, Fentiman IS (1999) Applied kinesiology for the treatment of women with mastalgia. International Symposium on Benign Breast Disease Abstract, Breast Care Campaign website www.breastcare.co.uk (accessed June 2001).

Henderson G (1998) The East Surrey breast cancer referrals guidelines project. Pulse, November.

Leinster SJ, Gibbs TJ, Downey H (2000) Shared Care for Breast Disease. Oxford: Isis Medical Media.

Minton JP, Abou-Isa H, Reiches M, Roseman JM (1981) Clinical and biochemical studies on methylxanthine related fibrocystic breast disease. Surgery 90: 229–304.

O'Reilly M, Patel K, Cummins R (2000) Tuberculosis of the breast presenting as carcinoma. Military Medicine 165(10): 800–2.

Thomson L (1999) Nurse led clinics will not solve all breast unit workload problems. Benign Breast Disease abstract: Breast Care Campaign website. www.breastcare.co.uk (accessed June 2001).

Ubhi SS, Shaw P, Wright S, et al. (1996) Anxiety in patients with symptomatic breast disease: effects of immediate v delayed communication of results. Annals of the Royal College of Surgeons of England 78: 466–9.

Woodward V, Webb C (2001) Women's anxieties surrounding breast disorders – a review of the literature. Journal of Advanced Nursing 33(1) 29–41.

CHAPTER FOUR
Diagnosing breast cancer

Breast cancer is diagnosed after screening (when the patient is asymptomatic) or when a patient presents with symptoms (symptomatic). Generally a lump of over 15mm can be found on self-examination although a clinician may find a lump on palpation of around 10mm. This is in contrast with tumours detected by mammography of 2–5mm (Mera 1997). Health care professionals now seek alternatives to surgical biopsies of lumps or mammographic abnormalities. In fact the number of screen-detected abnormalities found within the NHS Breast Screening Programme would make surgical biopsy of all of them impossible if this were to be the main diagnostic procedure (Poole 1997).

Triple assessment

Combined triple assessment as advised by the Cytology Sub-Group of the National Co-ordinating Committee of Breast Screening Pathology (1993) is the 'gold standard' for the diagnosis of breast cancer. Once the patient is in the breast unit, having been referred or having been through screening, the full diagnostic process will take place. This consists of clinical examination, imaging (mammography and/or ultrasound) and tissue diagnosis (fine needle aspiration or core biopsy).

Clinical examination

Undertaken properly, generally by the specialist breast surgeon, clinical examination is specific and sensitive, and is an important part of the diagnostic process. The examination must be carried out systematically. Inspection is important and both sides must be compared. The flat of the fingers is used to carry out palpation and all the quadrants of the breast must be covered. The area behind the nipple must be examined and any

51

discharge noted. The axilla should be examined although clinical assessment here is not accurate (Leinster et al. 2000).

The surgeon decides whether further investigations are necessary. Most
patients present as clinically normal and are discharged from the clinic
back to the care of their GP.

Imaging

Mammography (discussed in Chapter 3) and ultrasound are routinely used.
Both breasts will be examined by mammography even if a problem is detected only on one side – sometimes a cancer is found on the non-symptomatic
side. A benign tumour will look more regular and have regular margins
whereas a cancerous tumour will be more irregular in shape and often contain small foci of calcification (microcalcification), sometimes the only sign
of a malignancy (Mera 1997). Microcalcification can be associated with
breast cancer, DCIS or benign disease. Some forms of cancer, for example
medullary cancer, may look like a fibroadenoma. Stromal deformities are
mostly benign radial scars but small tubular carcinomas can look similar
mammographically. Further mammographic views may be carried out with
compression and magnification of the area and if the difference cannot be
ascertained further investigations must be carried out. Any mass visible on
a mammogram should have an ultrasound scan (Leinster et al. 2000).

Ultrasound (ultrasonography) is generally employed for the examination of dense breast tissue but does not detect microcalcification very well.
It is useful for identifying palpable masses, areas of nodularity or further
definition of masses detected on a mammogram. It can easily identify
benign breast cysts.

Cytology

Cells for laboratory analysis are obtained by fine needle aspiration, needle
core biopsy or surgical biopsy.

Fine needle aspiration

If a lump is clearly palpable a fine needle aspiration (FNA) can be taken.
FNA is quick, safe and inexpensive (Poole 1997). This is performed by
inserting a 21-gauge needle into the lump or suspicious area and evacuat-
ing cells and fluid. Ideally for a successful aspirate for cytology no aspirate
should show in the syringe. The contents are expelled onto a microscope
slide. These are then fixed by rapid air drying or by immersion in alcohol
and stained. Eosin and haematoxylin are used to stain air-dried slides and
alcohol-fixed slides are stained with Papinicolaou's stain. The slides are

then examined in the laboratory. The individual cells are evaluated according to their cytological characteristics. However, this method is not as accurate as histological diagnosis of intact tissue, for example core biopsy, or surgery (Mera 1997). Sometimes inadequate material is obtained – up to 20 per cent of cases. These are designated C1, inadequate for diagnosis (Leinster et al. 2000). Other classifications are:

C2 – definitely benign
C3 – suspicious, probably benign
C4 – suspicious, probably malignant
C5 – definitely malignant.

A C3 or C4 classification would warrant further investigation, usually a core biopsy or a surgical excision biopsy. It is likely that a suspicious lump would be surgically removed anyway.

Needle core biopsy

If a lump is clearly palpable and a FNA is inconclusive, a needle core biopsy can be taken without image guidance. It is less likely that an inadequate specimen will be obtained. Processing and reporting takes longer than for FNA but it is possible to distinguish between *in situ* and invasive carcinoma. If there is still a discrepancy formal excision biopsy will be carried out (Leinster et al. 2000).

When an abnormality is impalpable, for example microcalcification, it is necessary to carry out core biopsy under image guidance. This is undertaken when the clinician wishes to be absolutely sure that a sizable sample of lesion is obtained. Image-guided core biopsy of impalpable lesions is highly accurate. Up to 70 per cent of screening abnormalities are impalpable (Blamey et al. 2000). These may be localized by ultrasound or mammography. A local anaesthetic is used and the patient is positioned as if undergoing a mammogram. A nurse is present for support and to ensure that the patient remains still. The suspicious area is localized on the mammogram. The radiologist will make an incision into the skin of the breast. The narrow bore biopsy needle is inserted and the biopsy gun releases a mechanism attached to the needle and pushes the needle into the suspicious area. The spring mechanism makes a fairly loud sound and the patient should be warned about this. Up to five 'cores' are generally obtained. A core biopsy will ream out a core of tissue about 3mm wide and 10–15mm long (Lakhani et al. 1993). Core biopsies are X-rayed immediately to ensure that sufficient samples of calcification have been obtained. Care must be taken with small breasts not to traverse the full breast thickness (Evans et al. 1998).

An 11-gauge vacuum-assisted biopsy device, the mammotome, is now available. This provides more tissue and increases the diagnostic yield for the small number of lesions; neither FNA nor needle core biopsy provides a clear diagnosis (Blamey et al. 2000).

Patients find core biopsy quite acceptable (Evans et al. 1998). A small dressing is usually applied and the patient is advised that the area may be sore for 24 hours with a small amount of bruising. The patient's usual choice of mild analgesia can be used.

Needle core biopsy is reported as:

B1 – normal breast
B2 – benign breast tissue, for example fibroadenoma
B3 – equivocal, possibly potentially malignant
B4 – suspicious, for example atypical ductal hyperplasia
B5 – malignant.

The surgeon and radiologist work together closely at the breast clinic. They both assess the problem and decide independently on the significance of any abnormality. Their opinions are classified from 1 to 5.

1 Normal/no significant abnormality – no further investigations required. The patient is reassured and discharged.
2 Benign – a report of benign or normal breast tissue is acceptable.
3 Probably benign – applies to a definite discrete lump that shows benign features on clinical assessment and imaging but a cytological or histological diagnosis is required. To avoid a surgical biopsy a FNA must show unequivocally benign cells or a core biopsy must show a benign diagnosis. An equivocal FNA means that a core biopsy is necessary. 'Suspicious' or 'malignant' then indicates a surgical biopsy.
4 Probably malignant – this term is used for a definite lesion with features not compatible with a clearly benign diagnosis. FNA or core biopsy is performed to give a clear cancer diagnosis but diagnostic or therapeutic surgery is mandatory.
5 Malignant – unequivocal clinical or imaging signs of malignancy. Diagnosed with FNA, core biopsy or excision biopsy (Evans et al. 1998).

A specific category is decided for each lesion before FNA or any type of biopsy is carried out and therefore classification is not altered on receipt of the pathology report. These categories are as follows:

Category A – clinically and radiologically malignant. Operative biopsy required unless FNA or core biopsy shows cancer in which case the surgeon can offer therapeutic surgery.
Category B – definite lesion is present but clinically and on imaging it has benign characteristics. If no definite diagnosis is received on FNA or core biopsy the lesion is surgically removed.
Category C – a 'fail-safe' category. Clinically benign lesion in a patient of 25

years or under. Where there is a lumpy area and imaging is normal but the surgeon is not completely satisfied, FNA or core biopsy will be undertaken (Evans et al. 1998).

Essentially the effectiveness of FNA or core biopsy depends on the expertise of the operator to target the suspicious area of tissue (Poole 1997). However these non-surgical techniques offer increased efficiency of diagnosis at a lower cost (half that of a surgical biopsy) (Fine 1993). The accuracy of diagnosis remains equivalent to a surgical biopsy and there are negligible complications and less psychological trauma (Schmidt 1994).

Wire localization biopsy

Occasionally a core biopsy does not give enough information about the nature of a suspicious area or lump. An excision biopsy will be required to remove the area. The patient may be in hospital overnight or as a day case. If the abnormality is a mammographic finding rather than a palpable lump a wire localization biopsy may be performed. The radiologist uses a mammogram or ultrasound to insert a very fine wire, often with a needle on the end into the breast to pinpoint the area of suspicion. The radiologist may place more than one needle into the area having studied the mammogram first to ascertain where the needle will go (McGinn 1992). The wire is carefully taped to the patient and surgery is performed the same day. The surgeon follows the wire and excises the area around the needle. When the area is excised it will be X-rayed to ensure that all the correct area has been removed.

The patient is taken to the breast unit or X-ray department for the insertion of the wire and then returned to the ward to await surgery. This can cause much anxiety for patients as they are undergoing two procedures within a short time and facing the prospect of a biopsy. Women scheduled for breast biopsy experience heightened anxiety. The prevalence of benign breast disease in women and the anxiety caused by the prospect of breast cancer make these patients an important nursing concern (Deane 1997). To face a biopsy is to face the possibility of serious disease (McGinn 1992). It is good practice to avail these women of a contact number for the breast care nurse prior to the biopsy. The breast care nurse will probably not see every patient scheduled for biopsy or surgery for benign disease routinely but if they have a contact number any questions or anxieties can be discussed if necessary.

Until the 1990s women at the medical consultation were informed of a suspicious area within the breast requiring investigation in hospital. The patient was given a general anaesthetic and a biopsy analysed whilst the patient was still anaesthetized. Depending on the results of this frozen section the surgeon proceeded to a radical mastectomy. Consent for this was obtained beforehand so a woman did not know whether or not she would have a breast when she awakened. Therefore she suddenly had to cope with disfigurement and a life-threatening disease. Now women are offered the two-stage procedure of triple assessment and/or diagnostic biopsy before any surgery is considered (Batt 1994). Frozen section is still undertaken very occasionally when all other diagnostic biopsies are somehow inconclusive.

A new procedure, nipple endoscopy, is being undertaken in some centres. This involves the use of a 0.9mm camera inserted through the nipple so that the structure of the breast ducts can be seen and any areas of DCIS identified. These areas can then be marked and dissected.

BASO guidelines

The British Association of Surgical Oncology (BASO) have produced guidelines for surgeons working in breast cancer screening and diagnosis (BASO 1996). These quality objectives include:

- Women within screening will obtain rapid assessment and surgical opinion, a good cosmetic result and help from a breast care nurse.
- Surgeons must ensure that the majority of palpable and impalpable cancers receive a pre-operative tissue cancer diagnosis. Open surgical biopsies must be minimized where definitive histology proves benign.
- The time between excision and receipt of the specimen for X-ray or report in theatre should be less than 10 minutes.
- The surgeon should minimize the cosmetic effect of diagnostic biopsies.
- The accurate positioning of wires in wire localization biopsies should be maximized.
- More than 95 per cent of impalpable lesions should be correctly identified at the first localization biopsy (BASO 1996).

'One-stop' clinics

One-stop clinics offer same-day investigations of symptomatic breast problems and are becoming increasingly popular. In some units a FNA report is available within 30 minutes. Speedy diagnosis can reduce psychological distress for women with benign conditions but could be detrimental to those with cancer (Harcourt et al. 1999). The appropriate provision of psychological care warrants further research. Levels of distress at both types of clinic tend to be high at the first visit but Harcourt et al. (1999) found that eight weeks on, women with a speedy diagnosis of cancer were associated with higher levels of depressive symptoms.

Ubhi et al. (1996) studied immediate versus delayed communication of results via one-stop clinics, where the radiologist or cytologist provides the results of mammograms and/or ultrasound and FNA on the same day. In women with benign disease immediate communication of the results at the one-day visit was associated with a significant drop in anxiety post-consultation compared with returning a week later. Women with cancer were very anxious post-communication whether results were given immediately or not. Therefore it can be said that immediate reporting of results is beneficial in benign patients (Ubhi et al. 1996).

However, speedy diagnosis does not moderate the psychological impact of a cancer diagnosis. In some respects the stress is intensified when the results are provided quickly (Ambler et al. 1999).

Poole (1997) observes that the widespread use of fine needle techniques, whilst removing the process of a hospital stay and a general anaesthetic, has introduced the notion of the 'waiting-game'. Definitive results can be obtained within hours and this has led to diversification in the structure of diagnostic breast services. There has been a universal failure to address specifically the experience of women waiting for results of diagnostic tests. Some units can give results in as little as two hours. Further research must be done into the experiences of women undergoing non-surgical biopsy. The period of time waiting for results should be considered a distinct phase within the diagnostic interval (Poole 1997).

Giving the diagnosis – breaking bad news

A breast cancer diagnosis not only threatens an organ intimately related to self-esteem, femininity, sexuality and motherhood but is also a threat to life (Speigel 1990). Women, particularly those with a screen-detected cancer, are suddenly faced with the prospect of a life-threatening illness and possible death even though they are asymptomatic and feel well. People with cancer often search for their own explanation as to why they have developed it and may feel lonely and isolated. Cancer can involve many losses and can dramatically alter the person's life. However, individuals' reactions may vary – some may show a fighting spirit, others may become depressed and anxious (Morton 1996). Emotions tend to be strong in patients with breast cancer and health professionals need to be able to deal with these. They especially need to be aware of how to break the news that the patient's test results show that she has breast cancer.

The key task for the health professional is to establish the patient's information needs. The consultant breast surgeon usually delivers that news when the patient returns for her results. How the news is given depends on the patient's awareness of her condition. Patients who have no prior idea that they have cancer present a problem. To tell the news in a blunt fashion may lead to denial or overwhelming distress. The patient should be given a 'warning shot', given time to respond and then taken step by step until the word 'cancer' is mentioned. Time to assimilate the news should be given. Distress should be acknowledged and explored. Once information about diagnosis and treatment has been given, it is important that the health professional checks that the patient has understood what has been said. A family member or friend can be present or the patient can tape the consultation (Faulkner and Maguire 1994).

Questions about prognosis are almost inevitable. It is best to pitch the answer at an appropriate, realistic level. As this may elicit further concerns, time should be given to explore these. Treatment options should be given where possible. The patient may want to be fully involved or may want to leave the decision to the clinician. Patients' wishes should be followed wherever possible as this seems to affect their psychological adaptation (Faulkner and Maguire 1994).

Dr Robert Buckman (1999) advocates a six-step protocol for breaking bad news:

1 Getting started – it is important that the consultation takes place in a private setting with comfortable seating. The patient decides who is to accompany them. The consultant indicates that the conversation will be two-way; that is, asking the patient how they are feeling right now before any information is given.
2 Find out how much the patient knows – ask what they have already been told and what they understand. Note how technical their description is and what their emotional state is like.
3 Find out how much the patient wants to know – whether the patient wants every detail or a more general picture.
4 Share information – decide the agenda prior to seeing the patient, for example to cover diagnosis, treatment options, prognosis, support although in reality only diagnosis and treatment options will be covered at this consultation. Give information in small chunks, checking carefully that the patient has understood and has had a chance to ask questions. Long lectures are overwhelming. Ensure that the patient understands the language; do not use medical jargon.
5 Respond to the patient's feelings – identify her reaction and ask how she is feeling.
6 Plan the follow-through – outline a plan to be carried out and agree a contract with the patient when next to be seen, when the patient will undergo surgery, when the oncologist will see the patient if necessary, etc. Always give a contact number (Buckman 1999).

It must be acknowledged that there will probably be tears and distress; allow the patient to cry and provide tissues. The patient may not understand to begin with and may want to go over the information again and again. A single communication may not be sufficient for the patient who is shocked and anxious (Goldberg 1984). Also, doctors may think that they have communicated the news but the message may not have been received by the patient or the language may have been too technical (Ley 1982).

The patient should always receive bad news in person and not over the telephone except in exceptional circumstances. Eye contact and body language must be used to convey sympathy, encouragement, warmth and reassurance. Patients have a legal and moral right to accurate and reliable information and should be given the diagnosis honestly and in simple language. It is a good idea to inform the patient's GP about the patient's level of understanding so that the GP can offer additional support and information.

Sensitivity to the patient's culture, race, religious beliefs and social background is necessary. It may be necessary to use a family member to interpret if the patient does not speak much English. Some hospitals may have an interpreter or a contact number for one in the community.

Family or significant others should be present to provide support. In the case of breast cancer patients the breast care nurse is usually present at the consultation to provide support and reinforce the information following the consultation.

It is wise to avoid giving a prognosis with a definite timescale but a realistic, broad time frame can be given. Treatment options can be discussed and the patient assured that she will be involved at every stage of the decision making.

Help can be offered in telling family members the bad news. It is very difficult to inform children that their mother has breast cancer. Often the breast care nurse will visit the family at home where they are in familiar surroundings.

Everything relating to the consultation should always be documented in the patient's notes (Girgis et al. 1999).

Ultimately, patients who have been told their diagnosis can choose whether to deny what is happening or face it. People will develop their own ways of coming to terms with a cancer diagnosis. Reactions may include denial, anger and despair. For the health care professional, questioning, listening and responding are critical skills, required to discover how the patient perceives her situation. A careful choice of words is essential (Morton 1996). The breast care nurse has an extremely important role in supporting the patient who has been diagnosed with breast cancer and can offer back-up information, advice and counselling. She is also in a position to recognize signs of psychological morbidity in the form of a depressive or anxious state, which might develop in a newly diagnosed patient who cannot surmount certain psychological hurdles (Faulkner and Maguire 1994). (Psychological morbidity will be discussed in Chapter 11.)

Information needs at diagnosis and the breast care nurse's role

Whilst women with breast cancer are primarily concerned about their clinical treatment and chances of survival, it is important that the multidisciplinary team meet their other needs. Effective communication and respect for the patient's information needs are vitally important.

Information is an essential form of support following a cancer diagnosis (Bottomley and Jones 1997). Many women with breast cancer seek at least some information. Information seeking is one of the principal coping strategies used by people facing an adverse situation (Shaw et al. 1994). Providing women with breast cancer with the right type and amount of information is very important as a treatment choice may exist for many. Adequate information must be given as this decision is of utmost importance and providing a choice of treatment has been shown to be of benefit in terms of long-term adjustment. It also ensures that the patient feels comfortable in participating in the decision-making process. Health care professionals have a responsibility to provide specific information so informed decision making can take place (Leinster et al. 1989). Information must be full, prompt, clear and objective (NICE 2002).

It is also important to realize that a woman with a diagnosis of DCIS, although a non-invasive condition with a good prognosis, will share a similar response to a woman with invasive breast cancer (Bottomley and Jones 1997). It is vitally important, therefore to provide both these groups of women with clear, concise information.

Women need to be given an opportunity to share the impact of a cancer diagnosis and to discuss their information needs and that of their family, as their partners and families are also affected. The breast care nurse can arrange a home visit or an appointment for the patient and family to discuss their needs and address their fears and anxieties.

Information needs may vary for different age groups. Obtaining information may be difficult for the elderly women with breast cancer, who make up a large proportion of patients diagnosed with the disease. Older women tend to have less knowledge of the disease and risk factors and believe that they are less susceptible. They may also have more negative attitudes to screening (Mah and Bryant 1992).

A knowledge of what the patient wants to know can make the information-giving process worthwhile and effective. Nurses can play a key role in patient education, including providing useful and appropriate information to patients. Luker et al. (1995) undertook a study on information needs of women newly diagnosed with breast cancer. The information needs identified were:

1 How advanced the disease is and how far it has spread.
2 The likelihood of a cure.
3 How the treatment will affect social activities/hobbies.
4 How family/friends will be affected.
5 Information regarding diet, support groups, social worker, counselling.
6 Information on how body image will be affected.
7 Information on different treatment options, advantages and disadvantages.
8 Risk to family/family developing breast cancer.
9 Side effects of treatment.

The three most important needs for women were found to be the likelihood of cure, how far advanced the disease is and the different treatment options available. These three may well fall within the scope of the breast care nurse. She may act as facilitator, making medical colleagues aware of the patient's needs (Luker et al. 1995). Survival issues appear to be the priority at the time of diagnosis. Even though patients may say that they want to know everything, it may be appropriate to give high-quality information about specific issues identified by the patient rather than large amounts of general information (Luker et al. 1996). Providing information on other than survival issues may not be appropriate at diagnosis especially as memory is severely affected at this time.

The timing of giving information is important. The time when women are ready to receive information differs for each one and it may be required on an on-going basis (Brown et al. 2000). It is likely that much will not be remembered at first due to the shock of the diagnosis. It may be necessary to go over information several times. Information needs may change the further from diagnosis the patient gets. Also, as the patient will only be in hospital for a short time and then will be at home away from hospital staff, it is vital to give adequate information (Luker et al. 1995). Time is often limited in the hospital environment and the patient may want to know as much as possible about their care and treatment. Therefore, it is important to assess the priority needs of the patient and address those first.

Some women may have strong views on the way that health care professionals communicate. Some may prefer a positive, reassuring style, others prefer a style that fosters openness and honesty when information is given and also encourages questions. The surgeon may be seen as an important communicator (Brown et al. 2000). Sometimes, however, doctors and nurses may use minimizing language or behaviour to manage a difficult situation. Minimizing the size, severity and significance of the problem will limit distress but possibly only in the short term (Lawler 1991). NICE (2002) recommend that surgeons and oncologists undertake formal training in communication skills.

Some women at a consultation may wish to make notes or a tape recording. They are generally asked if they would like a friend or relative to be present for support and for remembering what has been discussed. Written information is usually provided as verbal information alone may not be sufficient. Pamphlets and other written information need to be readable and of a suitable level. Material in plain English with an easy to read format given out prior to treatment is preferable (Butow et al. 1998). It should be honest, relevant, user-friendly and timely (Mumford 1997). The information must be good quality and developed from the patient's perspective if it is to be effective. Good quality information is clearly communicated, evidence based and involves patients in the development process (Centre for Health Information Quality 2000).

The environment in which patients are seen is also important. The breast care nurse should be able to talk to the patient in a private and pleasant room where they will not be overheard. There should be enough space for the relative or friend accompanying her and there should be facilities for the provision of refreshments. The breast care nurse may wish to see patients in a room that contains the pamphlets and written information so that the patient can browse and take whatever seems to be appropriate for her.

Patients should be informed of sources of practical help, local support networks and benefits helplines. Some women with breast cancer may be entitled to aid from Macmillan Cancer Relief: the breast care nurse is in a position to identify these patients and provide information on this. Many women with breast cancer are over 65 years, many may live alone and require practical or financial help. Women with children or other dependants and carers may also require advice and support. Many units have a social worker who is attached to the unit and who can provide much assistance to these women.

Some women may also use the Internet for information and use on-line discussion groups and websites (Butow et al. 1998). Most of the breast cancer organizations now have websites with up-to-date information for patients, for example Breast Cancer Care, Breakthrough Breast Cancer.

Luker et al. (1996) found that women who were newly diagnosed felt that the most useful sources of information were the hospital consultant, the breast care nurse and the leaflets provided by the breast care nurse. Some felt that their GP, the ward nurses and the voluntary sector had been helpful.

For a patient with breast cancer the most important stage of psychological care is likely to be near the beginning of her cancer journey. The breast care nurse tends to become involved immediately after the patient has received her diagnosis or during the diagnostic consultation. Establishing a relationship prior to this offers a potential benefit (Ambler et al. 1999).

An advocacy style of intervention could reduce the stress of the consultation by directing it more towards the patient's needs. The main aims of the advocacy method are to increase the patient's sense of involvement, provide emotional support and promote better understanding of treatment outcomes and options. The breast care nurse meets the patient prior to the consultation and helps her compile a list of questions. She then accompanies the patient into the consultation and counselling continues afterwards (Ambler et al. 1999).

The breast care nurse is often the main source of information and support once the diagnosis is established. As well as receiving written and verbal information, the patient is provided with the telephone number of the breast care nurse so questions and fears can be addressed almost immediately. Time and privacy should be provided whether the consultation is via the telephone, in the breast care unit or at the patient's home. Adequate information and counselling should do much to help prevent physical and psychological problems at a later stage. The patient's primary care team should also have the contact number of the breast care nurse in case of future problems.

The specialist breast care nurse is becoming an increasingly important educational resource for patients (Luker et al. 1996). A major part of the breast care nurse's role is to support patients at the stressful time of receiving their diagnoses. Specialist breast care nurses ideally should complete the ENB A11, Advanced Breast Care Nursing (NHS Executive 1996) and hold an oncological qualification. Higher degree qualifications are desirable and should be in subjects that allow the individual to demonstrate their contribution to nursing knowledge (RCN 2002). Applicants for breast care nursing posts are generally appointed with the understanding that if they do not already possess a degree, they will be required to undertake one. The Royal College of Nursing Breast Care Nurses Forum (RCN 2002) recommend a standard of education and experience suitable for the role. Two years' experience in breast cancer care in any practice setting is advised along with the academic qualifications. Experience gained in practice is vital to demonstrate knowledge and skills to supplement theory. Teaching and assessing skills and counselling skills are extremely useful, although some may come into post without any training in counselling.

The RCN Forum sets out a proposed career continuum for advanced nursing practice roles in breast care culminating in the post of nurse consultant. At the moment there is only one such post in breast cancer care but it is hoped that future appointments will be made.

References

Ambler N, Rumsey W, Harcourt D, Khan F, Harcourt D (1999) Specialist nurse counsellor interventions at that time of the diagnosis of breast cancer comparing
'advocacy' with a conventional approach. Journal of Advanced Nursing 29(2),
445–53.

BASO (British Association of Surgical Oncology) (1996) Quality Assurance Guidelines
For Surgeons Working in Breast Cancer Screening. NHSBSP Publication no. 20.
Sheffield: NHS Breast Screening Programme.

Batt S (1994) Patient No More: The Politics of Breast Cancer. London: Scarlett Press.

Blamey RW, Wilson ARM, Patnick J (2000) ABC of breast diseases – screening for
breast cancer. British Medical Journal 321: 689–93.

Bottomley A, Jones L (1997) Breast cancer care: women's experiences. European
Journal of Cancer Care 6: 124–32.

Brown M, Koch T, Webb C (2000) Information needs of women with non-invasive
breast cancer. Journal of Clinical Nursing 9: 713–22.

Buckman R (1999) Robert Buckman's Six Step Protocol for Breaking Bad News. Ethics
in medicine website, http://eduserve.hscer.washington.edu/bioethics/topics/bad-
nws.html (accessed August 2001).

Butow P, Brindle C, McConnell D, Boakes R, Tattersall M (1998) Information booklets
about cancer: factors influencing patient satisfaction and utilisation. Patient
Education and Counselling 33(2): 129–41.

Centre for Health Information Quality (2000) Guidelines for producing health information. www.hfht.org/chiq/producers-guidelines.htm (accessed July 2001).

Cytology Sub-group of the National Co-ordinating Committee of Breast Screening
Pathology (1993) Guidelines for Cyto-Procedures and Reporting in Breast Cancer
Screening. NHSBSP Publication no. 22. London: NHS Breast Screening
Programme.

Deane K (1997) The role of the breast clinic nurse. The Association of Perioperative
Registered Nurses (AORN) Journal 66(2): 304–10.

Evans AJ, Wilson ARM, Blamey RW, Robertson JFR, Ellis IO, Elston CW (1998) Atlas
of Breast Disease Management: 50 Illustrative Cases. London: WB Saunders.

Faulkner A, Maguire P (1994) Talking to cancer patients and their relatives. Oxford:
Oxford University Press.

Fine R (1993) New breast biopsy improves outcomes, patient satisfaction. Same Day
Surgery 8(17): 95–7.

Girgis A, Sanson-Fisher RW, Schofield MJ (1999) Is there consensus between breast cancer patients and providers on guidelines for breaking bad news? Behavioural
Medicine 1999: 25(2) 69–77.

Goldberg RJ (1984) Disclosure of information to adult cancer patients: issues and
updates. Journal of Clinical Oncology 303: 1507–11.

Harcourt D, Rumsey N, Ambler N (1999) Same day diagnosis of symptomatic breast
problems: psychological impact and coping strategies. Psychology Health and
Medicine 4(1): 57–71.

Lakhani SR, Dilly SA, Finlayson CJ (1993) Basic Pathology: An Introduction to the
Mechanisms of Disease. London: Hodder Headline.

Lawler J (1991) Behind the Screens: Nursing, Somology and the Problem of the Body.
Melbourne: Churchill Livingstone.

Leinster SJ, Ashcroft JJ, Slade PD, Dewey ME (1989) Mastectomy versus conservative surgery: psychological effects of the patient's choice of treatment. Journal of Psychosocial Oncology 7(1/2): 179–92.

Leinster SJ, Gibbs TJ, Downey H (2000) Shared Care for Breast Disease. Oxford: Isis Medical Media.

Ley P (1982) Giving information to patients. In Eiser JR (Ed.) Social Psychology and Behavioural Medicine. Chichester: John Wiley & Sons.

Luker K, Beaver K, Leinster S, Owens RG, Degner L, Sloan J (1995) The information needs of women newly diagnosed with breast cancer. Journal of Advanced Nursing 22(1): 134–41.

Luker K, Beaver K, Leinster S, Samuel J, Owens RG (1996) Information needs and sources for women with breast cancer: a follow-up study. Journal of Advanced Nursing 23(3): 487–95.

McGinn KA (1992) The Informed Woman's Guide to Breast Health. Palo Alto, CA: Bull Publishing.

Mah Z, Bryant H (1992) Age as a factor in breast cancer knowledge, attitudes and screening behaviour. Canadian Medical Association Journal 146(12): 2167–74.

Mera S (1997) Pathology and Understanding Disease Prevention. Cheltenham: Stanley Thomas.

Morton R (1996) Breaking bad news to patients with cancer. Professional Nurse 11(10): 669–71.

Mumford ME (1997) A descriptive study of the readability of patient information leaflets designed by nurses. Journal of Advanced Nursing 26: 985–91.

National Health Service Executive (1996) Guidance for Purchasers. Improving Outcomes in Breast Cancer: The Research Evidence. London: HMSO.

National Institute for Clinical Excellence (NICE) (2002) Guidance on cancer services. Improving Outcomes in Breast Cancer. Manual Update. London: NICE.

Poole K (1997) The emergence of the 'waiting game': a critical examination of the psychosocial issues in diagnosing breast cancer. Journal of Advanced Nursing 25: 273–81.

Royal College of Nursing (2002) Advanced Nursing Practice in Breast Cancer Care. London: Royal College of Nursing.

Schmidt A (1994) Stereotactic breast biopsy. Cancer Journal for Clinicians 44(3): 172–91.

Shaw CR, Wilson SA, O'Brien ME (1994) Information needs prior to breast biopsy. Clinical Nurse Research 3(2): 119–31.

Speigel D (1990) Facilitating emotional coping during treatment. Cancer 66(6): 1422–6.

Ubhi SS, Shaw P, Wright S, et al. (1996) Anxiety in patients with symptomatic breast disease: effects of immediate vs delayed communication of results. Annals of the Royal College of Surgeons 78: 466–9.

CHAPTER FIVE

Surgery for breast cancer

The majority of treatments for breast cancer involve surgery in some form. It must be remembered that different surgeons have different theories and ideas, although all must adhere closely to national guidelines.

Surgery can be used to treat primary breast cancer, to reconstruct the breast following mastectomy (Chapter 6), to achieve palliation of local disease and prophylactically to treat high-risk women (Mera 1997). Surgery also has an important role in diagnosis when triple assessment and core biopsy are inconclusive. A lumpectomy (surgical removal of a lump) would be performed to remove the lump and establish a diagnosis. If benign, no further treatment would be ordered but if cancerous further definitive surgical treatment may be required. Surgery is also a method for staging breast cancer, a cancerous lump would indicate a second operation to remove axillary nodes to help with the staging process (The Breast Clinic online 2001).

Palliative surgery may be used where the patient has an ulcerating tumour with metastases. Cure is not possible but palliative surgery would help stop the problems of an ulcerating tumour.

Until the 1960s radical mastectomy was the only form of treatment. The rationale was that breast tumours spread rapidly to the surrounding lymph nodes so as much tissue as possible should be removed to minimize this. It is now recognized that micrometastases (which spread to other body parts) may have taken place by the time of diagnosis. Therefore, the emphasis is on local control supplemented by systemic adjuvant therapies.

Some tumours are viewed as inoperable, usually those fixed to the chest wall, where axillary nodes are fixed, or where there are advanced systemic metastases (Mera 1997). Around 70 per cent of patients with symptomatic breast lumps already have axillary lymph node metastases. Survival prospects can be improved by adjuvant therapies.

A multimodality approach to stage 1, 2 and 3 breast cancer is required. After a diagnostic biopsy treatment options should be discussed with the patient before selecting the therapeutic treatment. Local treatment is intended to maintain local control of disease and prevent recurrence (Dixon 1995). Characteristics such as grade and proliferative activity of the tumour are of value in making the final decision (Cancernet online 2001).

Types of breast surgery

Women are offered a choice whenever possible and the surgeon should fully explain the pros and cons of both procedures. Breast conservation surgery, together with radiotherapy, has been found to be as effective as a mastectomy in terms of overall survival for stages 1 and 2 breast cancer patients (Fisher et al. 1989). It was demonstrated that women who did not undergo radiotherapy following conservation surgery had a higher local recurrence rate than those who did. Various trials have demonstrated this, but research continues to determine whether certain groups of women, for example the elderly, can be spared radiotherapy (Veronisi et al. 1993, Fisher et al. 1995).

Many women still choose mastectomy although younger patients seem to choose breast conservation surgery. Breast conservation surgery is associated with better preservation of body image. However, not all women who wish breast conservation are suitable and a choice may not always be possible. The size of the cancer, the proximity of the cancer to the nipple and the presence of multifocal disease all govern the decision. The cosmetic result is always considered – if the breast is small and the area to be excised is large, the cosmetic result may be poor. The patient may be advised to have a mastectomy, although the final decision is hers.

The aims of surgery in general are:

1 to eradicate the primary tumour
2 minimize the chance of a local recurrence
3 achieve an acceptable cosmetic result
4 contribute to a good quality of life (West and Brown 1996).

Mastectomy

Localized breast cancers (about a third) that are unsuitable for breast conservation surgery can be treated by mastectomy and some patients choose a mastectomy as their first option (Sainsbury et al. 2000). Otherwise a mastectomy is carried out where the tumour is large, where the tumour is close to or underlying the nipple or where the breast is small and the tumour large (The Breast Clinic online 2001). Extensive malignant type calcifications, multiple primary tumours and failure to obtain tumour-free margins are also indications for mastectomy. Other reasons include physical disabilities that prevent the use of radiotherapy, for example the patient cannot lie flat or abduct the arm and any absolute contraindications for radiotherapy such as pregnancy, previous irradiation or systemic conditions such as scleroderma (Scarth et al. 2001).

The mastectomy generally carried out is a modified radical or Patey mastectomy. This may also be referred to as a total mastectomy with axillary clearance. The Patey mastectomy involves the removal of the breast and the dissection of the pectoral fascia from the pectoral muscles. The pectoralis minor muscle is either divided or removed. The pectoralis major muscle is left intact. The axillary contents are dissected and cleared. As long as the tumour is not fixed to the pectoralis major muscle, patients are usually considered suitable for this operation (West and Brown 1996).

Most methods of performing mastectomy have slightly different incisions, some horizontally across the chest wall, others more vertical. An ellipse is incised around the breast through which skin flaps are raised on either side. The surgeon dissects these down to the underlying pectoralis major muscle. The breast is then removed from the chest wall and the surgeon continues to dissect around to the patient's axilla. The axillary contents are then removed for staging. Two drains are inserted, one in the axilla and one under the lower breast skin flap. These are left in for variable amounts of time, generally about 5–10 days. The chest wall muscles are not removed unless the tumour has invaded the muscle (The Breast Clinic online 2001). Breast reconstruction can be carried out at the time of surgery or at a later date.

Radiotherapy is not usually necessary in patients undergoing mastectomy provided the patient has had a full axillary clearance, is at low risk of local recurrence or is node negative (Sainsbury et al. 1994). However, radiotherapy may be given if the tumour was close to the chest wall.

Simple mastectomy

This is removal of the entire breast without axillary node dissection or removal of the pectoral muscles. One or more nodes may occasionally be sampled when carrying out a simple mastectomy for DCIS (West and Brown 1996).

Subcutaneous mastectomy

The nipple and all the skin is preserved and an implant may be inserted. It cannot be guaranteed that all the breast tissue has been removed. The cosmetic effect is poor (Leinster et al. 2000).

Prophylactic mastectomy

One or both breasts are removed to prevent or reduce the risk of breast cancer. A total mastectomy is usually carried out to remove the breast and the nipple. This operation may be advised in women who have had cancer already to prevent it developing in the contralateral breast. Women with a strong family history or who have tested positive for the breast cancer gene may also opt for this. A recent study has shown that this procedure reduces the risk of cancer by up to 90 per cent in women who test positive for the BRCA1 gene (Kennedy et al. 2002). These women are at a 50–85 per cent risk of developing breast cancer.

Women who are diagnosed as having lobular carcinoma *in situ*, which may develop into breast cancer in one or both breasts, may also choose to have a prophylactic mastectomy. The risk of breast cancer can be reduced but no guarantee can be given as a small amount of breast tissue will be left. It is very important that the woman talks to the surgeon about the procedure and potential complications and that she also is offered counselling (The Breast Clinic online 2001).

Extended radical mastectomy

This involves removing the entire breast, the pectoral fascia and pectoral muscles, the ipsilateral axillary nodes and the internal mammary nodes. Intraplural dissection with removal of a portion of the ribs and sternum is carried out. This operation is rarely undertaken today: less extensive surgery is preferred.

Radical mastectomy

This is as above but leaves the internal mammary nodes and the ribs and sternum. Again, this is rarely carried out today (West and Brown 1996).

Mastectomy is usually performed for breast cancer but can be performed for a phyllodes tumour to remove the lesion from the body (The Breast Clinic online 2001).

Breast conservation surgery

All histological types of breast cancer can be treated by breast conservation surgery and radiotherapy. The rate of local recurrence is low and varies slightly with the technique used (for example lumpectomy, quadrantectomy, segmentectomy) (Weiss et al. 1992). However, multifocal disease is more likely to be treated by mastectomy. Breast conserving surgery is generally offered to patients with a single tumour less than 4cm in diameter as the cosmetic result following excision of large tumours is poor. A mastectomy with reconstruction may well give a better cosmetic effect in these cases. However, breast conservation can be possible in up to 80 per cent of patients with large operable breast cancers, and in about 25 per cent of patients with locally advanced breast cancer if a course of primary systemic treatment is given first to reduce the size of the tumour (Singletary et al. 1992). This neoadjuvant therapy usually consists of chemotherapy although hormonal treatment may shrink a tumour that has oestrogen receptors (Forrest et al. 1991).

Women over 65 years should not feel that age will be a determining factor for breast conservation surgery, these women benefit from survival and freedom from recurrence rates similar to those under 65 following lumpectomy and radiotherapy (Solin et al. 1995). However, young women with germ-line mutations or a strong family history may not be good candidates for breast conservation. The risk for contralateral tumours may be quite high for women who are positive for BRCA1 and BRCA2 mutations. Further evidence of breast conserving surgery success is needed for these women (Robson et al. 1998). Also young patients (less than 35 years) are 2–3 times more likely to develop local recurrence after breast conserving surgery. Young age appears to be an independent risk factor (Sainsbury et al. 2000). This may be because younger patients may have high-grade cancers with lymphatic vascular invasion and an extensive *in situ* component (Kurk 1992).

Wide local excision

The lump and a margin of surrounding breast tissue (usually 1cm although surgeons may vary in the size of margin that they take) are excised through an elliptical excision. Dissection is taken down as far as the pectoral muscle to ensure clearance below the tumour. Axillary clearance is often done at the same time through a separate incision for staging. The axilla contents are first to be removed to avoid theoretical seeding of tumour into a healthy site. Wide local excision is usually combined with radiotherapy to the remainder of the breast in case tumour cells are left in the breast but have not reached the axilla. Radiotherapy is used post-operatively to deal with these remaining malignant cells and to reduce the risk of primary tumours reforming in the breast (The Breast Clinic online 2001). The nipple is usually unaffected and if not damaged by radiotherapy the woman can possibly still breastfeed (Baum et al. 1994).

The outcome of this operation depends on how complete the excision is and the histology of the tumour. Certain features may indicate a risk of local recurrence, for example a grade 3 tumour or one with vascular/lymphatic invasion (Leinster et al. 2000).

Quadrantectomy/segmentectomy

Dissection of the tumour along with a whole quadrant or a segment of the breast with underlying tissue is carried out. Again the completeness of excision is the single most important factor that influences local recurrence. This operation may produce a poor cosmetic result so only retracted or dimpled skin overlying a localized breast cancer should be excised. Where a considerable volume of the breast has been removed the surgeon may consider a latissimus dorsi mini flap or a myocutaneous flap. Reduction surgery may also be carried out on the contralateral breast (Sainsbury et al. 2000).

Ductal carcinoma in situ

Mastectomy is virtually 100 per cent effective in curing DCIS but trials are underway to evaluate more conservative approaches (Mera 1997). Breast conservation surgery has been so successful for invasive cancer it is being extended to non-invasive (Fonesca et al. 1997). The National Surgical Adjuvant Breast and Bowel Project (NSABP) study B-17 (Fisher et al. 1998) compared women with localized DCIS and negative surgical margins who had excision and radiotherapy or no radiotherapy. The trial indicated that local excision and radiotherapy is acceptable for localized DCIS.

Axillary surgery

The axillary nodes lie beneath the axillary vein and can be divided into three levels:

Level 1   nodes up to the lateral border of the pectoralis minor
Level 2   nodes lie behind the pectoralis minor
Level 3   nodes lie between the pectoralis minor's medial border, the first
           rib and the axillary vein (Bundred et al. 1994).

There are approximately 20 nodes but these vary with each individual. A general idea of numbers in each level would be 13 in level 1, five in level 2 and two in level 3. Lymph drains from level 1 to 3. Very few patients have nodes involved at levels 2 and 3 without level 1 due to orderly drainage. However, there are lymph nodes present on the undersurface of the pectoralis major muscle so lymph can get to level 3 bypassing level 1. These 'skip metastases' are rare and occur in less than five per cent of patients with nodal involvement (Bundred et al. 1994).

It is generally agreed that determination of axillary node status by excising nodes and assessing them histopathologically is essential for staging breast cancer since nodal status is an important predictor of survival. It also treats the axilla. Metastases in lymph nodes indicate that cancer has spread and systemic adjuvant treatment is required. Involvement occurs in up to half of symptomatic and 10–20 per cent of screen-detected breast cancer patients (Bundred et al. 1994).

Axillary sampling is where four nodes are identified and removed for staging. Axillary clearance is an anatomical dissection of the axilla and removal of defined groups of nodes. The fascia is stripped from the axillary walls preserving the nerves if possible. The more radical the clearance the greater the chance of lymphoedema developing (Leinster et al. 2000).

A level 1 dissection (at least 10) provides information on whether or not metastases are present. A level 2 or 3 dissection provides more accurate information. A partial sampling (1 or 2 nodes only) cannot be adequate treatment as a single node metastasis at level 1 indicates a 12.5 per cent chance of level 2 involvement. Metastases at level 2 indicate a 50 per cent chance of level 3 involvement. Axillary radiotherapy can be given after a level 2 dissection but has more than a 30 per cent chance of causing lymphoedema (Bundred et al. 1994). Some surgeons will limit a dissection to level 2 as these patients will receive systemic therapy anyway. Most medical oncologists will give chemotherapy for tumours larger than 2cm and for tumours with poor prognostic factors. For these axillary dissection would appear to add little information and may cause some morbidity in the form of pain or swelling of the arm (Silverstein 1997).

Therefore for pre-menopausal patients with operable invasive breast cancer:

- axillary staging is mandatory for all patients
- level 3 dissection should occur for patients with palpable nodes and patients undergoing mastectomy and reconstruction
- all other pre-menopausal patients have the choice of level 3 dissection or axillary sampling.

Pre-menopausal patients must have a staging procedure and a level 3 clearance to identify who might benefit from aggressive systemic treatment. Removal of nodes at all levels is preferred after mastectomy as it prevents axillary radiotherapy.

For post-menopausal patients:

- level 3 dissection should occur for patients with palpable nodes
- all other post-menopausal patients with palpable breast cancer have the choice of level 3 clearance or axillary sampling
- patients with impalpable breast cancer of less than 1cm diameter have a choice of axillary sampling or a wait-and-see policy.

Post-menopausal patients should undergo some axillary surgery. After mastectomy, a level 3 clearance should be carried out. Axillary sampling can be done at the same time as a wide local excision of a screen-detected impalpable cancer. If diagnostic excision of such a cancer shows risk factors for nodal involvement, options are a full axillary clearance or axillary sampling (Bundred et al. 1994).

It has been found that assessment of the three to six firmest or largest nodes can lead to the detection of 93–98 per cent of node-positive patients and can give a correct qualitative assessment of node status in 96–99 per cent. Therefore sampling of these nodes seems to be a reliable alternative for the staging of symptomatic breast cancer. Prior to this, it has been believed that 10 nodes are usually necessary (Gabor 1999).

Complications of axillary surgery

Division of the sensory intercostobrachial nerve can cause damage to it. Many surgeons are careful to preserve it to minimize numbness down the inner aspect of the upper arm. One-third of patients develop a seroma after a level 3 clearance compared with less that five per cent of those who have four node sampling. This can restrict movement until it has been aspirated or is reabsorbed. Axillary surgery can also result in lymphoedema in around five per cent of patients who have had a level 2 or 3 clearance (Bundred et al. 1994).

Sentinel node biopsy

So it can be seen that important clinical decisions are based on the status of the axillary lymph nodes. It is routine to perform a complete or partial axillary dissection. With the development of screening many women who are seen are node negative. Extensive axillary surgery in these cases is difficult to justify as most gain no significant benefit and suffer considerable morbidity. Research has now focused on developing procedures to minimize morbidity by assessing axillary node status (Dixon 1998). This will lead to a significant change in breast cancer treatments.

The sentinel lymph node was discovered over 20 years ago by Cabanas as a specific draining lymph node. Cabanas confirmed that the sentinel node (the first node seen) was the first site of metastases and reported that often it was the only node that was affected (Cabanas 1977). Therefore, the histology of the first draining node could predict the histology of the rest.

In 1992, Morton et al. developed a method of identifying nodal areas at risk in patients with malignant melanoma called cutaneous lymphoscintigraphy. Therefore in breast cancer if malignant cells spread to a regional lymph node they should follow the lymph draining from a primary carcinoma. If the draining (sentinel) node is clear theoretically the others should be (Dixon 1998).

Pre-operative visualization of the draining node using a gamma camera is permitted by injecting a gamma emitting radiopharmaceutical around the primary tumour. In up to six per cent of patients the sentinel node is in the internal mammary chain (Krag et al. 1998). The surgeon can use a hand-held probe and locate the node with the highest uptake and excise the skin directly above it. Radioactivity can be identified in sentinel nodes 1–16 hours after injection by using different pharmaceutical agents. Technetium labelled albumin is very accurate, identifying sentinel nodes in all but three patients out of 241 in one study (Galimberti et al. 1998).

Another method is to inject a blue dye near to the breast tumour and track its path through the lymph nodes. The dye accumulates in the sentinel node (Cancernet online 2001). Blue dyes are used on a named patient basis only. Methylene blue is contraindicated as it can cause fat necrosis when injected subcutaneously.

These procedures would seem to have the potential to decrease morbidity without the cost of staging (Rubio et al. 1998).

It would be an advantage if the sentinel nodes could be assessed intraoperatively, then a patient with affected nodes could choose pre-operatively to proceed to a full axillary clearance if necessary. Routine frozen section examination can miss up to 30 per cent of metastases in sentinel nodes (Galimberti et al. 1998). A more accurate technique has been described but takes up to 40 minutes (Veronisi et al. 1998). This needs to be refined before intraoperative assessment of sentinel nodes can be undertaken. Also different surgeons need to produce a satisfactory rate of success in the identification of sentinel nodes (Dixon 1998).

The Medical Research Council (UK) has funded the audit phase of the ALMANAC trial (Axillary Lymphatic Mapping Against Nodal Clearance). This is ongoing and compares standard axillary management with sentinel node-guided axillary management. Various centres in the UK are taking part. The trial may stop if efficacy is definitely proved. It is envisaged that surgeons who have been involved in this trial will be a valuable training resource as they are trained to a specified, high standard and have been validated.

The National Cancer Institute in America has sponsored two large randomized clinical trials to compare sentinel lymph node biopsy with axillary node dissection for breast cancer. These trials are being carried out by the National Surgical Adjuvant Breast and Bowel Project (NSABP) and by the American College of Surgeons - Oncology Group (ACOS-OG).

The two techniques described previously can be used together. The surgeons in the trials will use either method or a combination of both. Both trials will examine the effect of sentinel node biopsy and full axillary dissection on disease-free and long-term survival. Side effects of each method will also be compared.

The NSABP will be studying whether sentinel node biopsy can replace axillary lymph node dissection in women with negative sentinel nodes and the ACOS-OG study is examining the same theory in women with positive sentinel nodes (National Cancer Institute 2000).

Nursing care of patients undergoing breast surgery

The information given as described previously can do much to reduce anxiety and aid with the decision making when choosing treatment options. The specialist breast care nurse assesses the patient's needs, priorities, fears and anxieties and sets realistic goals and objectives. The patient may be visited at home pre-operatively where she feels more relaxed and able to ask questions. The treatment options may be discussed with the family. Samples of breast prostheses may be examined if the woman is undergoing a mastectomy. Breast reconstruction may be offered at the time of diagnosis and planning for women undergoing mastectomy. Photographs available at the breast unit can be shown and women volunteers who have had the operation may be available to talk to patients and show their own reconstruction.

Post-operative care

Following mastectomy or breast conservation the patient will have two drainage tubes *in situ*, one medially and one laterally. Drainage from the axilla facilitates healing and helps prevent infection.

The drains are checked frequently for the first 24 hours and then at least twice daily. Bottles are changed as necessary and the amount and type of drainage carefully recorded. When the drainage over 24 hours falls to less than 50ml the wound drain is usually removed. If the drainage continues to be high the patient may be discharged with the drain in place. This can be monitored by the community nursing staff (West and Brown 1996.)

Seromas may form following an axillary clearance. This will require aspirating so it is important that the drain is not removed too early. The patient should be aware of this. Seromas can be aspirated by the surgeon or, at some units, the breast care nurse may do this. Seromas may continue to refill for 2–3 weeks and then will probably reabsorb. If left they will reabsorb eventually but will cause discomfort and restricted arm movements.

It is vital to mobilize the arm and exercises are commenced immediately. Exercises help the patient to regain the range of arm movements she had prior to surgery. Exercises help to control pain and aid tissue healing as more oxygen is supplied to the area during exercise (Breast Cancer Care 1999). The physiotherapist visits pre- and post-operatively and encourages these exercises to be carried out hourly as soon as possible after surgery. The arm is also observed regularly and adequate pain relief administered as prescribed. This also facilitates the exercises in the early days.

The patient is encouraged to continue with the exercises twice daily following discharge until she feels that she has regained a normal range of movement and can perform tasks such as hanging out washing or driving. Following radiotherapy the muscles can stiffen quickly and patients may be advised to continue with their arm exercises for up to two years afterwards (Breast Cancer Care 1999).

Examples of exercises include:

1 shrugging and circling the shoulders three times
2 lifting the elbow out sideways and down five times
3 lifting the elbow forward and up and down five times
4 brushing the hair
5 circling the elbow, three times forwards, three times backwards
6 gently swinging the arm forwards and back and side to side
7 back-drying with a towel
8 'walking' the hands up a wall, trying to reach higher each time.

Physiotherapists in each area will recommend exercises that may differ slightly.

The unaffected arm is used for blood pressure readings, injections, etc. to prevent lymphoedema. There is a high incidence following axillary clearance and nursing intervention to reduce the risk is very important (Williams 1992). Cuts, burns and insect bites must be avoided where possible to prevent infection. Electric razors are recommended for the removal of axillary hair. It is important to protect the arm against sunburn. If a cut is sustained the patient is advised to clean it with antiseptic and observe it closely. Tight fitting clothes and jewellery can also cause the arm to swell. Any redness, swelling or heat must be reported to the GP (West and Brown 1996). Lymphoedema will be fully discussed in Chapter 12.

Patients may be very reluctant to view the wound and should be given time to do so. The woman should be encouraged to look at it in her own time without being rushed or pressurized. Her husband or partner can be present if she wishes. (See Chapter 11 for psychological and psychosocial effects of breast surgery.)

A temporary prosthesis is fitted prior to discharge for mastectomy patients. This is done by the ward nurses or the breast care nurse. The breast care nurse may provide training to the ward staff in fitting a temporary prosthesis. Advice on how to care for this is given. The temporary prosthesis is usually very light so that it does not cause pressure on the wound. A permanent prosthesis is generally fitted around six weeks post-operatively. The patient is advised how to obtain one; often an appointment is given on discharge. The breast care nurse also advises on suitable bras. (Prosthetics and fitting will be covered in Chapter 10.)

The community nurse generally visits at home to check the wound and provide another means of support. Contact telephone numbers can be left. The community nurse can liaise with the breast care nurse if a problem arises. The patient will also have the breast care nurse's number. An appointment for the outpatient clinic will be given on discharge for the patient to obtain the results of her operation if these have not been given on the ward. These results consist of the histological details of the tumour and lymph node status. Adjuvant treatment will then be decided.

Complications of breast surgery

1 The usual short-term anaesthetic problems, for example nausea, vomiting, drug reactions.
2 Wound infection – can develop at any time until healing of the wound has taken place. The wound may appear red and inflamed, feel tender, swollen or warm or may discharge. The patient may feel unwell and feverish. Antibiotics should be prescribed.
3 Flap necrosis – if this occurs areas of necrotic skin need to be excised and skin grafts applied. Infection usually occurs secondary to this (Sainsbury et al. 2000).
4 Pain – more likely when the lymph glands have been removed. Analgesia and physiotherapy can help.
5 Cording – this is a pain which tends to be described as feeling like a tight cord running down the arm. Raised cord-like structures can be felt that reduce arm movement. This is due to hardened lymph vessels and is often noted a few weeks following surgery. Physiotherapy usually resolves this (Breast Cancer Care 1999).
6 Seroma formation – these occur in 33–50 per cent of patients, more commonly after axillary surgery. The fluid can be aspirated using a syringe and needle.
7 Haematoma – will eventually be reabsorbed but causes swelling and discomfort.
8 Pain and numbness on inside of upper arm due to division of inter-costabrachial nerve in the axilla during dissection (The Breast Clinic online 2001).
9 Lymphoedema due to axillary surgery.

Local recurrence

Tumours which are large, palpable and/or axillary node positive may need a more generous excision to avoid re-excision as there is a higher likelihood of finding persistent tumour on re-excision (Jardines et al. 1995). Recurrence means that treatment has failed. Factors related to local recurrence are:

1 completeness of excision
2 presence of an extensive *in situ* component defined as being more that 25 per cent of the main tumour mass being *in situ*, with cancer also being present *in situ* in the surrounding breast tissue (Christian et al. 1995)
3 lymphatic vascular invasion visible microscopically (Fisher et al. 1995)
4 high tumour grade (Dixon 1993)
5 under 35 years.

All invasive and non-invasive disease must be completely excised to minimize local recurrence after breast conservation surgery. It may be preferable to carry out a mastectomy with or without radiotherapy to the chest wall for patients at high risk of local recurrence (Sibbering et al. 1995).

Local recurrence following mastectomy is most common in the first two years and decreases as time passes. However, recurrence following breast conservation surgery occurs at a fixed rate each year. Follow-up should detect local recurrence whilst treatable and detect contralateral disease. Around 0.6 per cent per year develop this. Mammography should be performed regularly, annually or two-yearly depending on local and national guidelines, on one or both breasts. Scarring can appear as a stellate opacity following breast conservation so mammograms may be difficult to interpret (The Breast Clinic online 2001).

BASO guidelines

BASO Guidelines (1996) state that:

- Surgeons should ensure completeness of excision has been undertaken where breast conservation surgery has been performed and should minimize the number of re-excisions. Ninety per cent of operations with a proven pre-operative cancer diagnosis should not require a re-excision.
- All surgeons involved in the treatment of screen-detected cancers (and symptomatic) must offer treatment options wherever possible.
- Node status should be obtained on all invasive tumours either by clearance or sampling.

- Surgeons should be aware that a wide local excision is inappropriate for extensive DCIS.
- Ninety per cent of patients should be admitted within three weeks of being informed of the need for breast surgery.
- Yearly follow-up should be arranged. Recent NICE guidelines state that patients should be followed up for 2–3 years (NICE 2002).

Timing of breast surgery

It is believed that tumour cells are less likely to be disseminated when oestrogen is opposed by progesterone as occurs during the second half of the menstrual cycle. It has been suggested that timing surgery to coincide with this time may influence survival prospects (Mera 1997). Disease-free survival may be achieved for pre-menopausal women with breast cancer and positive lymph nodes if breast surgery is performed during this luteal phase (days 15–36) as opposed to the follicular phase (days 0–14) of the cycle (Veronisi et al. 1994). Studies are inconsistent but a trial is ongoing.

Early discharge

The average stay in hospital for breast surgery in the UK is seven days. Physical recovery is rapid but patients are required to have drains *in situ* to prevent seroma and therefore stay until drains are removed. Early removal often leads to seroma formation (Ball et al. 1992). Wound infection and decreased shoulder function can be further complications of early removal. Psychological adaptation may also be better with an extended stay (Bundred et al. 1998).

It has been found that when careful attention is paid to peri-operative care patients and families can manage the drain at home. In one study, patients, who had been discharged home after two days with drains *in situ*, were visited by the specialist breast care nurse and contacted every day by telephone. Information sheets and a 24-hour contact number were given. The breast care nurses liaised with and involved the community nursing staff. The early discharge was found to be safe with no adverse physical or psychological effects (Bundred et al. 1998).

Bonnema et al. (1998) also found that early discharge is safe and is well received by patients. It also seems to enhance social support within the family. In their study, patients were discharged with drains *in situ* after four days. Support was provided by the community nurses and the breast care nurse. Support from a specialist nurse reduces psychological morbidity

(McArdle et al. 1996) and therefore the patient may feel more confident and competent to manage the drain. It was found that the rates of complications or incidence of seroma formation were no worse in these patients who were discharged early from hospital. They were also highly satisfied with their community care. Early discharge translated into management policy could mean substantial savings in the UK.

Follow-up

Women who had undergone treatment for breast cancer used to be followed up in clinics for up to 10 years. Women would attend their yearly appointment for reassurance and support and the appointment itself often caused great anxiety. However, some women derived comfort from meeting other patients and gaining the reassurance of a mammogram.

NICE (2002) have now issued guidelines for follow-up after treatment for early breast cancer. Guidelines for follow-up of 2–3 years should be agreed by each of the cancer networks. The purpose of follow-up clinics is to detect and treat local recurrence at an early stage and to detect such side effects of treatment such as lymphoedema. However, intensive follow-up, looking for metastatic disease before symptoms present, does not benefit patients and can greatly increase anxiety.

All patients who have had treatment for breast cancer should have access to the breast care nurse indefinitely. The breast care nurse should provide a telephone advice service and can arrange a clinic appointment if there seems to be a problem. Counselling and advice should be provided to all patients, including those discharged from follow-up.

If the patient notices any new symptoms that could be a cancer recurrence she should contact the breast care nurse. Patients almost always notice the first symptoms themselves. Advice and information can be sought from the breast care nurse about what symptoms to report. Women should be informed and assured that there are no routine tests to detect recurrence as they are not necessary and do not improve survival.

Women in clinical trials will be followed up for longer, usually around 10 years. However, cancer networks should agree when to discharge women from routine follow-up and how often to undertake mammography on women who have been treated for breast cancer.

GPs should take over the care of the patient on Tamoxifen or other endocrine therapies and for stopping it after five years (NICE 2002). GPs should be able to refer back to the breast care team if there is any cause for concern.

Patients should be warned that lymphoedema can occur many years after treatment for breast cancer and should be given a contact number of the lymphoedema service along with advice on recognizing symptoms (NICE 2002).

Some areas may operate nurse-led clinics to follow-up patients who have had breast cancer treatment. This is a holistic, patient-focused service, which can enhance well-being and provide continuity of care. However some patients may prefer to see a doctor and resentment may be experienced from medical colleagues and peers. This extension of role needs time to achieve training and qualifications. Record keeping and documentation skills need to be of a high standard. The nurse must recognize her limitations and be aware of her accountability. There must be rigorous outcome measures and authority must be given by the employer. Employers should also provide supporting policies and procedures, a named assessor and clinical supervision. The nurse needs to maintain her skills and knowledge.

Reducing the intense routine follow-up and ending the long-term follow-up will release consultant and clinic time, making it possible for women with breast symptoms to be seen within the recommended two weeks (NICE 2002).

References

Ball ABS, Fish S, Waters R, et al. (1992) Radical axillary dissection in the staging and treatment of breast cancer. Annals of the Royal College of Surgeons, England 74: 126–9.

BASO (1996) Quality Assurance Guidelines for Surgeons in Breast Cancer Screening. NHS Breast Screening Programme. Pub. No. 20. April 1996.

Baum M, Saunders C, Meredith S (1994) Breast Cancer: A Guide for Every Woman. Oxford: Oxford University Press.

Bonnema J, van Wersch AMEA, van Geel AN, et al. (1998) Medical and psychosocial effects of early discharge after surgery for breast cancer: randomised trial. British Medical Journal 316: 1267–71.

Breast Cancer Care (1999) Post-operative problems following breast surgery. Factsheet 10. London: Breast Cancer Care.

Bundred N, Morgan DAL, Dixon JM (1994) ABC of breast diseases: Management of regional nodes in breast cancer. British Medical Journal 309: 1222–5.

Bundred N, Maguire P, Reynolds J, Grimshaw J, et al. (1998) Randomised controlled trial of effects of early discharge after surgery for breast cancer. British Medical Journal 317: 1275–9.

Cabanas RM (1977) Lymph node metastases, indicators, but not governors of survival. Archives of Surgery 119: 1067–72.

Cancernet online (incorporating PDQ online) (2001) Breast Cancer Treatment (Health Professionals). http://www.cancernet.nci.nih.gov/cancerinfo/pdq/treatment/breast/healthprofessional (accessed August 2001).

Christian MC, McCabe MS, Korn EL, et al. (1995) The National Cancer Institute Audit of the National Surgical Adjuvant Breast and Bowel Project protocol B-06. New England Journal of Medicine 333: 1456–61.

Dixon JM (1993) Histological Factors predicting breast recurrence following breast conserving therapy. Breast 2: 197.

Dixon JM (1995) Surgery and radiotherapy for early breast cancer. British Medical Journal 311: 1515–16.

Dixon JM (1998) Sentinel node biopsy in breast cancer. British Medical Journal 317: 295–6.

Fisher B, Redmond C, Poisson R, et al. (1989) Eight year results for a randomised clinical trial comparing total mastectomy and lumpectomy with or without irradiation in the treatment of breast cancer. New England Journal of Medicine 320(8): 22–8.

Fisher B, Anderson S, Redmond CK, et al. (1995) Reanalysis and results after 12 years of follow up in a randomised clinical trial comparing total mastectomy with lumpectomy with or without irradiation in the treatment of breast cancer. New England Journal of Medicine 333(22): 1456–61.

Fisher B, Dignam J, Wolmark N, et al. (1998) Lumpectomy and radiation therapy for the treatment of intraductal breast cancer – findings from the National Surgical Adjuvant Breast and Bowel Project B-17. Journal of Clinical Oncology 16(2): 441–52.

Fonesca R, Hartmann LC, Petersen IA, et al. (1997) Ductal carcinoma in situ of the breast. Annals of Internal Medicine 127(11): 1013–22.

Forrest APM, Anderson EDC, Gaskill D (1991) Primary systemic therapy for breast cancer. British Medical Bulletin 47: 357–71.

Gabor C (1999) The reliability of sampling three–six nodes for staging breast cancer. Journal of Clinical Pathology 52(9): 681–3.

Galimberti V, Zurrida S, Zucali P, Luini A (1998) Can sentinel node biopsy avoid axillary dissection in clinically node negative patients? The Breast 7: 8–10.

Jardines L, Fowlde B, Schultz D, et al. (1995) Factors associated with a positive re-excision after excisional biopsy for invasive breast cancer. Surgery 118(5): 803–9.

Kennedy RD, Quinn JE, Johnston PG, Harkin DP (2002) BRCA1: Mechanisms of inactivation and implications for management of patients. Lancet 360(9338): 1007.

Krag DN, Asikaga T, Harlow SP, Weaver DL (1998) Development of sentinel node targeting technique in breast cancer patients. The Breast 4: 67–74.

Kurk JM (1992) Factors influencing the risk of local recurrence in breast cancer. European Journal of Cancer 28: 660–6.

Leinster SJ, Gibbs TJ, Downey H (2000) Shared Care for Breast Disease. Oxford: Isis Medical Media Ltd.

McArdle JMC, George WD, McArdle CS, et al. (1996) Psychological support for patients undergoing breast cancer surgery: a randomised study. British Medical Journal 312: 813–16.

Mera S (1997) Pathology and Understanding Disease Prevention. Cheltenham: Stanley Thornes.

Morton DL, Wen DR, Wong JH, et al. (1992) Technical details of intraoperative lymphatic mapping for early stage melanoma. Archvies of Surgery 127: 392–9.

National Cancer Institute (2000) Cancer Facts. Questions & Answers about NCI's Sentinel Node Biopsy Trials. Factsheet 7.44. http://cis.nci.nih.gov/fact/7.44.htm.

National Institute for Clinical Excellence (NICE) (2002) Follow-up after treatment for early breast cancer. Guidance on Cancer Services. Improving Outcomes in Breast Cancer. Manual update. London: NICE.

Robson M, Glewski T, Haas B, et al. (1998) BRCA – associated breast cancer in young women. Journal of Clinical Oncology 16(5): 1642–9.

Rubio IT, Korourian S, Cowan C, et al. (1998) Sentinel lymph node biopsy for staging breast cancer. American Journal of Surgery 176 (6): 532–7.

Sainsbury JRC, Anderson TJ, Morgan DAL, Dixon JM, et al. (1994) ABC of breast diseases: Breast cancer. British Medical Journal 309:1150–3.

Sainsbury JRC, Anderson TJ, Morgan DAL (2000) ABC of breast diseases: Breast cancer. British Medical Journal 321: 745–50.

Scarth H, Cantin J, Levine M, et al. (2001) Clinical practice guidelines for the care and treatment of breast cancer. Guideline 3 – mastectomy or lumpectomy? The choice of operation for clinical stages 1 & 2 breast cancer. CMJA 158(3 Suppl.): S1521.

Sibbering DM, Galia MH, Morgan DAL, et al. (1995) Selection criteria for breast conservation in primary operable breast cancer. Breast 4: 232–3.

Silverstein MJ (1997) Diagnosis and treatment of early breast cancer. British Medical Journal 314: 1736–9.

Singletary SE, McNeese MD, Hortobagyi GN (1992) Feasability of breast conservation surgery after induction chemotherapy for breast cancer. Cancer 69: 2849–52.

Solin LJ, Schultz DJ, Fowlde BL (1995) 10 year results of the treatment of early stage breast carcinoma in elderly women using breast conserving surgery and definitive breast irradiation. International Journal of Radiation Oncology, Biology, Physics 33(1): 45–51.

The Breast Clinic online (2001) Surgery. www.thebreastclinic.com (accessed August 2001).

Veronisi U, Luini A, Del Vecchio M, et al. (1993) Radiotherapy after breast preserving surgery in women with localised cancer of the breast. New England Journal of Medicine 328(22): 1587–91.

Veronisi U, Luini A, Manani L, et al. (1994) Effect of menstrual phase on surgical treatment of breast cancer. Lancet 343 (8912): 1545–7.

Veronisi U, Zurrida S, Galimberta V (1998) Consequences of sentinel node in clinical decision making in breast cancer and prospects for future studies. European Journal of Surgical Oncology 24: 93–5.

Weiss MC, Fowlde BL, Solin LJ, et al. (1992) Outcome of conservative therapy for invasive breast cancer by histologic subtype. International Journal of Radiation Oncology, Biology and Physics 23(5): 941–7.

West N, Brown H (1996) Surgery for breast cancer. In Denton S (Ed.) Breast Cancer Nursing. London: Chapman & Hall.

Williams AE (1992) Management of lymphoedema – a community based approach. British Journal of Nursing 1(8): 383–7.

CHAPTER SIX
Breast reconstruction

Introduction

Since the early 1990s, the number of breast reconstructions undertaken following mastectomy have increased. Breast reconstruction is an alternative for almost every woman who is about to undergo or who has undergone a mastectomy. Age should not be a contraindication; neither should metastatic disease if quality of life is going to be improved. The increase is due to the unequivocal demonstration of the procedure's oncological safety and the availability of reliable methods of reconstruction. It is undertaken in the treatment for cancer of the breast, in the management of treatment failure following breast conservation surgery and radiotherapy and after prophylactic mastectomy in high-risk patients. Women who have prophylactic mastectomy for family history may choose to have a bilateral procedure as breast reconstruction can yield very natural results. Many options exist – breast reconstruction can be achieved with a variety of autogenous tissue techniques or the insertion of a prosthetic implant. Breast reconstruction is a safe and acceptable procedure following mastectomy for cancer. There is no evidence that it has adverse oncological consequences (Malata et al. 2000).

Patient selection is important to optimize results, improve quality of life and minimize complications whilst fully treating the malignancy. The breast surgeon should explain all the options available to the patient as every type of reconstruction may not be available in every centre. Close cooperation between the breast reconstruction surgeon and oncologist is vital to achieve these objectives (Malata et al. 2000).

Women should be given sufficient information and education in order to make informed choices so that the correct procedure is chosen for the individual. Before the mastectomy is the best time to start thinking about reconstruction to decide whether an immediate or delayed reconstruction is best for that patient. It should be emphasized that results vary. It is impossible to achieve a perfect match with the other breast but the result can be perfectly acceptable and give an equal appearance in a bra. However, it may have less droop and sensation will be reduced (Cancer Bacup 2001). Breast reconstruction is a major surgical procedure and can involve a series of operations for a satisfactory result. Surgery may also be carried out on the contralateral breast to create a balanced appearance (Harcourt and Rumsey 2001). It is vital that the patient's expectations are realistic.

It can be argued that breast reconstruction is cosmetic only as there is no reconstructive technique available to restore the breast to its original function of providing milk for the newborn. However, a second and very important function is to provide symmetry. We expect to feel and see in ourselves an overall sense of balance. Patients can feel 'one-sided' following mastectomy. Some women cannot feel symmetrical with only an external prosthesis (University of Iowa online 1995). The purpose of the operation is to reconstruct a breast mound and restore symmetry. It can reduce the psychological trauma of the change in body image experienced after mastectomy (Watson et al. 1995).

Breast reconstruction can be performed any time after mastectomy but some options offer better results when carried out at the time of the initial surgery. The best way to address this is to discuss all possible options with the breast care team. It may be possible to show the patient photographs and put her in touch with someone who has already undergone a reconstruction (Breast Doctor online 2001).

Breast reconstruction requires taking into account the amount of skin remaining on the chest and its quality. Excess scarring or changes due to radiotherapy may necessitate a reconstruction that brings volume and skin to the area. A mature breast will require a reconstruction that mimics the normal droop of the breast as the new breast needs to look as if it belongs there for the best cosmetic effect. Again, it is important to be aware of all the options so that an informed decision can be made.

Timing of surgery

In the past it was felt that breast reconstruction should be delayed in order to enable the woman to grieve for and to accept the loss of a breast and then make a decision so that she would accept the reconstructed breast more readily (Winder and Winder 1985). Delayed reconstruction was thought to facilitate adjustment to the cancer diagnosis and altered body image.

Breast reconstruction following mastectomy has now become an integral part of the holistic treatment of breast cancer (LaRossa 1997). Immediate reconstruction is now often thought to be preferable as it indicates positive adjustment to the diagnosis and offers greater psychological benefits (Rowland et al. 1995). The patient who has an immediate reconstruction will wake up with a breast mound and this is extremely important to some women. Also the surgeon can work with undamaged tissue. There is no fibrosis, scar tissue or damage from radiation or other adjuvant treatments.

Delayed reconstruction is often performed when there has not been an opportunity for immediate reconstruction due to logistical problems, lack of local expertise or the patient not having decided (Breast Doctor online 2001). The main advantage of delayed reconstruction is that the patient has more time to consider the options. Some may find that an external prosthesis is more suitable after all.

In a study by Al-Ghazal et al. (2000a) it was found that 95 per cent of patients who had immediate reconstruction preferred this and 77 per cent of patients who had delayed would have preferred immediate. Depression and anxiety were decreased and body image, self-esteem, feelings of attractiveness and better psychosocial well-being were significantly superior in the immediate reconstruction group.

Some women may be advised to wait, especially if the breast is being reconstructed in a complicated procedure involving tissue transfer. Women with other health conditions such as high blood pressure, obesity or smokers may also be advised to wait.

There may be other problems that are influencing decision making, for example body image, sexual problems, mental health problems, marriage problems. It is important that this is explored pre-operatively and the patient is referred on for specialized help if this is the case.

The appropriate time, therefore, for a woman to undergo reconstructive breast surgery depends on the disease – size, type, spread of the cancer, whether there is a reconstructive surgeon available in the patient's area and how the patient feels. Some may prefer to wait, others may wish surgery to be undertaken immediately (Parker 1996). Decisions on timing will be made by the patient in conjunction with the breast care team and the oncologist.

Psychological aspects

Reconstructive surgery can lessen the psychological impact of breast cancer surgery and the resulting disfigurement. It is intended to offer psychological benefits following mastectomy for breast cancer, for example improved body image, less anxiety and depression, improved quality of life. The women who opt not to recreate a breast shape tend to be in the minority. Many will opt for a temporary external prosthesis, although these can act as a reminder of the cancer and its treatment (Harcourt and Rumsey 2001). Although an external prosthesis may mask the loss of the breast to the outside world, it does not always help the patient address the sense of deformity and altered body image (Al-Ghazal et al. 2000b). Some women may find it harder than others to accept the loss of their breast. In most cases a woman's breasts affect how she feels about herself, sexually and emotionally. Even if her partner feels the same way about her following surgery it does not necessarily follow that the woman herself will feel the same. It is ultimately her feelings that count. Women who are not in a relationship may be especially concerned about meeting someone new and explaining about their cancer. Reconstructive surgery may help to make her feel more comfortable forming a new relationship (Breast Cancer Care 2001).

A study by Al-Ghazal et al. (2000b) showed that women who had immediate reconstruction recalled less psychological distress than those who underwent simple mastectomy only without reconstruction. This may be because these women did not feel the self-consciousness that goes with the loss of a breast.

The NHS Executive (1996) recommended that the possibility of reconstruction should be discussed with all women considering a mastectomy. This is very important as few patients realize until it is mentioned at consultation that reconstructive surgery is possible during the same procedure as a mastectomy. Awaking with a new breast can cause the perception that surgery can have a favourable outcome, which encourages psychological and emotional adjustment. The patient has the care of the new breast to focus on rather than focusing on the loss of the cancerous one (Fournier and Schafer 2001).

Although age is not a barrier women who pursue reconstruction tend to be younger, are of higher socio-economic status, are more likely to be married and may have actively sought information regarding reconstructive surgery (Rowland et al. 1995). However, at any age a woman may be motivated by the need to restore wholeness and improve self-confidence and femininity. Some may, however, wish to avoid further surgery.

Occasionally, a woman may choose to pass the decision of whether to undergo breast reconstruction back to the health professionals. The breast care nurse needs to be able to offer psychological support and help her to make an informed choice without actually dictating the outcome. The decision should be entirely that of the woman. The support women receive when making decisions about their primary treatment should extend to the decision about reconstruction (Harcourt and Rumsey 2001). Even with a reconstructed breast, women may still have difficulties adjusting to the loss of a natural breast through breast cancer.

Implants

Implants are the most straightforward option for breast reconstruction. The silicone implant (a silicone shell filled with a set amount of silicone) is inserted under the chest wall muscles (pectoralis major and parts of the serratus anterior and rectus abdominus). This is known as a subpectoral reconstruction. The surrounding tissues are sutured to hold the implant and prevent lateral or upward movement (Parker 1996). This operation tends to give satisfactory results only if the patient has small breasts.

When a larger or a ptotic breast needs to be developed, a tissue expander may be used. This may be carried out at the time of operation or as a delayed procedure. The expander is a fluid filled sac that can be inflated over weeks or months to stretch the skin and muscle to match the other breast. A double lumen expander may be used. The outer lumen is a silicone sac and the inner lumen is the expander that is partially filled with saline at the time of operation. Expansion continues as an outpatient every week or maybe 2–3 weeks depending on the preference of the surgeon, who can precisely adjust the volume of the implant. The inflation is done by injecting saline through the filler port, which is placed subcutaneously at the time of surgery. To achieve a natural ptosis of the breast it is necessary to over-inflate the expander. When the patient is happy with the size the expander is over-inflated then some saline withdrawn to achieve a natural droop. The port can then be removed under a local anaesthetic (Parker 1996). Another option is to remove the expander once the size is correct and replace it with a permanent implant.

The patient should be made aware that she will appear asymmetrical whilst inflation is underway and may wish to be fitted with a temporary partial prosthesis until the breast is of the required size.

If a patient has had chest wall radiotherapy, tissue expansion may not be recommended. Radiotherapy can cause fibrosis in the chest wall muscles and in the overlying skin. It may be difficult to achieve satisfactory expansion and therefore a myocutaneous flap may be preferable. However, if a tissue expander is already in place, post-operative radiotherapy can be carried out if necessary (Watson et al. 1995). This must not take place until inflations are complete as radiotherapy reduces the skin's ability to stretch and delays healing (Parker 1996). Preferably, women who need radiotherapy are usually advised to wait at least a year before having reconstruction to give the skin a chance to recover from the effects of radiotherapy (Breast Cancer Care online 2001).

A subcutaneous reconstruction may be carried out in women who are having prophylactic mastectomy because of a strong family history of breast cancer. The breast tissue is removed but the skin, nipple and areola are left. An implant is placed beneath the skin. As the surgeon would be concerned about the risk of recurrence in the preserved nipple and skin, this would probably not be carried out for a patient with breast cancer.

Concurrent treatment with immediate breast reconstruction and adjuvant chemotherapy appears feasible and safe. It does not increase acute surgical complications or chemotherapy side effects and does not require any changes in dose intensity or timing of inflations (Caffo et al. 2000).

Complications

Discomfort may be experienced to the chest wall as skin and muscle are stretched. Inflammation and swelling will settle. All implants are recognized as foreign by the body and some scar tissue forms around them. The formation and subsequent contraction of this fibrous capsule is known as capsular contraction. This results in hardening and deformity of the breast mound causing pain and embarrassment for the patient (Watson et al. 1995). Over-expansion is thought to reduce the risk of capsular contraction. The patient is allowed to bath or shower once the dressings are off and is encouraged to massage the skin with cream or lotion to reduce the risk of capsular contraction. The implant usually has to be removed if this occurs.

The saline in a tissue expander may 'leak' due to rupture, valve failure or the implant coming to the end of its life. It will need to be removed if this occurs.

Infection can occur in a small percentage of patients necessitating removal of the implant. Removal of the implant for whatever reason may cause the patient great distress as she decides whether or not to pursue further attempts at reconstruction. The breast care nurse has an important role in supporting the patient in her decision.

Silicone implants obscure X-rays making follow-up mammography slightly difficult. The radiographer needs to be informed that a patient has breast implants as it is possible to get a good mammogram of a breast containing an implant (Cancer Bacup 2001).

The long-term cosmetic outcome of breast implants is unknown. Capsular contraction contributes to a poor cosmetic appearance. However, patients without capsular contraction can still show signs that the cosmetic outcome is deteriorating. A possible cause is late asymmetry produced by the failure of both breasts to undergo symmetrical ptosis with ageing (Clough et al. 2001). Losing or gaining weight can also alter the appearance.

It is very important that the patient is made aware of all possible complications and is given the chance to discuss all concerns thoroughly with the breast care team. Women tend to vary in the amount of information they require. They should be aware of what to expect on return from surgery, for example drains, intravenous infusions, pain and the extent of scarring. The patient undergoing tissue expansion may become frustrated as the procedure takes time to complete (Parker 1996).

Following surgery, the patient may need time to adjust to her new breast – the breast care nurse can discuss fears and anxieties and offer support.

The incidence of contralateral breast cancer after unilateral breast reconstruction is low. In most cases contralateral breast cancer presents at an earlier stage compared with the initial breast cancer and the prognosis is good. In patients who develop a contralateral breast cancer after mastectomy and unilateral breast reconstruction, there is no reason why reconstruction of the second breast should not be offered to provide optimal breast symmetry and a better quality of life. The best result is obtained when similar methods and tissues are used on both sides (Chang et al. 2001).

Health risks

Rupture of the implant is a major concern for patients. Silicone implants have always been very popular until recent reports of ruptures and leaks. No worldwide studies have demonstrated systemic health risks from silicone but some women develop local reactions causing pain, deformity and capsular contraction. Gel from a silicone implant can 'bleed' into the periprosthetic space and silicone can travel to the lymph nodes in a very small percentage of women. There is no concrete evidence that this causes diseases in women but some women with silicone implants do get some rheumatoid diseases (Breast Doctor online 2001). There is no evidence to show that silicone is carcinogenic (Watson et al. 1995).

Most problems appear to have been associated with silicone injections where the compound is injected straight into the breast rather than implants. These injections are now banned in the UK and USA.

The Department of Health has concluded that there is no good evidence of an abnormal immune response to silicone and no evidence for a link with connective disorders. All breast implant operations should be recorded and adverse effects reported (Cancer Bacup 2001).

A nationwide study undertaken in Sweden compared 7000 women with breast implants, either for cosmetic reasons or after breast cancer surgery, and a control group of over 3000 women who had undergone breast reduction surgery only. No excess risk for connective tissue disease was found. Direct comparison of the two groups showed that those with implants had a slightly lower risk of connective tissue disease, therefore it was concluded that there is little likelihood of a connection between connective tissue disease and breast implants (Nyren et al. 1998).

The patient should discuss all health concerns with the surgeon and be aware that breast implants are very effective and safe for the majority of women (Breast Doctor online 2001).

The Department of Health withdrew implants called Trilucent implants in 1999. These consisted of a silicone elastomer shell with a lipid filler derived from soya bean oil. A small number of women reported local complications. These included reports of swelling associated with rupture. This may have been due to a local inflammatory response. There was no evidence of permanent harm. Not enough is known about soya bean oil and its possible effects on the body. Women who have these implants are advised to discuss with their surgeon whether or not to remove them (Department of Health 1999).

Myocutaneous tissue reconstruction

Pedicle and free flaps

Saline implants are not always suitable for every woman requiring breast reconstruction. Patients with radiation changes, excessive skin scarring or damaged chest wall muscles are prone to complications when implants are inserted without adequate soft tissue coverage. In these cases it is necessary to move the patient's own healthy tissue to the area. The techniques include (1) moving muscle, (2) moving muscle and skin, or (3) moving muscle with fat and skin. Tissue can be transferred on a set of blood vessels – a pedicled flap – or as a free flap where the blood vessels are cut and reattached near the chest. Free flaps are more flexible in that tissues from all parts of the body can be brought to the chest wall to construct a breast. Pedicled flaps tend to be more restrictive due to the blood vessels remaining attached to supply the flap with nutrients. Both are used to provide the chest with healthy tissue. Sometimes an implant has to be used in addition to provide the required volume (Breast Doctor online 2001).

Pedicled flaps tend to have a higher complication rate than free flaps but they tend to be more easily dealt with. These complications can include localized tissue loss and wound healing problems. These occur when the blood supply is inadequate for the tissue volume and can be corrected by surgery. However, flap necrosis will occur in around 10 per cent of pedicled TRAM (transverse rectus abdominus myocutaneous) flaps (Watson et al. 1995).

Free flaps tend to be more robust. The number of complications is lower but can be more severe. When the blood vessels are cut and reattached using microsurgery there is the possibility of blood flow problems at the sites of the vessel anastomoses. These can result in the death of the flap if not noted in time. Eight per cent of free flaps will require further surgery and five per cent will result in loss of the flap. Therefore, patients undergoing this type of flap tend to be hospitalized for longer and are nursed initially in Intensive Care. Problems can also occur at the donor site due to excess scarring; this can be surgically removed. Free flap surgery should only be undertaken by very experienced microsurgeons (Breast Doctor online 2001).

A free tissue flap:

- is where tissue is cut completely from the donor site and moved to a new site anywhere on the body
- is where the blood supply is cut and the veins and arteries are reconnected in the new site
- can be moved anywhere that allows the blood supply to be reattached
- includes fat, muscle and skin
- gives a good cosmetic result
- is a long, technically difficult operation, which can only be performed by a microvascular surgeon
- has fewer complications but these are more complicated to deal with.

A pedicle tissue flap:

- is where skin, fat and muscle is cut free from the donor site and moved nearby
- does not have its blood supply cut as the flap remains attached to the original site by the blood vessels
- can only be moved as far as the blood supply allows
- gives a good cosmetic result
- is not as technically difficult as a free tissue flap, and can be performed more quickly
- has more complications but these are easier to deal with (Breast Doctor online 2001).

The myocutaneous flaps used require the movement of the latissimus dorsi muscle with overlying skin or the lower abdominal fat and skin based on the rectus abdominus muscle (transverse rectus abdominus myocutaneous flaps – TRAM flaps). Latissimus dorsi flaps require a prosthesis between them and the chest wall to create a breast mound. TRAM flaps do not usually require an implant to be inserted. They can be performed as a pedicled flap based on the superior epigastric artery or a free flap using a microsurgical anastomosis. All are substantial operations (Watson et al. 1995).

TRAM flaps

The abdomen has two paired muscles running from the costal cartilages of the fifth, sixth and seventh ribs to the top of the pubic bone – the rectus abdominus muscle. It is a superficial muscle supplied by the superior and deep epigastric arteries. If one of these is used for breast reconstruction the woman's activities will not be affected. If both are used weakness of the abdominal muscles will make sitting up from lying down more difficult.

The rectus muscle is used to carry fat and skin from the abdomen to the chest for the construction of a breast mound.

A piece of abdominal wall skin with the underlying fat is cut out and freed from the rest of the abdominal wall except the abdominus rectus muscle, to which it remains attached. Large blood vessels within the rectus muscle feed the muscle and fat to keep it alive. The entire flap is rotated under the skin of the lower chest so it comes out of the hole in the skin where the breast used to be. The flap is cut to size and shape and then sutured. It can be transferred as a free or pedicled flap (Breast Doctor online 2001). A free flap requires microsurgery to remain viable and is less common.

The scar is identical to the one following abdominoplasty. The belly button is left attached to the abdominal wall and when the skin of the upper abdomen is stretched to close the wound the belly button is repositioned to an anatomic location. Several drains are inserted to control the accumulation of fluid and blood.

A TRAM flap may be unsuitable for women with a diminished microcirculation, for example diabetics, the obese, smokers, or those who had previous surgery or radiotherapy carried out on the area of the flap or blood supply (Parker 1996).

The first 24 hours post-operatively are critical and the patient requires vigilant care and monitoring. The viability of the flap is easily compromised and the patient who has had a TRAM flap remains in Intensive Care for 24–48 hours to monitor the blood supply (Fournier and Schafer 2001). The flap is checked for temperature, colour and capillary refill. It should appear pale pink – a dusky or bluish colour could indicate venous congestion leading to necrosis. Skin should be warm – any coolness may indicate a problem with blood perfusion. The nurse can assess capillary refill by applying gentle pressure to the flap with a finger. The colour should return a few seconds after the tissue blanches – if not venous congestion could be indicated (Parker 1996).

The flap must also be protected from pressure, kinking and stretching. The patient is generally allowed to lie on the non-affected side, which elevates the newly constructed breast and improves drainage (Williams 1998).

Signs of infection must be watched for, that is, erythema, tenderness, pyrexia or discharge, as this may compromise the viability of the flap.

At least two closed wound drains will be inserted into the reconstructed breast area. There is a greater risk of haemorrhage following immediate reconstruction due to the removal of the breast and axillary lymph nodes (Parker 1996). Drains should be observed for patency and can be removed when drainage appears to be minimal. The wound should be observed for haematoma formation – small haematomas will probably reabsorb, although surgical intervention may be necessary for large ones. Drainage of the wound and prevention of haematoma formation is very important as the survival of the transplanted graft depends on the growth of blood vessels in the area into which the tissue is transplanted. Prevention of exudates ensures that a satisfactory 'bed' is provided for the new graft (Williams 1998).

Pain relief may be initially administered through a continuous infusion. Adequate analgesia will be required in order for the patient to be able to carry out the appropriate post-operative arm exercises as given by the physiotherapist.

A supportive mesh is generally inserted to reduce the risk of herniation. Removing the rectus abduminus muscle weakens the abdominal wall and herniation may occur in 10 per cent of women (Watson et al. 1995). However, patients usually look on the use of the abdominal fat and skin as a bonus, as it is identical to a 'tummy tuck'. Patients are usually asked to wear a girdle for six weeks post-operatively to support the abdomen.

Tight dressings should be avoided. Patients are generally advised to wear a sports bra and to avoid underwired bras. TRAM flaps require 4–6 weeks to heal before the abdominal wall is comfortable, it may take up to three months for the patient to recover properly. Walking and gentle exercise is encouraged, as is gentle swimming. Exposure to the sun is to be avoided.

The TRAM flap should look and feel natural, and will conform to weight and age changes (Fournier and Schafer 2001).

Radiotherapy after TRAM flap reconstruction

Pathology of breast tumours and the extent of nodal involvement determine whether radiotherapy is given after mastectomy for breast cancer. The long-term effect of radiotherapy on the outcome of breast reconstruction with the free TRAM flap is still unclear. For patients who need post-operative radiotherapy the timing of TRAM flap reconstruction is controversial. A study compared the outcome of delayed and immediate free TRAM flap reconstruction in patients who received post-mastectomy radiotherapy. Patients who received immediate TRAM flap reconstruction before radiotherapy were compared with patients who had radiotherapy before the TRAM flap was performed.

Early complications included vessel thrombosis, partial/total flap loss, mastectomy skin flap necrosis and local problems with wound healing. Late complications included fat necrosis, volume loss and flap contracture of free TRAM breast mounds.

The incidence of early complications did not differ much between the two groups. However the incidence of late complications was higher in the group who had undergone immediate reconstruction than in the delayed group.

The conclusion was that reconstruction should be delayed until radiotherapy is complete in patients who are candidates for free TRAM flaps (Tran et al. 2001).

Latissimus dorsi flap

This flap is useful for patients who cannot have a TRAM flap. The latissimus dorsi flap uses the upper back muscles and skin to reconstruct a breast mound. This is a good option for small to medium breasts. However the skin on the back has a different colour and texture to that of breast skin. The latissimus dorsi muscle is one of the largest muscles in the body, located on the back. It arises from the lower six vertebrae, the lumbar fascia and the crest of the ileum and inserts into the bicipital groove of the humerus. The majority lies subcutaneously and is therefore easily accessible. It can be transferred as a pedicle flap to provide coverage for an implant. Either the muscle alone or muscle and skin can be transferred. Part of the muscle, an area of overlying skin and its blood supply are dissected, rotated on a pedicle and then tunnelled beneath the skin under the arm to be placed on the anterior chest wall (Parker 1996). It covers the implant and is joined to the skin and muscle already present. The skin attached to the muscle will become the skin of the new breast.

An implant is always required for appropriate breast volume. The latissimus dorsi muscle is thin and not enough can be brought to the front to give sufficient volume to the new breast. The donor scar runs diagonally across the back, which may be covered by a bra but may be noticeable in a swimsuit or summer clothing. Everyday activities are not affected too much but women who ski will notice weakness when pushing off. Heavy patients may notice weakness when using their arms to arise from a low chair (Breast Doctor online 2001). Sometimes a twitch due to the severed nerves can be a problem.

A latissimus dorsi flap is unsuitable for patients who have a damaged latissimus dorsi muscle, or who have very large breasts.

Post-operative care of the patient and observation of the latissimus dorsi flap is as the TRAM flap (above) but the patient does not go to Intensive Care. The patient may also recover more quickly.

Gluteal flaps

These are not as commonly used as the others described. Only women with sufficient extra tissue in the gluteal (buttock) area are considered. The blood vessels for this type of flap are short so gluteal flaps are always free flaps. The short blood vessels are cut and a microscope is used to sew the vein and artery of the gluteal muscle and its overlying skin and fat to a vein and artery in the chest wall. These flaps are generally used as a last resort (Breast Doctor online 2001).

The nipple

A nipple can be reconstructed after the reconstruction has healed and settled into its final position and shape, then the nipple can be positioned accurately. The time interval may be 3–4 months following the reconstruction. A nipple may be reconstructed from grafted skin tissue from suitable areas of the body, for example top of the inner thigh. 'Tattooing' of the areola after the reconstruction may be used but does not produce a shape. It will not function or have the same sensation as a natural one (Cancer Bacup online 2001). Prosthetic companies make prosthetic nipples, which are usually 'stick-on' and can be positioned by the wearer.

Some hospitals may have a prosthetic technician who will make prosthetic nipples for each individual patient. The patient generally has an appointment to decide on shape, size and colour and a mould is made of the remaining nipple so that it can be matched up. This is then used to make a silicone nipple, which the technician colours to match the other one. At the second appointment the nipple is fitted and the patient can decide if it is satisfactory. The mould is always kept and the patient can contact the technician when a further one is required. For a bilateral reconstruction the patient and technician have to decide on a suitable shape, size and colour without the remaining one as a guide. Patients are, in general, extremely pleased with these. Often the technician and breast care nurse obtain the patient's consent to have photographs taken by the medical illustrator. This enables other women considering the procedure to get some idea of the finished effect.

Discharge home

Post-operatively and following discharge nurses need to monitor the woman's mood and feelings, observe for signs of depression and anxiety, how she views her reconstruction and how supportive her home situation is. The community nurse is in an excellent position to monitor the patient psychologically and physically. It is important that arm exercises are carried out at home, referral to a physiotherapist may be made to help with this. The patient may feel more able to discuss her feelings in her home surroundings. It can be seen if her expectations have been met: however she may be disappointed at first if the breast does not appear to be how she envisaged, especially if surgery to the contralateral breast is to be undertaken at a later date or if she is undergoing inflation of a tissue expander. It is important that she understands that time is needed for healing. This depends largely on the patient's age, nutritional status, state of health, stress levels and any pre-existing conditions (Williams 1998).

The future

In October 2000 the Royal College of Surgeons announced a joint training scheme for breast surgeons and plastic surgeons so that more women can have reconstruction following mastectomy. Performing the two operations immediately after each other should spare the woman the psychological trauma of losing a breast and the pain and trauma of another procedure at a later date. This also has financial implications, avoiding duplicated surgery and consultations. The college held a masterclass for breast and plastic surgeons to learn more about oncoplastic surgery. As breast reconstruction becomes increasingly popular in the UK, more surgeons are required to undertake the latest techniques in surgery. At the time of the announcement there were only 300 breast surgeons and 190 plastic surgeons in the country, of whom just over a quarter carry out breast reconstruction work (Woodman 2000).

The Royal College of Surgeons held a further training course in October 2002 – breast cancer awareness month – in breast reconstruction for surgeons training in oncoplastic surgery. The latest scarless surgical techniques were demonstrated and also the psychological needs of women undergoing this surgery were addressed. Four patients who had undergone reconstructive surgery shared their experiences with the surgeons learning the new skills. The objective was that an oncoplastic surgeon can remove the tumour and rebuild the breast at the same time. Approximately 40 per cent of breast reconstructions are performed at the time of mastectomy and similar uptakes are reported when this is offered to patients in the UK. The Department of Health now funds 10 oncoplastic surgeon posts in England. This is hoped to ensure that women are offered the latest in treatments to help them make an informed decision that is right for them (Royal College of Surgeons 2002).

References

Al-Ghazal SK, Sully I, Fallowfield L, Blamey RW (2000a) The psychological impact of immediate rather than delayed breast reconstruction. European Journal of Surgical Oncology 26(1): 17–19.

Al-Ghazal SK, Fallowfield L, Blamey RW (2000b) Comparison of psychological aspects and patient satisfaction following breast conservation surgery, simple mastectomy and breast reconstruction. European Journal of Cancer suppl 1: 25–9.

Breast Cancer Care online (2001) Reconstruction. http://www.breastcancercare.org.uk (accessed November 2001).

Breast Doctor online (2001) Breast Cancer. http://www.breastdoctor.com (accessed 2001).

Caffo O, Cazzoli D, Scalet A, Zani B, et al. (2000) Concurrent adjuvant chemotherapy and immediate breast reconstruction with skin expanders after mastectomy for breast cancer. Breast Cancer Research and Treatment 60(3): 267–75.

Cancer Bacup (2001) Understanding Breast Reconstruction. www.cancerbacup.org.uk (accessed November 2001).

Chang DW, Kroll SS, Dackiw A, et al. (2001) Reconstructive management of contralateral breast cancer in patients who previously underwent unilateral breast reconstruction. Plastic and Reconstructive Surgery 108(2): 352–8, Discussion 359–60.

Clough KB, O'Donoghue JM, Fitoussi AD, et al. (2001) Prospective evaluation of late cosmetic results following breast reconstruction: 1. Implant reconstruction. Plastic and Reconstructive Surgery 107(7): 1702–9.

Department of Health (1999) Withdrawal of oil-based breast implants. Message from Dr Jeremy Metters, Deputy Chief Medical Officer. London: DoH.

Fournier J, Schafer SL (2001) TRAM flap surgery: Vigilant care promotes healing and is cost-effective. American Journal of Nursing 101(suppl): 16–18.

Harcourt D, Rumsey N (2001) Psychological aspects of breast reconstruction: a review of the literature. Journal of Advanced Nursing 35(4): 477–81.

LaRossa D (1997) Breast Reconstructive Surgery Options. Oncolink website www.oncolink.com (accessed November 2001).

Malata CM, McIntosh SA, Purushotham AD, et al. (2000) Immediate breast reconstruction after surgery for cancer. British Journal of Surgery 87(11): 1455–72.

NHS Executive (1996) Improving Outcomes in Breast Cancer: The Manual. London: DoH.

Nyren O, Yin L, Josefsson S, McLaughlin JK (1998) Risk of connective tissue disorders among women with breast implants: a nationwide retrospective cohort study in Sweden. British Medical Journal 316: 417–22.

Parker JM (1996) Breast reconstruction. In: Denton S (1996) Breast Cancer Nursing. London: Chapman & Hall.

Rowland JH, Drosso J, Holland JC, et al. (1995) Breast reconstruction after mastectomy: who seeks it, who refuses? Plastic and Reconstructive Surgery 95: 812–22.

Royal College of Surgeons of England (2002) News Room, 13 February 2002. More Surgeons to be Trained in Breast Reconstruction. http://rcs.niss.ac.uk/public/pns/DisplayPN.cgi?pn_id=2002_0014 (accessed September 2002).

Tran NV, Chang DW, Gupta A, et al. (2001) Comparison of immediate and delayed TRAM flap breast reconstruction in patients receiving post-mastectomy radiotherapy. Plastic and Reconstructive Surgery 108(1): 78–82.

University of Iowa online (1995) Plastic Surgery – Breast Reconstruction, www.surgery.uiowa.edu (accessed November 2001).

Watson JD, Sainsbury JRC, Dixon JM (1995) ABC of breast diseases: Breast reconstruction after surgery. British Medical Journal 310: 1117–21.

Williams L (1998) Nursing management of adults undergoing cosmetic or reconstructive surgery. In: Beare PG, Myers JF (eds) Adult Health Nursing. 3rd edn. London: Mosby.

Winder AE, Winder BD (1985) Patient counselling: clarifying a woman's choice for breast reconstruction. Patient Education and Counselling 7: 65–75.

Woodman R (2000) UK surgeons to offer more women immediate reconstruction after mastectomy. OBGYN.net publications. Reuters Health Information online www.obgyn.net/reuters (accessed November 2001).

CHAPTER SEVEN

Chemotherapy for breast cancer

Chemotherapy can be used for cure, control or palliation. The very mention of the word chemotherapy is frightening for patients. They envisage months of hair loss, nausea, fatigue and infections. The options and the drug names are confusing. However, the combination of drugs depends on the characteristics of the tumour and the medical oncologist will decide the most effective drug combination and dosage for each individual patient. The short-term side effects can be managed (apart from hair loss) through supportive medication and lifestyle changes.

Women with early breast cancer are given adjuvant chemotherapy as an 'insurance policy' after surgery to eradicate micrometastases. This does not apply to women with metastatic disease where the aim is not to cure but to control or shrink a tumour to improve quality of life. The side effects should not outweigh the benefits. Metastatic disease will be discussed in Chapter 15.

Often chemotherapy is given prior to surgery if the tumour measures 3cm or more (neoadjuvant chemotherapy). This may make it possible for a patient to have a lumpectomy rather than a mastectomy, or to have an immediate reconstruction following mastectomy.

Chemotherapy agents are also called antineoplastic or cytotoxic agents. The role of these drugs is to slow and hopefully halt the spread of the neoplasm. Most tumours respond better when treated with a combination of drugs. There are three goals associated with the use of the most common chemotherapy drugs:

1 To damage the affected cells' DNA. Selectivity is the ultimate goal but it is not always possible to be selective.
2 To inhibit the synthesis of new DNA strands to stop the cell from replicating – the replication of the cell allows the growth of the tumour.
3 To stop the mitotic processes of a cell. Mitosis is the splitting of the cell into two new ones. Stopping mitosis stops cell replication (division) of the cancer and may ultimately halt its progression (Altruis Biomedical Network online 2000).

The cell cycle

The cell cycle includes all the processes necessary for nuclear and cell division. It is the continuous process from one mitotic division to the next. The cell cycle can be divided into phases: interphase (during which DNA replicates), mitosis (cell divides), and cytokinesis (cytoplasmic division – cytoplasm is all the material within the cell outer boundary but excludes that within the nuclear membrane) (Brooker 1996).

A knowledge of the cell cycle in 'normal' and malignant cells is necessary when planning the use of cytotoxic drugs. Thus, the multidisciplinary team can choose the correct cytotoxic drug for the patient and plan a course of treatment that offers maximum benefit with minimum side effects.

Interphase and DNA replication

The cell is in the GO (Growth O) phase initially – this is a resting phase and chemotherapy will not work.

Interphase is the stage during which all day-to-day metabolic processes of cells occur. It is also the stage between two mitotic divisions when the cell prepares the materials and structures for division. The interphase can be divided into three stages:

1 G1 phase (Growth 1) – the cell takes on energy and nutrients. Proteins are synthesized. Chemotherapy and radiotherapy are effective in this phase. Two centrioles lying close to the nucleus replicate and each resultant pair moves to opposite poles of the cell to form the mitotic spindle. This is formed from protein strands consisting of microtubules.
2 S phase (Synthetic) – the cell prepares for division. The DNA in the chromatin replicates. The two new cells resulting from mitosis will have identical genetic material. The triggers for cell division and DNA replication are not well understood. During replication the two strands of DNA unravel (DNA has two strands coiled into a double helix). Other enzymes cause two new strands to be formed using the existing separate strands as templates. Once replication is complete the double set of DNA joins with proteins to form new chromatin strands.
3 G2 phase (Growth 2) – the cell rests but gathers energy and nutrients needed for mitosis. Chemotherapy drugs can affect this delicate process and prevent cell division (Brooker 1996).

Mitosis (M phase)

The cell splits into two. This is a continuous process but usually consists of four stages.

1 Prophase – the chromatin (a substance containing the genetic material

or chromosomes of the cell) changes and forms visible chromosomes. A double set of chromosomes result from DNA replication during interphase. Each half of this double chromosome is known as a chromatid. The nucleoli break down and the nuclear membrane disappears. Each pair of centrioles move to opposite poles of the cell where they form the mitotic spindle.

2 Metaphase – the double chromosomes move to the middle of the cell so that their centromeres are arranged along the equator of the mitotic spindle.

3 Anaphase – the double chromosomes split at the centromere, each becoming a complete chromosome. The fibres of the mitotic spindle contract, causing a chromosome from each new pair to be pulled to the opposite pole of the cell (Brooker 1996).

4 Telephase – the set of chromosomes at each pole uncoils to form the chromatin. The nuclear membrane reforms, the mitotic spindle disappears and the nucleoli reform.

One cell will differentiate and one will stay as a stem cell (the basis of all cells), which goes into the GO or resting phase until stimulated. Cells in the GO phase are temporarily out of the cell cycle for several hours to several years depending on the type of cell. When it is signalled to reproduce it moves into the G1 phase. Damage to an organ stimulates the cell out of the resting phase. Cancer cells develop as various DNA mutations occur in cells exposed to a carcinogenic agent or if a cancer gene already present is activated.

How chemotherapy works

Chemotherapy disrupts the cell cycle. The chemotherapy drug causes the cell's death. Cells that are vulnerable are dividing or preparing to divide. Current research is looking at ways to target cancerous cells without damaging healthy cells. The majority of drugs are not specific and lead to many of the side effects associated with chemotherapy. However, some drugs are most cytotoxic during a specific phase of the cell cycle and are called cycle-specific drugs. These are very effective in malignancies with a large number of actively dividing cells. They are best administered over a long period to allow the cells to reach the phase when the drug will act.

Drugs that disable resting cells and cells preparing for division are called cell cycle non-specific agents. These damage the cell but death does not occur until the cell attempts to divide. These drugs tend to be more dose-dependent; that is, the number of cells killed is in direct proportion to the amount of drug given (Beare and Myers 1998).

Most drugs affect rapidly dividing cells so cells in the resting phase may remain viable and reproduce causing recurrence of disease. Repeated courses of chemotherapy must be given to achieve disease remission because it must be assumed that cancer cells remain behind even when all diagnostic methods show the patient to be disease free.

Chemotherapy cannot distinguish between normal and abnormal cells therefore both types of cells are affected. The normal cell population recovers much more quickly than the cancer cell population. This difference in rate of repair can be exploited by scheduling chemotherapy precisely so that only normal cells have time to recover.

As previously mentioned, most tumours respond best to a combination of drugs. Combination approaches are developed using the following principles:

- Only drugs that are definitely known to be partially effective when used on their own should be selected for combination use.
- Drugs that have differing toxic effects are selected to decrease a potentially lethal effect that could result from repeated insults to one organ.
- Optimal doses are used.
- The combination of drugs is administered as frequently and consistently as possible while allowing normal tissue to recover between cycles (Beare and Myers 1998).
- Cell death is increased due to the synergistic action of the drugs.
- Cell death is increased by using drugs that act at different phases of the cycle.
- There is a reduced risk of drug resistance developing.

Classification of chemotherapeutic agents

Cytotoxic drugs are usually classified according to their antineoplastic action.

Alkylating agents and antitumour antibiotics comprise drugs that are cell cycle non-specific (damage DNA in resting and dividing cells). Alkylating agents produce breaks and cross-links in the strands of cellular DNA – these impair DNA synthesis preventing the cell from replicating. An example is nitrogen mustard, a very early chemotherapy drug. Antitumour antibiotics (anthracyclines) bind directly to DNA hindering replication and work throughout the cell cycle (Beare and Myers 1998). Examples include Doxorubicin (adriamycin) and Epirubicin. A combination of drugs including an anthracycline is generally considered to give a higher response rate especially in pre-menopausal women.

Antimetabolites and vinca alkaloids are cell cycle specific. Antimetabolites are specific to the S phase of the cell cycle. The cell mistakenly incorporates an antimetabolite into the DNA during DNA synthesis resulting in disruption of cell replication. Examples are Methotrexate and Fluorouracil (which is often used in breast cancer). Vinca alkaloids are derived from plants and and are specific to the M phase of the cell cycle. They stop the formation of microtubules needed for the formation of the mitotic spindle. The cell is stopped at metaphase, it cannot divide and so dies. Examples are Vincristine, Vinblastine, Paclitaxel (Taxol) and Vinorelbine (Navelbine).

When is chemotherapy administered?

A cycle of chemotherapy refers to the one administration of the drugs. A course refers to all the cycles in the treatment. Any number from four to eight cycles may be given in any course. Adjuvant chemotherapy (systemic therapy) is a whole body treatment.

Many factors are taken into account when deciding to give a patient chemotherapy, for example tumour size and grade, lymphatic/vascular invasion, rate of tumour cell growth, hormone receptor status (patients with hormone receptor negative tumours are generally given chemotherapy, hormone receptor positive are often given hormone therapy), oncogene expression and lymph node involvement. Factors such as age, general health of the patient, location of the tumour, whether or not axillary lymph nodes are enlarged are all taken into consideration along with menopausal status, stage of disease and the risk/benefit of treatment. The wishes of the patient are also carefully listened to.

Chemotherapy is not recommended for non-invasive *in situ* cancers which have almost no risk of metastasizing. More aggressive treatments are given to women who have invasive breast cancer and who are premenopausal. If lymph nodes are involved chemotherapy is recommended regardless of menopausal status or tumour size (Breast Cancer Org. online 2001).

Chemotherapy is also given to pre-menopausal women who have an invasive tumour that has not spread to lymph nodes and is 1cm or more in size. It would be considered in a post-menopausal woman who has these factors.

It may be recommended in women who are pre-menopausal with a tumour confined to the breast, smaller than 1cm but has one or more unfavourable characteristics, for example is oestrogen receptor negative. In many women chemotherapy and hormone therapy may be combined.

For node positive women there is a 25 per cent improvement in relapse rate and a 15 per cent greater chance of a cure. For node negative women, as the prognosis is better, these figures will be in the region of 15 per cent and 10 per cent. This means that many women will receive no benefit from chemotherapy because they are cured anyway, or the tumour will return despite chemotherapy. As breast cancer is so common, however, if chemotherapy is given to all patients many lives will be saved (Cancernet.co.uk online 2002).

The multidisciplinary team consider each patient individually and decide together on the best course of treatment for each taking into account all of the above. The surgeon, medical oncologist, pathologist and breast care nurses are all involved at every step.

Chemotherapeutic drugs in common use

All breast cancer centres will vary slightly in the drugs that they use and, as research is ongoing, the following are examples only. Side effects will be mentioned below as they apply to most or all treatments but will be discussed in more detail later.

All chemotherapy drugs can cause nausea so anti-emetics are given prior to chemotherapy and for a few days afterwards. Appetite may be reduced. If the white blood cell count falls, the patient is very prone to a severe infection and must telephone the unit if experiencing fever, pyrexia or is feeling at all unwell. If the haemaglobin is low the patient may complain of headaches, fatigue and palpitations. Nosebleeds, bleeding or bruising show that the platelet count is low and the patient again must contact the unit. The mouth may become sore and ulcers may develop. Not all the chemotherapy drugs will cause hair loss but patients will be able to obtain a wig and the loss is generally temporary. If the patient is pre-menopausal her periods may be affected. This may be temporary or permanent causing menopausal symptoms. Fatigue can be a major problem. During the administration of chemotherapy veins may become damaged. They may become hard and 'cord-like'. This is caused by a superficial thrombosis and can take a few months to resolve. The insertion of a PICC line (Peripherally Inserted Central venous Catheter) or Hickman line may overcome this problem.

Extravasation is when the drugs leak out of the vein causing irritation and tissue damage. All nurses involved in the giving of chemotherapy are fully trained and know what to do. There may be pain, stinging or burning at the injection site along with redness or swelling. The unit should be contacted immediately (Cancernet.co.uk online 2002).

Adriamycin/Cyclophosphamide (AC)

Adriamycin/Cyclophosphamide (AC) is given every three weeks as a slow injection. The blood count is taken prior to treatment and if low, treatment is delayed. Adriamycin is red so the patient may find that the urine is coloured red, this is normal. AC will cause hair loss. This will occur 3–4 weeks after the first course and all hair may be lost including body hair, eyelashes and eyebrows. Constipation may be a problem. AC is given with dexamethasone to help prevent sickness, however steroids also have side effects including weight gain, fluid retention and agitation.

Adriamycin can (rarely) damage the heart. A cardiac function test may be done prior to or during chemotherapy. The risks are very small if the dose is correct and not exceeded. Patients are advised to stop smoking.

Intravenous Cyclophosphamide/Methotrexate/Fluorouracil (CMF)

This is probably the most common regime for adjuvant treatment for breast cancer. It is administered as follows.

Methotrexate (intravenously) days 1 and 8
Fluorouracil (intravenously) days 1 and 8
Cyclophosphamide (intravenously) days 1 and 8.

This is repeated every 28 days. The blood count is taken one day before each cycle. Hair loss is less common, but it may become thinner, with 20 per cent of patients experiencing considerable thinning (Cancernet.co.uk online 2002). Diarrhoea may occur.

Cyclophosphamide used to be given as a tablet daily for 14 days but the intravenous administration is now more common.

5 Fluorouracil, Epirubicin and Cyclophosphamide (FEC)

This is given once every three weeks intravenously. Hair loss will occur. Patients may report a sensitivity to light and sore hands and feet. Epirubicin will colour the urine red. It is necessary to monitor cardiac function as epirubicin can cause cardiac damage. The patient may also complain of a sore mouth.

Epirubicin/Cyclophosphamide (EC)

This is given once every three weeks intravenously. It will cause hair loss.

Mitomycin C, Methotrexate and Mitrozantone (MMM)

Methotrexate and Mitrozantone are given every three weeks intravenously and Mitomycin C is given every six weeks. Tamoxifen must not be prescribed as kidney function may be damaged. The urine may be coloured blue.

The following chemotherapy drugs are not used in the adjuvant setting but are given for metastatic disease.

Capecitabine (Xeloda)

Capsules taken orally as an adjuvant treatment for breast cancer. These are taken for two weeks then a break of a week. Hair loss is uncommon. (Capecitabine is discussed in more detail in Chapter 15, see pp 256–7).

Taxotere (Docetaxol)

Given every three weeks as an intravenous infusion for an hour. Hair loss will occur and the nerve endings may be irritated. There may be some discolouration in nail colour and skin may be dry. Dexamethasone is given as a pre-medication on the day before treatment, on the day and the day after treatment to prevent anaphylactic shock. Corticosteroids also reduce the leg oedema that may occur. Palmar and plantar syndrome may also be experienced. There is a trial in progress to give Taxotere as an adjuvant treatment (TACT trial) but this is not yet standard practice.

Taxotere and Adriamycin

Taxotere is given as an intravenous infusion three weekly. Adriamycin is given as a single IV injection. Hair loss will occur. Cardiac function tests will be undertaken.

Taxol (Paclitaxel)

Given via an IV infusion via a cannula over three hours. The patient is very carefully monitored. Usually 4–6 cycles are given. Blood tests and scans are done after the third and sixth cycle to monitor response. The patient will have hair loss. An allergic reaction is possible on the first and second infusion. Taste may be altered and diarrhoea may occur. The patient may complain of aching joints and muscles (Cancernet.co.uk online 2002). Premedication with a corticosteroid, an antihistamine and a histamine H2-receptor antagonist is recommended to prevent anaphylaxis.

Taxol is a famous chemotherapy drug due to the reports in the media during 2000 about 'postcode lotteries'. However, Taxol is now in general use. It has been approved for the treatment of breast cancer that has spread to the lymph nodes following surgery and a doxorubicin (Adriamycin) containing chemotherapy. It benefits patients with receptor negative tumours.

Taxol is also given if breast cancer has metastasized and a combination of other drugs had not been effective, or where there has been a relapse of breast cancer within six months of adjuvant chemotherapy.

Taxol is derived from the bark of the Pacific yew tree. This was found to have anti-tumour properties in 1963. In 1971 the active ingredient was found to be Paclitaxel, however problems were encountered in producing, extracting and processing it. By 1989 patients with advanced ovarian cancer were found to be showing a 30 per cent response rate to Taxol. Problems were due to supply shortages. In 1992 Taxol was approved for use after first line or subsequent treatment for advanced ovarian cancer. By 1994 clearance had been given for use in advanced breast cancer and by 1999 approval had been given for the production of semi-synthetic Taxol (Taxol.com online 1998).

High dose chemotherapy

This is still under investigation in the UK, clinical trials are taking place. It is based on the theory that the larger the dose of chemotherapy the greater the chance of destroying all cancer cells present. High dose chemotherapy would probably be used if the patient had more than 10 lymph nodes involved or if initial chemotherapy had shrunk a tumour but there was a high risk of recurrence. It is not suitable for all women.

Before chemotherapy is given healthy bone marrow or stem cells (blood cells at the earliest stages of development) are removed and stored as bone marrow cells left in the body could be severely damaged. Intensive treatment is then given for a few days. The bone marrow or stem cells are then returned to help revive the immune system. Alternatively donor marrow can be used usually from a sibling or unrelated donor who is a good match. The blood count becomes very low and the patient is monitored very closely as an inpatient (Breast Cancer Care 1999).

Administration

Chemotherapy is prescribed by specialist non-surgical oncologists who work with expert pharmacy and laboratory support. Nurses who have had additional training in chemotherapy administration deliver the chemotherapy. Expertise is needed in both methods and problems of administration. The nurse needs a thorough understanding of the management of drug delivery devices, specific drug actions, side effects, toxic effects and dosage ranges. Patient teaching is given for the recognition and self-management of side effects. Intravenously is the most common route but drugs can be administered via peripheral and central venous access devices. The chemotherapy nurse must always be aware of the toxicity of the drugs and take precautions when handling both the drugs and the excreta of patients (Beare and Myers 1998). Chemotherapy is administered on an oncology ward or at designated day care facilities.

A Hickman line may be inserted into the subclavian vein to make chemotherapy easier and more comfortable. This is done as a simple procedure that does not require a general anaesthetic. A chest X-ray will confirm the correct position of the line. This negates the need to find a vein every time chemotherapy is given. It may also be used when the patient is having chemotherapy continuously via a pump.

A PICC (Peripherally Inserted Central venous Catheter) line may be used instead of a Hickman line. This is inserted into a vein in the arm near to the antecubital fossa then follows the route of this vein leading to the larger veins which lead to the heart. Not all patients are suitable for this. The PICC and Hickman lines are also used to obtain blood samples and need to be flushed regularly to maintain patency – this can be done by the patient after teaching or by the district nurse.

Side effects of chemotherapy

Side effects result from the damage to normal cells alongside the malignant cells. In some cases the side effects prevent the course of chemotherapy from continuing. Rapidly dividing cells are most vulnerable so it is bone marrow, gastrointestinal tract, hair follicles and gonadal cells that suffer the most impact. Some people have few or no side effects; others have severe reactions.

Neutropenia

The compromise of the immune system by chemotherapy can lead to overwhelming infections. Neutropenia is the most important factor that predisposes patients to infection. As the neutrophil count falls the risk of infection rises. A rapid decline or persistent neutropenia will increase the risk. It usually caused by chemotherapy-induced reduction of the white blood cells in the bone marrow.

The signs and symptoms of infection may be very subtle at first and nursing and medical staff need to be alert. In the compromised patient a fever may be the only sign of a life threatening septicaemia. Patients are informed of what to be aware of and must contact the unit if there is any problem 24 hours a day. For example:

- any redness of the skin, any rash, lesions or skin breakdown
- any lesions, redness, tenderness or coating of the mouth
- cough, cold symptoms or pleuritic pain. Patients are instructed not to treat themselves for a cold but to report it
- any pain, itching or burning in the perineal area.

The patient will be admitted for intravenous antibiotics, swabs, blood cultures and symptomatic care (Beare and Myers 1998).

If the patient is thought to be in any way prone to infection, Granulocyte Colony Stimulating Factor (GCSF or trade name Neupogen, for example) can be given. This is a naturally occurring growth factor that increases the number of infection fighting white blood cells. It helps to maintain adequate numbers of granulocytes, which destroy bacteria. GCSF can now be made in the laboratory. It is a clear colourless liquid that can be given subcutaneously, usually with the second cycle of chemotherapy if the patient is prone to infection with the first cycle. The incidence of febrile neutropenia and hospital admission is reduced.

Anaemia

Anaemia may not be life threatening but can severely affect the quality of the patient's life. The patient is educated about the specific symptoms, for example lethargy, dizziness, breathlessness and fatigue. A full blood count is done and a blood transfusion may be required.

Bleeding

Chemotherapy-induced thrombocytopaenia is a common cause of bleeding. As the platelet count decreases, problems with clotting arise and the risk of bleeding increases. The patient is again informed of the possibility of problems and must report any headaches, bruising or nosebleeds. If possible, physical activity and trauma should be avoided. Treatment consists of assessment, observation and possibly a platelet infusion.

Oral complications

In normal circumstances the mouth needs to be clean, moist and comfortable. Chemotherapy affects the epithelial cells in the oral mucosa, which slough and become denuded as a result of the cytotoxicity of the drugs. This can cause lesions, ulcers and inflammation (mucositis, stomatitis) (Beare and Myers 1998). The patient is also susceptible to thrush and herpes simplex if the white cell count is low. Treatment includes using a soft toothbrush, saline or a prescribed mouthwash, a prescribed oral gel if appropriate, Vaseline to lips, clear fluids through a straw and ice to suck. Patients are advised to try soft foods and small, frequent meals. Alcohol and tobacco are to be avoided (Cancernet.co.uk online 2002).

Alopecia

The loss of hair can have a devastating effect on the patient's body image. The scalp hair is most commonly affected but other body hair may become thin, depending on the individual. Because the hair follicles are metabolically active they are susceptible to the effects of certain chemotherapy drugs. This is temporary – hair will grow back once treatment is completed but may be changed in colour and texture – a patient may find that she has a head of wavy or grey hair after treatment!

Prevention can be attempted. Cooling the scalp during some chemotherapy regimes has been shown to prevent or reduce total hair loss. The small blood vessels surrounding the hair follicles are constricted and the cells are prevented from taking up the chemotherapy (Peck et al. 2000). Cooling the scalp to a temperature of 17°C to achieve a subcutaneous temperature of 20°C constricts the blood supply and diminishes their perfusion. The coldness itself also reduces the availability of cytotoxic drugs (for example Doxorubicin, which is temperature dependent) to the cells of the follicles by reducing their metabolic rate (Cancernet.co.uk online 2002). It is the combined effect of both these mechanisms that prevents or reduces alopecia.

Not all breast cancer centres use scalp cooling as the evidence is inconclusive. However, in some circumstances reducing alopecia contributes towards improvement in self-esteem. Commercially available systems use cooled air blown over the scalp, frozen gel caps or a liquid coolant circulated through a refrigeration unit (Peck et al. 2000). Tolerance is variable especially as the course of chemotherapy progresses. The time in the unit is lengthened, for example the cold cap is put on 15 minutes prior to treatment and left on for 1–2 hours afterwards. Some clinical trials show success with the cold cap system when used with Taxotere, Taxol, Epirubicin and Cyclophosphamide. However, it may not work on all patients (Cancernet.co.uk online 2002).

Patients are often worried about hair loss above all else so coping strategies must be explored. These may include: using a soft hair brush, having hair cut shorter, using a gentle shampoo, not having a perm or colour, using cotton pillowcases, letting hair dry naturally instead of using a hairdryer, not using tongs or heated rollers. Scarves, hats and baseball caps are often worn to great effect. Patients may be able to access HEADSTART through the oncology unit or breast care nurse; this is a national organization (part of Breast Cancer Care), which supplies headwear to patients undergoing chemotherapy. It is run by trained volunteers who sell hats, scarves and turbans, and give advice on how to wear them. A wig can be organized at the start of treatment by the unit, free if an inpatient or if on benefits.

Nausea and vomiting

This is possibly the most famous side effect of all but not all drugs cause it and not all patients will experience it. Control promotes quality of life during treatment and helps towards maintaining nutrition and patient compliance. Nausea and vomiting may be acute, chronic or anticipatory. Many cytotoxic agents cause the epithelial cells lining the gastrointestinal tract to become stimulated or the 5-HT3 receptors in the vomiting centre in the medulla. However, anticipatory nausea occurs before a treatment and has often been termed a Pavlovian response based on the patient's previous negative experience of chemotherapy (Beare and Myers 1998). The patient may be very anxious or sometimes even the sight of the hospital can trigger it. Very severe cases may require the help of a psychiatrist or psychologist.

Anti-emetics are vital. These can be given orally the day before treatment and for a few days afterwards, and intravenously with the chemotherapy. Further IM injections may be carried out at home by the community nurses if the problem is severe. Examples of anti-emetics include Prochlorperazine, high-dose Metaclopramide, Domperidone, Cyclizine and Hyoscine. Dexamethasone may also be given. The group of drugs 5-HT3 receptor antagonists, for example Ondansetron, Granisetron, has greatly increased the potential to control and limit nausea and vomiting (Cotton 1996).

Again it is vitally important that the patient has advice on coping strategies. Complementary therapies such as relaxation, visualization and hypnotherapy may help with anticipatory nausea. Other measures include sipping cold, clear fluids slowly, trying jellies/sorbets, ginger/mints, herbal/peppermint tea, small frequent meals, dry foods. Spicy, fatty or very sweet foods should be avoided. The patient could try cold foods if the smell of cooking is a trigger. Fresh air and wearing loose fitting clothes may help.

Fertility

Chemotherapy does not appear to damage a woman's eggs but can cause changes within the ovaries that stop eggs being released. Younger women are more likely to retain their fertility. Factors include the type and dose of drug given. The alkylating agents are most likely to cause infertility, one of which is most commonly used in combination with other chemotherapy drugs. Women over 40 years develop amenorrhoea following a much lower dose than women under 40 years (Breast Cancer Care online 2001). Younger women can also restart their periods months after chemotherapy has finished.

It can be difficult to diagnose infertility following chemotherapy. The specialist will test whether the ovaries are working again by looking at factors such as the periods restarting, hormone levels and the evidence of menopausal symptoms. However, eggs could be produced even if periods do not restart so it is wise to continue with contraception to prevent pregnancy. The pill is not usually recommended as it is possible that the hormones in it could stimulate any remaining breast cancer cells. The medical oncologist will advise when it is safe to conceive following treatment.

Various techniques are possible to preserve fertility although some are not widely available. The patient would need to discuss this with the specialist team. Procedures involve freezing embryos (although hormone injections are given and may stimulate growth of breast cancer cells; also chemotherapy would be delayed). Eggs can be frozen but this is only available privately. Egg donation is another option but this also involves taking hormones. The freezing of ovarian tissue is also being researched (Breast Cancer Care online 2001).

Infertility is extremely difficult for the patient to cope with especially when facing breast cancer as well. She and her partner (if applicable) will require much support from the breast care nurse and specialist staff to whom she may be referred. Support groups may be useful.

If chemotherapy has interfered with the functioning of the ovaries the patient may experience menopausal symptoms such as hot flushes, night sweats and vaginal dryness. The patient is advised to wear cotton clothing and use layers of cotton bedclothes that can be removed. A cool room and electric fan may help. It is important to maintain fluid intake and avoid hot or spicy foods. Gentle exercise, relaxation and complementary therapies may help. Taking phytoestrogens in the form of linseeds, soya products or supplements can lower the rate of hot flushes (Cancernet.co.uk online 2002). However, a normal balanced diet containing fruit and vegetables will provide phytoestrogens. Advice should be taken from the breast care nurse or dietitian as it is unclear whether large doses have an oestrogenic effect. Breast care and oncology nurses have a central role in informing and supporting these women.

Fatigue

Cancer treatment related fatigue is a very prevalent and distressing symptom of cancer therapy. Reaction to the cancer diagnosis, health and nutritional status and symptom distress can all influence fatigue during chemotherapy. Interventions are required to minimize this fatigue and improve quality of life. A study examined the relationship between exercise and fatigue in women undergoing chemotherapy in the first three cycles of CMF or AC for breast cancer. It was found that exercise significantly reduced fatigue. (Schwartz et al. 2001). It is important that the patient works out a moderate exercise programme that is within their limitations, and that this is balanced with rest.

Another study suggests that changes in skeletal muscle size and strength can occur during adjuvant chemotherapy for breast cancer. This increase does not seem to diminish the subjective experience of fatigue and may lead to potential muscle damage if exercise is not moderate. Further research is needed in this area (Kaspar and Sarna 2000).

It has also been suggested that exercise is necessary to prevent 'sarcopenic obesity'. This is a common problem among patients receiving adjuvant chemotherapy but overeating is not the cause. It is indicative of weight gain in the presence of lean tissue loss or absence of lean tissue gain. Exercise is recommended especially for the lower body to prevent weight gain (Demark-Wahnefried et al. 2001). Exercise increases muscle strength, gives better flexibility, promotes restful sleep, increases the sense of well-being and gives a greater sense of control. Some women will gain a significant amount of weight especially pre-menopausal women. This is a distressing condition especially as the cause is not overeating – in fact the patient may suffer from nausea. Nurses must be aware of the possibility of weight gain and include this when educating and informing the patient on other aspects (McInnes and Knobf 2001). Nurses must also acknowledge that fatigue is a symptom and address the cause with simple measures wherever possible.

Interventions include advice on diet, sleep, rest, attention restoring activities, anti-depressants if appropriate, energy conservation, stress management, psychosocial support and possibly blood transfusion if the patient is anaemic.

Insomnia and fatigue can also be related to depression, which can in turn severely affect quality of life. Staff on the oncology unit may use questionnaires such as the HAD Scale for monitoring anxiety and depression. This is a tool devised by St James' Hospital, Leeds and the higher the score the greater the depression, although a high score for anxiety may be considered normal especially on the first and subsequent visit. This may be done on the first visit and every three months, but units will vary.

Psychosocial aspects

Women diagnosed with stage 1 or 2 breast cancer undergo rigorous multimodal treatments. The period of time from the diagnosis through initial treatments is often six months or longer and can be followed by five years of hormonal therapy. Women have to incorporate the physical and psychological demands of treatment into their lives. Chemotherapy along with surgery, radiotherapy and hormone treatment places these patients at risk from cancer related fatigue (Woo et al. 1998).

Patients may experience many other symptoms when undergoing chemotherapy. Skin problems, constipation, diarrhoea, cystitis, taste alteration and sensitivity to the sun may be reported. Some patients report difficulties in their ability to remember, think and concentrate. Health care professionals must be aware of the need for informed consent, counselling and psychosocial support (Brezden et al. 2000). The goal must always be the holistic management of each individual patient.

As well as providing physical care to the patient undergoing chemotherapy, the multidisciplinary team must be aware that the patient is coming to terms with the diagnosis as well as coping with the treatment. The oncology and breast care nurses have an important role in listening to and supporting the patient throughout. Chemotherapy can affect body image deeply and the various side effects, if experienced, can affect the patient's home and working life considerably. The needs of the partner and family must be taken into consideration and referrals made to other disciplines if necessary, for example family therapy or social services, to assist with practical and financial advice. Many units have a specialist social worker attached who will help and support the patient and family. Units may also offer alternative therapies to women undergoing chemotherapy for breast cancer such as massage, yoga, aromatherapy, counselling, etc.

A study found that men whose wives were having chemotherapy for breast cancer felt unsure and unprepared as to how to act. They wanted to be present at appointments, access information services and to be emotionally supportive. They also needed to be treated with respect and have their views taken into account. They relied on health professionals to give information and support. Being informed involved learning about the cancer, supporting their wives' decisions and informing family, children and friends. Family life also had to be kept going amid the disruption and stress of the illness. Most men were challenged by trying to keep routines going especially for the children. Men had to rely on others to undertake family and childcare activities. They felt overwhelmed and stretched especially when helping around the home was unfamiliar. Managing finances was an added problem. Most coped by putting their needs second and adapting their work life. They found that they were strengthened by their wives' positive attitudes. However, the couples tended to protect each other by not sharing emotions and anxieties (Pearce 2001). This illustrates the need for the oncology, breast care and community nurses to be aware of the problems faced by the family of the patient undergoing chemotherapy for breast cancer.

Clinical trials

Clinical trials are research studies that look at different aspects of patient care. Trials are a routine part of specialist breast cancer centres. They may be instigated by The Research Council, a pharmaceutical company or as an investigational study. Many different types of chemotherapy trials are carried out to look at improved ways of giving existing treatments. All trials have strict guidelines so not all patients are eligible to take part. Patients who are not eligible should be reassured that they will receive the best care and treatment.

The unit will have a clinical trials co-ordinator or research nurse who, along with the oncologist, discusses with the patient exactly what is involved in a trial. This may include the type of treatment, side effects, benefits and extra investigations. Written information is provided and the patient is given time to make a decision. Informed consent is obtained and the patient can withdraw from the trial at any time. It is emphasized that the trial is voluntary.

A committee oversees the trial and if it becomes clear that one treatment is significantly better than another the trial will be stopped and all the patients offered the most effective treatment. The research nurse is available to contact at any time and will carry out a home visit to discuss the trial if necessary. The research nurse liaises with hospital departments to arrange scans, X-rays, etc., collects data, monitors the patient at each visit and ensures that quality-of-life questionnaires are given to each patient. Any problems are recorded on serious adverse effect forms.

Each new drug is rigorously tested prior to being given to patients. Laboratory tests are undertaken first, then three phases of testing patients in clinical trials, before being routinely used (Breast Cancer Care online 2001).

Phase 1 trials

The drug is given to a small number of patients. In breast cancer it may be given to patients who have not responded to standard treatment. It is observed for how much can be given and how often. Side effects are noted. The main aim at this stage is not to effect a cure but the cancer may show some response to the drug.

Phase 2 trials

When the maximum dose and side effects have been established the phase 2 trials begin. Larger numbers are required for these. The aim is to fine tune the dose and establish if there is enough response for it to be an improvement on previous treatments.

Phase 3 trials

The drug is now tested on a much larger group of patients. It is compared with the best current or standard treatment. Sometimes it is the length of a treatment that is tested. These are usually randomized trials. Patients are divided into two groups who receive different treatments. The groups need to be similar so it can be established that the treatment is having an effect, not because one group is different. Patients are told that they may be in the standard group.

The benefits of being part of a trial are:

- the patient may be the first to benefit from a new treatment
- the patient is taking an active role in the treatment plan
- it is an opportunity to help research and improve future treatment
- the patient is seen much more frequently by medical staff for various tests during treatment so that effects can be monitored. The follow-up is much longer, which can be very reassuring to some patients.

The drawbacks are:

- the patient may be in the standard group
- there may be unexpected side effects
- the drug may not be more effective
- it may not work for all patients
- the extra hospital visits may be inconvenient or a too frequent reminder of the illness – follow-up may go on for 10–15 years (Breast Cancer Care online 2001).

The field of chemotherapy is changing constantly and there are many drugs in use. Women may be extremely anxious when they learn that they are to undergo chemotherapy. The treatments and their effects have physical and psychological effects and can have great impact on the patient and the family. It is important for health care professionals to be aware of changing treatments and their effects so that women undergoing chemotherapy for breast cancer can be adequately informed and supported.

References

Altruis Biomedical Network online (2000) www.chemotherapies.net (accessed January 2002).
Beare PG, Myers JL (1998) Adult Health Nursing, 3rd edn. New York: Mosby.
Breast Cancer Care (1999) Fact sheet 4, sections 1–3. Chemotherapy. London: Breast Cancer Care.
Breast Cancer Care online (2001) www.breastcancercare.org.uk/Breastcancer/Treatment/Chemotherapy (accessed January 2002).

Breast Cancer Org online (2001) www.breastcancer.org (accessed January 2002).

Brezden CB, Phillips K, Abdolell M, et al. (2000) Cognitve function in breast cancer patients receiving adjuvant chemotherapy. Journal of Clinical Oncology, July 14: 2695–701.

Brooker C (1996) Nursing Applications in Clinical Practice: Human Structure and Function. 2nd edn. London: Mosby.

Cancernet.co.uk online (2002) www.cancernet.co.uk/chemotherapy.htm (accessed January 2002).

Cotton T (1996) Chemotherapy for breast cancer. In Denton S (Ed.) Breast Cancer Nursing. London: Chapman & Hall.

Demark-Wahnefried W, Peterson BL, Winer EP, et al. (2001) Changes in weight, body composition and factors influencing energy balance among pre-menopausal breast cancer patients receiving adjuvant chemotherapy. Journal of Clinical Oncology, May 1: 2381–9.

Kaspar CE, Sarna LP (2000) Influence of adjuvant chemotherapy on skeletal muscle and fatigue in women with breast cancer. Biological Research for Nursing 2(2): 133–9.

McInnes JA, Knobf MT (2001) Weight gain and quality of life in women treated with adjuvant chemotherapy for early stage breast cancer. Oncology Nursing Forum 28(4): 6675–84.

Pearce S (2001) Men's experiences of coping with their wives' breast cancer involved focusing on the cancer and treatment and focusing on family life to keep going. Commentary on Hilton BA, Crawford JA and Tarko MA, Men's perspectives on individual and family coping with their wives' breast cancer and chemotherapy. (Western Journal of Nursing Research 2000 22: 438–59.) Evidence Based Nursing 4(1): 31.

Peck HJ, Mitchell H, Stewart AL (2000) Evaluating the efficiency of scalp cooling using the Penguin cold cap system to reduce alopecia in patients undergoing chemotherapy for breast cancer. European Journal of Oncology Nursing 4(4): 246–8.

Schwartz AL, Mori M, Gao R, et al. (2001) Exercise reduces daily fatigue in women with breast cancer receiving chemotherapy. Medicine and Science in Sports and Exercise 33(5): 718–23.

Taxol.com online (1998) www.taxol.com (accessed January 2002).

Woo B, Dibble S, Piper B, et al. (1998) Differences in fatigue by treatment methods in women with breast cancer. Oncology Nursing Forum 25: 915–20.

CHAPTER EIGHT

Radiotherapy for breast cancer

Introduction

Radiotherapy is the use of high-energy X-rays in the treatment for cancer. It is commonly used in combination with surgery to treat early breast cancer. It is given following breast conservation surgery to the remaining tissue to eradicate any remaining cancer cells and minimize the risk of local recurrence. Breast conservation surgery with radiotherapy is an effective and safe alternative to mastectomy in patients with early breast cancer (Ragaz et al. 1997). There is little difference in disease-free or overall survival for patients with early stage breast cancer treated by either breast conservation surgery or mastectomy (Deutsch and Flickinger 2001). Several studies have shown that all patients should receive radiotherapy to the breast after quadrantectomy or wide local excision. A level 2 trial has shown that radiotherapy significantly reduces the risk of local recurrence and consequent mastectomy (Gelber and Goldhirsch 1994).

Radiotherapy may also be used prior to surgery along with chemotherapy to shrink a tumour, on fungating wounds to shrink the tumour and reduce exudates, and for elderly patients instead of surgery.

The patient who is reluctant to undergo radiotherapy needs to weigh the benefits of avoiding the inconvenience and side effects against the risk of local recurrence and a possible future mastectomy. A group at such low risk of local recurrence to allow breast conservation surgery without radiotherapy has not been fully defined. However, the patient's wishes must be taken into account – it may be appropriate to omit it after full discussion with the individual patient. Sometimes it is omitted in frail, elderly women.

Radiotherapy after mastectomy

Radiotherapy may be given after mastectomy but only if the patient is at high risk of local recurrence. Patients who display any two of the factors associated with increased risk should be given post-operative radiotherapy (Sainsbury et al. 1994). The patient will generally also have other adjuvant treatment. Various trials have shown that locoregional irradiation after mastectomy combined with systemic treatment improves local control and survival compared with systemic treatment alone in both pre- and post-menopausal women at high risk of relapse (Kunkler 2000). If chemotherapy is planned as well as radiotherapy, irradiation can be delayed until chemotherapy is complete provided that the risk of residual disease in the breast and regional nodes is low. A compromise may be to give 3–4 cycles of chemotherapy, suspend it during radiotherapy, then resume and complete the chemotherapy (Langmuir et al. 1993).

The breast surgeon will offer the patient a choice of treatment wherever possible. This will depend on certain factors:

1 Patient choice – some patients worry about recurrence after breast conservation surgery. However, with proper selection and treatment the risk is no greater than that of chest wall recurrence following mastectomy. Some women alternatively wish to conserve their breast at all costs.
2 Breast size – a small breast may have a significant defect following breast conservation surgery and a poor cosmetic outcome if a relatively large amount of tissue is removed to obtain clear margins. A larger breast may be less deformed but large and pendulous breasts may present technical difficulties for radiotherapy and the cosmetic outcome may be poorer.
3 Size and location of the tumour – for example a large tumour in a small breast as above. Patients with a tumour behind the nipple are generally advised to have a mastectomy as cosmetic outcome and prosthetics would be unsatisfactory.
4 Pathology – multiple tumours, extensive DCIS (Langmuir et al. 1993).

Not all patients will have the lymph node areas treated; this depends on the level of axillary surgery performed. If a complete axillary clearance is carried out post-operatively, then radiotherapy to the axilla will be avoided to prevent lymphoedema. Treatment to the axilla may be considered for positive axillary nodes or high-grade tumours.

How radiotherapy works

Radiation deposits energy in cells resulting in ionization. This causes physical and chemical reactions that result in the water molecules in the cell breaking up and damaging the DNA in the cell nucleus. Radiation-induced damage is greatest during mitosis when intracellular DNA is doubled and during the G2 phase of the cell cycle. The damage can result in breaks in either the single or double strands within the DNA. Single strand breaks tend to be ineffective in cancer treatment as the cells can repair this type of break. Double strand breaks are more difficult to repair and the cell can be irreversibly damaged. Interactions with the DNA affect the cells' ability to divide or cause the cell to die instantly (Holmes 1996a). As all the cells do not die instantly the effects of radiation build up over time and can carry on after treatment is complete.

As the treatment is not selective normal cells are also affected, therefore the total dose of radiation is delivered in fractions to allow normal and malignant cells to attempt to repair between successive fractions. The area to be treated may be known as the 'target tissue'. The cells that are killed by radiation are those undergoing mitosis and cell division, known as radiosensitive. Once these cells have been killed the rest will be radioresistant; that is, at a stage in the cell cycle that is not sensitive to radiation. However, within 24 hours other cells will be progressing through the cycle and there will be a new supply of radiosensitive cells. Therefore, if the same amount of radiation is given the next day the same percentage of cells will be killed, and this will continue each time the same dose is given. The tumour re-population is minimized by limiting breaks in the treatment. Completion of the course of radiotherapy within the prescribed time is vital for the patient to receive the best outcome from her treatment.

Ionizing radiation in the form of electromagnetic radiation (X-rays and gamma rays) are used in radiotherapy.

How radiotherapy is given

The maximum tolerated dose of ionizing radiation will be delivered precisely to the part of the body affected. The principle underlying radiotherapy to the breast area is to irradiate the chest wall, any remaining breast tissue, plus node bearing areas in the axilla (unless axillary clearance has been undertaken), the supraclavicular fossa and the internal mammary chain (Oliver 1996).

The roentgen is the accepted unit of measurement for the energy in a beam of radiation. However, in therapeutic radiotherapy it is the energy absorbed by tissue that is important. This used to be termed the radiation absorbed dose (rad). The accepted term of measurement is now the gray (Gy). One gray is equal to a radiation dose of 1 joule per kilogram; one hundreth of a gray (centigray) = 1 rad (Oliver 1996).

Teletherapy

Teletherapy is also known as external beam therapy. This is the commonest method of giving radiotherapy for breast cancer. Teletherapy is the delivery of an accurate dose of radiation energy to a specific body part from a machine at a distance (Oliver 1996). It comprises high-energy X-rays produced by linear accelerators. These are machines that produce X-rays of increasingly greater energy. The rays can be used to destroy cancer cells deep in the body or on the surface depending on how much energy they possess. The higher the energy of the X-ray beam the deeper the rays go into the target tissue (Oliver 1996). Teletherapy is most often given on a linear accelerator at energies of 6, 8 or 10MeV. A linear accelerator is skin sparing, therefore in a patient who has had a mastectomy the dose would be brought up to the skin surface using a tissue equivalent material. This is generally either 0.5cm or 1cm thick and is laid over the area, therefore avoiding damage to underlying structures by the X-rays.

Gamma rays from cobalt units and lower energy X-rays may be used. Gamma rays are produced spontaneously as elements such as uranium, radium and cobalt 60 release radiation as they decay. Each element decays at a specific rate and gives off energy in the form of gamma rays and other particles. Gamma rays and X-rays have the same effect on cancer (National Cancer Institute online 1992).

In external beam therapy the machines are sited in protected rooms with concrete walls. An 8MeV linear accelerator requires 7ft thick concrete walls to attenuate the radiation produced when the machine is on. The entrance is angled; that is, a 'maze' is walked through to reach the treatment area, as radiation cannot turn corners and the walls and entrance are shielded. Radiotherapy units, therefore, tend to be in larger hospitals and cancer units. This is also due to cost – a linear accelerator costs £1–1.5 million.

The planning session

Healing is generally adequate 2–4 weeks after surgery to allow treatment to commence. The volume of tissue to be irradiated and the number of fields to be used are decided at the planning session. Two or more treatment fields are used in breast cancer, directing the radiation beam at the patient from different angles (Oliver 1996). The most common field arrangement for breast irradiation is known as a 'tangent pair'. Two parallel opposing fields are positioned to skim tangentially across the breast from both medial and lateral directions to irradiate the breast uniformly. The whole field extends from the midline to the mid-axillary line and from 1.5cm below the inframammary crease up to the level of the supraclavicular joint (Langmuir et al. 1993). This is necessary as microscopic breast tissue extends beyond the breast mound. Careful simulation and field placement are required to minimize the volume of underlying heart and lung tissue irradiated. Additional fields may be used to irradiate the main lymph drainage areas.

The patient attends the radiotherapy unit for the first time for the planning session. Thorough explanation is given of all the treatment and procedures backed up by written information. The patient lies on the treatment simulator, which is a direct mock-up of a therapy machine, but the X-rays taken are only for the planning and are low energy – similar to normal diagnostic X-rays. The exact area to be treated is decided on. The machine is positioned at the correct field sizes and angles for each patient and all measurements are very accurately checked and recorded for each beam. The use of computers allows treatment to be planned in three dimensions. The patient has to lie very still whilst this is being done, usually positioned with the elbow on the affected side raised to shoulder level. There is a support on the couch for the patient to grip to enable her to keep the arm in the correct position. The patient needs to have continued with arm exercises prior to radiotherapy. Some centres use a specially designed board which positions both arms up above the head. This can be more comfortable than the traditional position but the patient needs to have regained a wide range of arm movements. Marks are drawn on the skin to outline the fields to be irradiated. In some cases up to five small tattoos (the size of a pinhead) are made to give a permanent record of the measurements (Cancernet.co.uk online 2002). Each patient will have a different treatment plan.

Once the measurements are taken the oncologist and physicist or radiographers decide on the best way of delivering the amount of radiation required and the type of machine to be used. The simulator also provides an X-ray image to confirm how much lung is included in the fields to be treated, and modified if necessary.

The treatment

The patient is given her first appointment after the planning session. The treatment machine is like the simulator but larger. Treatment usually only takes a few minutes and is painless. Radiographers operate the machines to deliver the treatment. The patient is left alone but the radiographers watch her constantly on a video camera and in some centres use an intercom to communicate. Otherwise the patient is asked to raise a hand if she is having problems and the radiographers can be with her straightaway.

Radiotherapy regimes may vary at different centres but some regimes may be:

- 15 treatments of 40Gy over three weeks (Mon–Fri)
- 20 treatments of 45Gy over four weeks (Mon–Fri)
- 25 treatments of 50Gy over five weeks (Mon–Fri).

The patient adopts the exact position decided on at the planning session. A special armrest may be provided. The exact area to be treated is identified using the planning marks and narrow laser beams ensure the patient is correctly aligned and light beams ensure that the energy beam is correctly positioned. The patient is left alone whilst the machine is functioning – it may be quite noisy. The main discomfort may come from lying still on a hard table. The patient may also be anxious about being left alone but this anxiety may be reduced by detailed explanation and the chance to see the machine before the start of treatment.

Contraindications

1 Serious pulmonary disease that may be compromised by an otherwise small amount of lung irradiation is a consideration.
2 Severe uncontrolled diabetes and collagen vascular disease are contraindications as tissues in these cases tolerate irradiation poorly.
3 Serious cardiac disease is a consideration if the tumour is on the left side.
4 The patient must be able to lie still during planning and treatment and be co-operative. Patients with dementia and severe psychiatric disorders are usually unsuitable for radiotherapy (Langmuir et al. 1993). It may be successful but the individual patient must be carefully assessed.

Boost therapy

Many centres may use a boost to raise the dose to 60Gy to treat the scar area and therefore the dose is brought up to the skin surface. This is given when treatment is complete and may be a single small field of electron beam therapy, iridium wire insertion (Oliver 1996), or the use of an orthovoltage machine. The boost will include the entire breast scar and tumour bed. Therefore, it is important that the scar is located directly over the tumour (Langmuir et al. 1993). The indications for boost irradiation are not well defined. However, failure to provide a boost in patients who have a positive margin of resection has been associated with a 30 per cent recurrence rate (Ryoo et al. 1989). With tumours less than 1cm wide and clear margins following wide local excision, it may not be necessary to give a boost.

Travel

Often patients have to travel daily to the radiotherapy unit as it may be situated in a hospital some distance from their home. Transport can be provided if necessary but can be a problem, so patients are encouraged to find their own transport wherever possible. Help with travel fares may be obtained from Macmillan Cancer Relief or from the DSS if on a low income. A course of radiotherapy can last from three to five weeks and the disruption of travelling every day can affect family life and social activity.

If travel is not possible the patient may be admitted Monday to Friday, perhaps staying in hostel accommodation, and going home at the weekends. This means long periods away from home and probably few visitors. The patient may feel quite well in herself and treatment only takes a few minutes each day, so a sense of frustration may set in.

Side effects

Radiotherapy affects normal cells as well as cancer cells in the treated area. The side effects will vary with each individual.

Fatigue

Fatigue is a common complaint of patients receiving radiotherapy for breast cancer. Fatigue tends to increase over the course of radiotherapy treatment, being highest at around two weeks after the end of treatment, then improving until gone at around three months. Fatigue tends not to be influenced by age, length of time since surgery, stage of disease, weight or length of time since diagnosis. It can be related to symptom distress and psychological distress (Irvine et al. 1998). Fatigue has a negative impact on the patient's quality of life and this is evident by the end of treatment. Patients are given a careful explanation of the possibility of fatigue prior to treatment and can therefore be prepared for it. The nurse can help by reiterating this and advising of the need to rest as much as possible although light exercise can be beneficial in those patients fit enough to undertake it. The patient is also advised to eat a nutritious diet and take plenty of fluids. If the patient lives a distance away from the unit the fatigue may well be compounded by the daily journey to the hospital for treatment.

Skin reaction

With new machinery and the delivery of smaller fractions the radiotherapy dose delivered to the skin is minimized. This has reduced the incidence of immediate skin reactions (Sainsbury et al. 1994). However, a radiation skin reaction will occur in the majority of patients undergoing radiotherapy for breast cancer with varying degrees of severity (Porock and

Kristjanson 1999). It tends to be more severe in those patients who have had chemotherapy and in large-breasted women. It is most likely to show in the area being treated as a mild erythema developing around two weeks after treatment has begun. Some flaking or peeling of the skin may occur as treatment progresses, which may result in the area becoming inflamed, moist and sore. Treatment may vary between units but patients are often given aqueous or E45 cream to be used twice daily from the start of treatment as radiotherapy will dry the skin initially. Some centres may allow the use of pure aloe vera but there have not been any clinical trials undertaken. One per cent hydrocortisone cream may be given for mild erythema but not for moist desquamation. The skin is monitored daily by the radiographers. A more severe breakdown of the skin may require assessment and dressing from the community nurses.

Breast care and community nurses can help the patient to care for the skin and be aware of potential problems. The patient may use lukewarm water for washing, simple or baby soap and no additives during a bath or shower. Extremes of temperature should be avoided. Underarm deodorant should be avoided along with perfumes, lotions and creams. Unperfumed baby powder may be used sparingly on the underarm area and the area must be washed and dried gently. The patient is advised to expose the area to the air each day if possible for 20–30 minutes and to wear comfortable loose clothing in natural fibres such as crop tops or camisoles. Tight clothing and underwired bras should be avoided to reduce trauma to the area. The skin will be sun sensitive from now on, not just for the duration of treatment, so it is advisable to keep out of the sun or to use a high-factor sun cream.

If dressings are required for broken skin (moist desquamation) the community nurses can liaise with the radiographers to ensure that the correct treatment is being carried out.

Nausea and dysphagia

Not all patients will feel nauseous. When radiotherapy is administered the toxic results of cell breakdown are excreted by the body by normal processes of metabolism (Oliver 1996). Toxic waste materials may stimulate the chemoreceptor trigger zone in the brain or the patient may find the journey and feelings of lethargy cause travel sickness. However, feeling nauseous may be due to apprehension and nerves and patients are often advised that the actual treatment should not make them sick.

The patient is advised on a balanced diet and may prefer to eat bland foods if dysphagia is a problem. Paracetamol suspension may be prescribed before meals. The patient is also advised to increase oral fluids to facilitate the excretion of waste products.

Other temporary side effects include local oedema and epilation of axillary hair if the axilla has been treated.

Some side effects can occur months or years after treatment and are quite rare.

1 Fibrosis – the breast may be smaller or a different shape due to a build-up of scar tissue.
2 Transient cough – due to the effects of radiotherapy on the lung near to the affected area.
3 Telangectasia – 10 per cent (or possibly less) of patients will develop dilation of the capillaries in the breast. Not painful but the area tends to be a red/purple colour (Cancernet.co.uk online 2002). This is much less common now due to the skin sparing linear accelerator.
4 Weakening of the underlying ribs leading to fractures.
5 Lymphoedema due to a combination of surgery and irradiation of the axilla if the axilla is to be treated. This can also be caused by severe fibrosis blocking lymph drainage of the arm.
6 Cardiac problems – only a small part of the left anterior descending artery and small fraction of lung tissue are now routinely included in radiotherapy fields so the risk of cardiac damage is low (Sainsbury et al. 1994). The increasing replacement of older machines with ones that have greater technical capability to shield critical structures helps.
7 Radiation induced brachial plexus neuropathy and arteritis of large vessels – uncommon delayed complications of local radiotherapy. Arteritis with ulcerated plaque formation at the subclavian-axillary artery junction can develop consistent with radiation induced disease. Nerve damage may present as upper arm pain, weakness, tingling, numbness and loss of function (Rubin et al. 2001).

These side effects are rare and it is generally agreed that the benefits of radiotherapy outweigh the risks of these potential side effects.

Brachytherapy

The radiation dose is delivered close to the tumour site. This is provided by a sealed radioactive source where the radioactive isotope is contained within a 'shell' (Holmes 1996b). These take the form of needles, pellets, wires, ribbons, tubes or capsules, for example. Brachytherapy is generally used for easily accessible sites near the surface of the body or in or near a body cavity. The 'shell' is implanted into breast tissue under general anaesthesia or is loaded into previously inserted inert tubes. After-loading is carried out manually or by a remote controlled after-loading device such as the Selectron machine (Oliver 1996). Patients undergoing brachytherapy are sources of radiation for as long as treatment continues. Strict precautions must be taken by staff and all must adhere to statutory regulations.

Time, distance and shielding are the keys to staff safety. The longer the exposure, the greater the amount of radiation absorbed, and the further away the individual is from the source the smaller the dose (Holmes 1996b). The patient is nursed in a designated room or area. Shielding using lead aprons or screens should be employed according to local policy. Visitors and staff should be controlled. Radiation signs should be prominently displayed and all staff should wear radiosensitive film badges. Long-handled forceps and a lead container must be available in case the source becomes dislodged – it must be retrieved only with forceps and placed in the lead container (Holmes 1996b). Advice and guidance are given by a designated radiation protection officer.

This therapy can only be given in specialized units. The patient may feel alone and isolated especially when visitors are restricted. Sensitive, well-planned nursing care is needed to ensure that members of staff do not appear to be in a constant hurry to leave the patient, thus maintaining a sense of well-being.

Particle beam radiotherapy

The effect of radiotherapy depends on the ability of cells to repair damage and also on the rate of energy loss in different types of radiation as they pass through tissue (linear energy transfer – LET). X-rays and gamma rays are low LET radiation so matter is ionized only sparsely. Higher LET radiation (particulate radiation) causes more damage to cells (Holmes 1996b). This is particle beam radiation and involves the use of subatomic particles to treat localized cancers. A very sophisticated machine is required to produce and accelerate the particles required for the procedure. These particles deposit more energy along their path through tissue than X-rays or gamma rays causing more 'direct hits' (National Cancer Institute online 1992).

Palliative radiotherapy

Locally advanced breast cancer recurrence in the breast or on the chest wall can cause fungation, ulceration and haemorrhage. When surgery can no longer eradicate the disease therapy is aimed at locoregional control. A course of external beam radiotherapy can dry ulcers, stop bleeding and lessen disfigurement, thereby improving quality of life. If a good response is obtained surgery may be carried out, depending on the individual. Full-dose irradiation of about 50Gy to the breast with external beam is sometimes carried out along with interstitial implantation. Regional nodes are also treated (Langmuir et al. 1993).

Intraoperative radiotherapy

This is a new, experimental procedure. A special probe, encased in lead to protect deep structures is placed into the cavity left by the tumour during breast conservation surgery. The probe delivers a beam of radiation to the normal breast tissue around the cavity edges. The probe is attached to an electron generator and accelerator and the procedure takes around 40 minutes, negating the need for post-operative radiotherapy. This could reduce the workload of radiotherapy units considerably.

Problems with delivery of radiotherapy

A study has shown that in breast cancer there is a direct link between treatment delay and survival (Richards and Westcombe 1999). The government target of reducing deaths by one-fifth over the next decade could be achieved by providing adequate radiotherapy facilities to deliver proved clinical treatments (Burnet et al. 2000).

A two-week interval to plan and start curative radiotherapy is considered reasonable by the Joint Council of Clinical Oncology but may not always be achieved. Waiting lists need to be reduced as delay may allow progression of the tumour stage, which is associated with worse survival (Christensen et al. 1997). At many UK centres a 14-week wait is typical and introducing an additional delay of four weeks before planning and starting treatment must prejudice outcomes as more tumour cells are present when treatment starts (Burnet et al. 2000). However, it is thought to be imperative only for patients undergoing neo-adjuvant therapy, for patients who have had surgery centres are taking the view that it is mainly a 'back-up' treatment.

Gaps in radiotherapy need to be avoided. Only about one-third of patients complete their treatment in the prescribed time, the remainder take longer due to interruptions (Joint Council for Clinical Oncology 1993). This could worsen outcome. Missed fractions can be compensated for by treating twice a day but this requires additional linear accelerator capacity. Patients can be treated at a weekend but this has implications for staff salary costs (Burnet et al. 2000).

More than one fraction per day could be given. Hyperfractionation involves increasing the number of fractions and reducing the dose per fraction. Randomized controlled trials have shown improvements in outcomes. Lack of resources means that this is not generally implemented.

New linear accelerators are being purchased by centres but these replace old machinery, few are additional. Funding is also required for extra staff – radiographers, physicists and oncologists. An overall relative improvement in cancer cures of about 35 per cent could be achieved with adequate radiotherapy facilities (Burnet et al. 2000).

Follow-up

The oncologist and radiographers review the patient at each visit. Patients are then seen about six weeks following the end of treatment. Contact numbers are always given and the breast care or community nurse can also be contacted. Regular follow-up continues for five years.

Patients may fear radiotherapy as they may not understand it and have several weeks of treatment to face. Nurses need to be aware of the need for continuing assessment of the patient and for accurate, timely information. They are required to have a sound knowledge base with understanding of the aims of radiotherapy, its potential hazards and side effects (Oliver 1996).

Despite the problems mentioned previously, modern radiotherapy planning and delivery are improving cancer treatment, outcomes and quality of life. Radiotherapy is now an essential part of cancer care either used alone or as part of a combined modality therapy. Nurses who have an understanding of radiotherapy and its delivery will be able to provide appropriate education and information for those patients offered radiotherapy and will be able to prepare them for the lengthy process ahead (Nicolaou 1999).

START trial (standardization of breast radiotherapy)

This was a phase 3 trial, which ran from 1999 to 2002. It evaluated the safety and efficacy of radiotherapy fraction sizes greater than 2Gy. A total of 4000 patients were recruited. Patients were randomized to three or five weeks of radiotherapy. There were also associated studies of quality of life, blood sampling, photographic assessment and family history questionnaires.

References

Burnet NG, Benson RJ, Williams MV, Peacock JH (2000) Improving cancer outcomes through radiotherapy. British Medical Journal 320: 198–9.
Cancernet.co.uk online (2002) Radiotherapy to the breast. www.cancernet.co.uk/rxt-f.htm (accessed February 2002).

Christensen ED, Harvald T, Aggestrup S, Petterson G (1997) The impact of delayed diagnosis of lung cancer on the stage at the time of operation. European Journal of Cardiothoracic Surgery 12: 880–4.

Deutsch M, Flickinger JC (2001) Shoulder and arm problems after radiotherapy for primary breast cancer. American Journal of Clinical Oncology 24(2): 172–6.

Gelber RD, Goldhirsch A (1994) Radiotherapy to the conserved breast: is it avoidable if the cancer is small? Journal of the National Cancer Institute 86: 652–4.

Holmes S (1996a) Making sense of radiotherapy: curative and palliative. Nursing Times 92(23): 32–3.

Holmes S (1996b) Making sense of radiotherapy: delivery and safety. Nursing Times 92(27): 42–3.

Irvine DM, Vincent L, Graydon JE, et al. (1998) Fatigue in women with breast cancer receiving radiation therapy. Cancer Nursing 21(2): 127–35.

Joint Council for Clinical Oncology (1993) Reducing Delays in Cancer Treatment: Some Targets. London: Royal College of Physicians.

Kunkler I (2000) Adjuvant irradiation for breast cancer. British Medical Journal 320: 1485–6.

Langmuir VK, Qazi R, Poulter CA, et al. (1993) Breast cancer. In Rubin P (Ed.) Clinical Oncology: A Multidisciplinary Approach for Physicians and Students. 7th edn. Philadelphia, PA: WB Saunders.

National Cancer Institute online (1992) Cancer Facts: Radiotherapy. cis.nci.nih.gov/fact/7-1.htm (accessed February 2002).

Nicolaou N (1999) Radiation therapy treatment planning and delivery. Seminars in Oncology Nursing 15(4): 260–9.

Oliver G (1996) Radiotherapy for breast cancer. In Denton S (Ed.) Breast Cancer Nursing. London: Chapman & Hall.

Porock D, Kristjanson L (1999) Skin reactions during radiotherapy for breast cancer: the use and impact of topical agents and dressings. European Journal of Cancer Care 8(3): 143–53.

Ragaz J, Jackson SM, Le N, et al. (1997) Adjuvant radiotherapy and chemotherapy in node positive pre-menopausal women with breast cancer. New England Journal of Medicine 337(14): 956–62.

Richards MA, Westcombe AM (1999) Influence of delay on survival of patients with breast cancer: a systematic review. Lancet 353: 1119–26.

Rubin DI, Schomberg PJ, Shepherd R, et al. (2001) Arteritis and brachial plexus neuropathy as delayed complications of radiation therapy. Mayo Clinic Proceedings 76(8): 849–52.

Ryoo MC, Kagan AR, Rollin M, et al. (1989) Prognostic factors of recurrence and cosmesis in 393 patients after radiation therapy for early mammary cancer. Radiology 172: 555–59.

Sainsbury JRC, Anderson TJ, Morgan DAL, Dixon JM (1994) ABC of breast diseases: Breast cancer. British Medical Journal 309: 1150–3.

Chapter nine

Endocrine therapies

Introduction

Adjuvant therapy is used to treat micrometastases before they are clinically detectable. Patients at high risk of metastatic recurrence are treated with systemic adjuvant therapy following surgery for the primary tumour. As has already been discussed, chemotherapy is used for this purpose. The other adjuvant therapy is hormonal or endocrine therapy. It is also used as a primary therapy in elderly women who are unfit or are unwilling to have surgery.

The hormone oestrogen produced by the ovaries stimulates the proliferation of breast and endometrial cells and is considered a promoter for breast and endometrial cancers. This has led to breast cancer being described as a hormone-dependent tumour. The varying proportions of the different oestrogens in the bloodstream may affect breast cancer risk (Baum et al. 1994). Progesterone, also produced by the ovaries, may play a protective role in counteracting the stimulatory effect of oestrogen.

The levels of oestrogen fall at the menopause and the risk of breast cancer reduces but then increases again later. Endocrine therapy uses the body's own mechanisms to fight breast cancer and is less toxic than other methods. It cannot cure the disease but leads to a slowing of its progression.

The endocrine system

The endocrine system consists of endocrine glands which secrete hormones directly into the bloodstream. Hormones are proteins or chemical messengers that circulate in the bloodstream and then exert a specific effect on certain organs – the target organs. Hormones regulate many of the biochemical reactions that take place within cells and therefore exert influences on a range of cellular processes. New reactions are not initiated;

131

hormones modify the rates of those already taking place. Examples of typical hormones are oestrogen, progesterone, thyroid hormone, follicle stimulating hormone and growth hormone.

Steroid hormones derive from cholesterol which is present in large quantities within the cell. They are small and lipid soluble and pass directly through the cell membrane of the target organ cell. They include hormones produced by the ovaries, testes in men and the adrenal cortices. Steroid hormones are synthesized and released when the gland is stimulated. The synthesis of steroid hormones is dependent on a large number of enzyme-driven steps and as each enzyme is synthesized under the direction of a different gene there is potential for genetic error.

Hormones are not fully functional until they have been released by the cells which synthesize them. In the ovaries the theca interna and externa are the two layers of connective tissue stroma which surround the follicles containing immature eggs. The inner layer of a follicle is made up of granulosa cells. The eggs mature and are released at ovulation, for which luteinizing hormone (LH) is responsible. The hypothalamus produces luteinizing hormone releasing hormone (LHRH), which stimulates the pituitary gland to release LH and follicle stimulating hormone (FSH). The theca interna synthesizes androgens under the influence of luteinizing hormone and these are converted to oestrogen by the granulosa cells. Follicle stimulating hormone stimulates the growth of these follicles and the secretion of oestrogen. Oestrogen is then released by the ovary into the circulation. When a mature ovum from the ovarian follicle is released, FSH stimulates the follicle to develop into the corpus luteum, which produces progesterone.

Two types of oestrogen are produced, oestradiol and oestrone, these synthesize oestriol, a weaker hormone which appears in the circulation. A very small amount of oestrogen is also produced by the adrenal glands. Oestrogens are essential for the development of female organs and secondary sexual characteristics, for example the ductile system of the breast. As already mentioned above, progesterone is also secreted by the ovaries and is responsible for the development of the secretory cells of the breast. At the menopause ovarian function reduces and ovulation ceases.

Most hormone release tends to be regulated by a negative feedback mechanism. The endocrine gland is stimulated to release the hormone. That hormone then causes a physiological response that reverses the stimulant, leading to a decrease in hormone output. Hormone levels, therefore, remain relatively low. Positive feedback mechanisms operate in a small number of cases. The pre-ovulatory surge of oestrogen from the ovaries leads to a rise in LH and FSH, which stimulate a further increase in oestrogen.

In post-menopausal women the main source of oestrogen is not through the ovaries but through the conversion of androgens from the adrenal glands into oestrogen. This is done by aromatase, an enzyme. The conversion process is known as aromatization and happens mainly in fatty tissues (Cancer Bacup online 2001).

Steroid hormone receptors

The sensitivity of a tissue to a hormone depends on the receptors to which the hormone molecules can attach. Most receptors are on the surface membranes and there may be up to 100,000 receptors per cell. Hormone receptor sites were first discovered in the late 1950s when radioactively labelled oestrogens were taken up selectively by hormone-dependent organs in the body. Therefore, it was deduced that oestrogen receptor sites exist in hormone responsive tissue. Progesterone sites have also been demonstrated (Fenlon 1996).

Some receptors, however, are within the target cell, for example receptors for steroid hormones are within the nuclei as membranes are very permeable to steroid hormones. They pass through the cytoplasm into the nucleus where they bind with the receptor.

Oestrogen is released by the ovary, circulates in the blood and has its effect on other body cells that possess oestrogen receptors. Many breast cancer cells have oestrogen receptors (termed ER+ or ER positive) and the presence of these receptors on the breast cancer cells has an influence on the aggressiveness of a particular cancer. An oestrogen receptor is like a 'lock' on a cell's surface. The 'lock' is the same shape as an oestrogen molecule and therefore the oestrogen is like a 'key' to fit that lock. When oestrogen fits the receptor the cell's growth is stimulated and the breast cancer continues to grow. Receptors are most often found in invasive lobular carcinoma (Mera 1997). The presence of oestrogen receptors on a breast tumour can influence the patient's chance of a cure.

Oestrogen receptors are measured in femtomoles per milligram of cytoplasmic protein from 0 to more than 1000. If the concentration is more than 10Fmol/mg it is ER+ (Osborne 1985). ER status is decided by histochemical or biochemical methods. Up to 75 per cent of post-menopausal and 50 per cent of pre-menopausal tumours are ER+ or PR+. Depriving a breast cancer of oestrogen has been shown to cause the tumour to regress. ER+ tumours seem to be less aggressive than ER- ones. They are more common in post-menopausal women as the incidence of receptor positivity increases with age. Patients with ER+ tumours survive longer as their response to endocrine therapy is better. Relapse-free survival also appears to be associated with the presence of progesterone receptors (Mera 1997).

The presence of oestrogen and progesterone receptors therefore shows a good correlation with patient response to endocrine therapy and the determination of receptors may be used as a basis for the selection of patients for endocrine therapy. Not all the cancer cells will be killed as cancer comprises a mix of cells, some which are hormone sensitive and others that are not. Therefore, the cells that are not sensitive could grow and the cancer will recur. Also a source of oestrogen may be eradicated but another may take over and cause cancer to recur. However, if one hormone treatment is not effective on all cells another may still cause a response by attacking a different group of cells or by cutting an oestrogen supply (Fenlon 1996).

Hormone therapies

Hormone therapies can be given prior to surgery to shrink a tumour or after surgery to reduce the risk of recurrence. Generally one treatment is given at a time but in certain cases more than one may be given. The drugs given either lower the levels of oestrogen and progesterone or block their effects.

Hormone therapies work in three ways: (1) block the production of oestrogen, (2) down-regulate the production of oestrogen by the pituitary gland, (3) block the oestrogen receptors on cell walls.

Blocking oestrogen production

In pre-menopausal women this is ovarian ablation and is often offered to pre-menopausal women with metastatic breast cancer. This procedure can improve survival by up to 25 per cent in these women. Women who do not want chemotherapy may also be offered ovarian ablation. It is associated with considerable side effects due to the abrupt early onset of the menopause. Ovarian ablation can be achieved in a number of ways:

1 surgical removal of the ovaries
2 radiotherapy delivered electively to the pelvis in high-risk menopausal women
3 Zoladex (goserelin) – a monthly or three-monthly injection of a slow-release pellet via a large needle subcutaneously. Zoladex is a LHRH analogue and blocks the hormone produced in the anterior pituitary gland that instructs the ovaries to produce oestrogen. The production of luteinizing hormone and follicle stimulating hormone is blocked, therefore it is a luteinizing hormone release hormone (LHRH) blocker. The injection of 3.6mg is generally given monthly into the abdomen on alternate sides by the district nurse, practice nurse or GP. The three-monthly dose is not yet licensed for breast cancer (Cancer Research UK online 2002). The side effects may include menopausal symptoms such as hot flushes and sweats, lethargy, nausea and indigestion and weight gain. (See pp 139–41 for coping with menopausal symptoms.) The first treatment

may cause bone pain due to a surge in LH and FSH levels initially creating an increase in oestrogen production. Initially Tamoxifen may be given for the first two weeks to prevent this (Cancernet.co.uk online 2002). Zoladex is reversible apart from where the patient is close to the menopause. Within three weeks of commencing Zoladex oestrogen will be at a similar level to that of a post-menopausal woman. It can be given for pre-menopausal women with early breast cancer and post-menopausal women with secondary breast cancer (Breast Cancer Care online 2002a).

4 In post-menopausal women the adrenal glands are still producing some oestrogen. Some drugs called aromatase inhibitors block the production of oestrogen from the adrenals, but they only work in post-menopausal women, for example Arimidex (anastrazole), Letrozole (Femara), Exemestane (Aromasin). These drugs are generally given for metastatic breast cancer although Arimidex is being trialled for use in primary breast cancer. Aromatase inhibitors are given to women who have not responded to Tamoxifen or progesterone. They have various menopausal-like side effects including hot flushes, vaginal dryness, nausea, bowel problems, fatigue, headaches and temporary hair thinning (Cancer Research UK online 2002).

(a) Arimidex (anastrazole) – blocks aromatization and prevents the chemical change into oestrogen. The main side effects are hot flush-es and sweats but no weight gain. Trials are ongoing looking at Arimidex as a neo-adjuvant therapy and also as a first line therapy, comparing it with Tamoxifen. Arimidex causes fewer adverse effects, for example less blood clotting and vaginal bleeding than Tamoxifen. Results of three large international trials published in 2001 showed that Arimidex delayed progression of breast cancer longer than Tamoxifen in women whose tumours were ER+ and PR+ (National Cancer Institute online 2002b).

(b) Exemestane (Aromasin) – an irreversible steroid inhibitor. In the body exemestane suppresses oestrogen and when the drug is stopped oestrogen levels are still low. It is an aromatase inactivator; it destroys the enzyme site and inactivates it. It is generally given to patients whose disease has recurred or progressed on Tamoxifen. An ongoing trial is looking at whether it is better to give Exemestane to post-menopausal women with primary breast cancer after 2–3 years on Tamoxifen rather than giving the standard Tamoxifen for five years.

(c) Letrozole (Femara) stops the production of oestrogen from the adre-nal glands in post-menopausal women. It can be given to women who cannot take Tamoxifen or for whom Tamoxifen does not work. It may be the treatment of choice as a primary therapy in the elderly. Yet another trial is comparing Letrozole given after five years of Tamoxifen to post-menopausal women with primary breast cancer rather than Tamoxifen alone.

(d) Aminoglutethamide tablets are another option but are rarely used now as natural steroid production has been stopped and are associated with a range of toxicities. Aminoglutethamide was the first aromatase inhibitor.
(e) Tamoxifen remains the standard of care for now but aromatase inhibitors could change that very soon (National Cancer Institute online 2002a).

Down-regulation of the pituitary gland

Progesterone may be used for secondary breast cancer. The drug fools the signal pathway between the pituitary gland and the ovaries by increasing the blood levels of another hormone produced in the ovaries. Thus, the pituitary thinks the ovaries are producing too many hormones including oestrogen, and switches off the signal by itself. The level of oestrogen on the blood is reduced. Drugs given for this purpose include Medroxyprogesterone acetate (Provera) and Megestrol acetate (Megace) (Cancernet.co.uk online 2002). Megace has a direct effect on a tumour via its own progesterone receptors. Stimulation of these receptors causes the cell to slow its growth.

These can be given to control the growth of breast cancer cells if they stop responding to Tamoxifen. Side effects include nausea, reduced appetite, fluid retention, muscle cramps, rashes, fatigue, insomnia and tender breasts. They tend to be less effective than some of the aromatase inhibitors. A formal assessment of response is usually carried out 2–3 months before continuing indefinitely.

Blocking oestrogen receptors

The oestrogen receptor on the cells is blocked with Tamoxifen, a drug developed 20 years ago. Tamoxifen is a receptor antagonist also known as a SERM – a selective oestrogen receptor modulator. It blocks the oestrogen receptors on the breast cancer cells so that the cells will not be able to respond to the circulating oestrogen in the body. Adjuvant hormonal therapy in the form of Tamoxifen in ER+ patients for five years is associated with highly significant reductions in the annual rates of recurrence and death. Tamoxifen is used most often in post-menopausal women with invasive breast cancer or after chemotherapy in pre-menopausal women with ER+ tumours. The overall results of available studies suggest that if chemotherapy is given in addition to Tamoxifen in post-menopausal women with ER+ disease a small but significant advantage is gained (National Cancer Institute online 2002b). Some women will be given both even if ER- as some trials have shown that Tamoxifen is effective in ER- women, also giving a small, significant advantage. The worldwide overview of adjuvant trials suggests that the combination of chemotherapy and Tamoxifen may have a greater effect on mortality in women over 50 years than Tamoxifen alone (Early Breast Cancer Triallists' Collaborative Group 1992). Tamoxifen does not destroy cancer cells but prevents their growth if they have an ER concentration on their cell surface that suggests that they require hormonal stimulation to grow.

The most benefit is in women with positive lymph nodes but those with negative nodes will benefit too. In a 10-year trial, the 10-year mortality outcome in over 30,000 randomized women with invasive breast cancer showed an increase in survival in the patients who received adjuvant Tamoxifen; that is, Tamoxifen for 10 years produced a 6.2 per cent increase in the chance of survival (Early Breast Cancer Triallists' Collaborative Group 1992).

Tamoxifen is usually taken orally as 20mg daily; 10mg and 20mg tablets are available. Tamoxifen is also available in liquid form. It can protect against osteoporosis as it has an oestrogen-like effect on bone. Tamoxifen also influences a favourable lipid profile to protect against heart disease. Furthermore, it is associated with a reduction in the risk of contralateral breast cancer (National Cancer Institute online 2002b). However, it may increase the risk of endometrial cancer and uterine sarcoma in women who have not had a hysterectomy.

Side effects can include hot flushes, menstrual problems, vaginal irritation and discharge, fluid retention, depression and rashes. Many women also complain of weight gain. Tamoxifen may bring on the menopause if the patient is near that age. Ophthalmic problems may also be reported. Rarer side effects include allergic reactions, hair thinning, flaking nails and voice changes.

Since the 1960s, the National Surgical Adjuvant Breast and Bowel Project (NSABP) in the USA has been involved in breast cancer trials to improve breast cancer treatment. A recent study (Protocol P-1, the Breast Cancer Prevention Trial) was a prospective double blind trial that compared Tamoxifen to a placebo in healthy women. Women on the trial were at greater risk than the normal population of developing breast cancer. This breast cancer risk was determined by a computer calculation based on the following:

1 how many first-degree relatives of the woman had been diagnosed with breast cancer
2 whether the woman had ever been pregnant or how old she was at first delivery
3 how many previous benign breast biopsies she had had, especially if atypical hyperplasia had been diagnosed
4 if 60 years or older qualification was on age alone
5 if the woman had had previous LCIS
6 her age at first menstrual period.

The trial ran from June 1992 to September 1997 and included 13,388 participants. The group of patients taking Tamoxifen had a significant decrease in the number of women being diagnosed with breast cancer – a 50 per cent reduction in the incidence of invasive and non-invasive breast cancer in this high-risk population. The greatest benefit was seen in those over 60 years with 112 diagnosed with ER+ tumours in the placebo group and 38 in the Tamoxifen group. Tamoxifen also reduced the incidence of tumours in those patients with a previous biopsy that showed LCIS or atypical ductal hyperplasia.

There was a reduction in the incidence of fractures and a cardiac protection function was noted. However, there was an increase in the incidence of endometrial cancer in the Tamoxifen group (women over 50 years) – 33 cases versus 14 in the placebo group. There also appeared to be an increased risk of DVT and pulmonary embolus in the Tamoxifen group on the trial (NSABP 1998).

The Early Breast Cancer Triallists' Collaborative Group performed a study, published in 1998, which included information on 37,000 women in 55 trials of adjuvant Tamoxifen. Women with ER+ tumours were found to benefit and a 50 per cent decrease in the incidence of contralateral breast cancer in patients on Tamoxifen regardless of the primary tumour's ER status was found. The benefit of Tamoxifen for ER+ pre-menopausal women was also confirmed. Women under 50 years obtained a degree of benefit from five years of Tamoxifen similar to that obtained by older women (Early Breast Cancer Triallists' Collaborative Group 1998).

Other trials looking at Tamoxifen for prevention of breast cancer in high-risk women were ongoing until 2003. Results published in February 2003 showed that women at high risk of developing breast cancer taking Tamoxifen were less likely to be diagnosed with benign breast conditions than women who were at equal risk but took a placebo. Women treated with Tamoxifen had 29 per cent fewer biopsies than those taking the placebo. The overall risk for developing benign breast disease was 28 per cent. This was seen mainly in pre-menopausal women. The results seem to suggest that Tamoxifen works on early breast abnormalities that are subsequently associated with the development of breast cancer. The Tamoxifen group also had reduced rates of atypical hyperplasia, which is associated with an increased risk of developing invasive breast cancer. This trial was undertaken as the result of the Breast Cancer Prevention Trial did not really answer whether Tamoxifen prevented breast cancer developing or simply treated very small breast cancers (Tan-Chui et al. 2003). Another study, the International Breast Cancer Intervention Study (IBIS) is ongoing until 2005. However preliminary results were published in 2002. These also showed that Tamoxifen can reduce the incidence of breast cancer in women at increased risk from the disease. IBIS involves 7000 healthy women in Australia, New Zealand and four European countries. Participants will continue to be followed to see if a particular group at high risk can be identified for whom the benefits of Tamoxifen outweigh the risks (National Cancer Institute online 2002b). The American Society of Clinical Oncology recommends that women aged 35+ with a five-year projected breast cancer risk of more than 1.66 per cent be considered candidates for Tamoxifen.

Another SERM, Raloxifene (Evista), is currently being studied in the USA. The STAR trial compares Tamoxifen and Raloxifene to see how Raloxifene compares in reducing the incidence of breast cancer in post-menopausal high-risk women. Raloxifene was originally approved as a drug to prevent osteoporosis but studies show that women taking Raloxifene developed fewer breast cancers than those taking a placebo. STAR began in 1999 and will continue for 5–10 years. This will be a very large trial, recruiting 22,000 women.

Coping with menopausal symptoms

Ovarian ablation for breast cancer will cause an early menopause in pre-menopausal women. Tamoxifen may halt periods but these will restart when therapy ceases, but if the woman is near to the menopause, this may not be the case. Tamoxifen will not protect against pregnancy and women are advised to use effective contraception as it is not advisable to become pregnant whilst taking Tamoxifen. An early menopause and infertility brought on by hormonal therapies can be very difficult for the woman to cope with. She requires much support from the breast care nurse, and from the community or practice nurse in the case of the woman receiving Zoladex. Feelings of isolation and loss, especially if the woman has no children and wishes to have a family, can be overwhelming. This can have a huge impact on the patient's partner and relationship. She may also be experiencing problems such as weight gain, vaginal dryness, stress incontinence, vulval itch, pain on intercourse and loss of libido, any of which will also impact on her relationship with her partner. The nurse needs to be aware of her own limitations when caring for these women and know when to refer on for specialist help for advice and counselling on sexual and fertility issues.

The psychological effects can also be difficult to deal with. It may not always be clear which are menopausal symptoms and which are symptoms as a consequence of a breast cancer diagnosis. The patient may be emotional and anxious with a low sex drive and mood swings. The realization of the enormity of the diagnosis and treatment, often including surgery, radiotherapy, chemotherapy and hormone treatment can have a great effect on a woman's psychological state. This coupled with the physical effects described above can be devastating. It may make her relationship with her partner and family more difficult as they may not know how to approach her and do not want to upset her. This can create a circle where the woman feels even more anxious and loses her self-esteem. It is vital that these women receive the appropriate support and advice from health care professionals. Talking to the breast care or community nurse, a counsellor or a support group may enable a woman to cope better with mood swings. Referral to complementary therapies for example can often open new doors for the patient, involving new activities, relaxation, aromatherapy and many more. Studies are ongoing to determine whether there is a connection between hot flushes and stress and whether relaxation is helpful in this case.

There are various ways to treat menopausal symptoms, which may go some way to restoring a woman's self-esteem and help her to cope with the treatment. Symptoms experienced are given below.

Hot flushes and sweats

These can completely disrupt the patient's life, making it difficult to socialize and especially to sleep. Advice given may include:

1 Wear cotton clothing in layers so that some can be removed. Layers of bedclothes are preferable to a duvet so some can be removed in the night.
2 Try not to have the room too warm. A fan may help as may the use of cool sprays and wipes to the skin.
3 Try gentle exercise and relaxation. Yoga and meditation may help.
4 Avoid tea, coffee and spicy foods. Avoid alcohol.
5 Stop smoking.
6 Try splitting the dose of Tamoxifen, 10mg morning and evening or changing the brand.
7 Homeopathic remedies – sage, rhubarb root extract, sulpha and graphites for example (Breast Cancer Care 2002).
8 Aromatherapy and herbal remedies – can be useful but the patient or therapist needs to check with the cancer specialist first. Evening Primrose oil may help some women. Herbal remedies are not clinically tested as they are classed as foodstuffs; therefore there may be inconsistences in dosages and preparations.
9 Phytoestrogens in the form of soya products, seeds, grains and various supplements available. However, it is not absolutely clear if these increase the risk of recurrence (Breast Cancer Care 2002).
10 Progesterone in low doses, norethisterone 5–20mg or medroprogesterone 10–20mg daily (Marsden and Sacks 1997).
11 Clonidine 50–100mcg twice daily – this is effective but may soon wear off. Side effects include dry mouth and headache.
12 HRT in some circumstances (see later).

13 A recent study suggests that Fluoxetine (Prozac) and some of the other new antidepressants may be effective for hot flushes (Loprinzi et al. 2002).

Vaginal dryness

Vaginal moisturisers can be used, for example Replens, KY jelly. Oestrogen pessaries are available but their use needs to be discussed with the patient's cancer specialist – the amount used is very small so may well not affect any part of the body (Breast Cancer Care 2002).

Frequency of micturition may also be a problem. The nurse may be able to recommend a specialist nurse to discuss this and provide advice on pelvic floor exercises and other strategies.

Psychological effects

Some women may find that they become forgetful, which can be extremely distressing – the patient may feel that she is losing control of her mind and her body. Making lists may help. Relaxation, yoga, meditation and complementary therapies may help her to keep calm. These will also help mood swings and anxiety. The contact with a patient support group can be of great benefit to some women. The breast care nurse can also be available for the patient's partner and family for extra support and refer on for specialist help if necessary.

Osteoporosis

General aches and joint pains may be experienced but the patient may be at risk of osteoporosis when undergoing the menopause. Regular weight bearing exercise especially walking is recommended to protect against bone density loss. Exercises to strengthen the back muscles may improve the support to the spine and minimize the risk of fractures. The National Osteoporosis Society recommends a calcium-rich diet, for example dairy products, nuts, fish, leafy green vegetables and calcium supplements. Again, HRT may help in certain women. Raloxifene can be used for osteoporosis instead of HRT but can cause flushes and vaginal dryness. Raloxifene is a selective oestrogen receptor modulator or SERM. Trials have been undertaken to investigate its role (Cancer Bacup online 2000).

Heart disease

To reduce the risk of heart disease the patient is given advice about diet and exercise and strongly advised to stop smoking if applicable.

Breast cancer and HRT

Research continues into the link between hormone replacement therapy (HRT) and breast cancer. Some research shows that use long-term is associated with a slightly increased risk, some shows the opposite. Anyone diagnosed with breast cancer who is taking HRT will most likely be asked to stop as a precaution.

The evidence on the use of HRT increasing the risk of developing breast cancer is inconclusive. The most significant factor appears to be the duration of usage. HRT taken after the menopause, if used for less than five years, does not significantly increase the risk of breast cancer (Colditz et al. 1995). After five years the relative risk increases especially in post-menopausal women over 60 years (Colditz et al. 1993). This risk is reduced after stopping HRT and has disappeared after stopping it for five years. A history of benign disease does not appear to alter risk. Also in relation to taking HRT, some studies show that women with a family history of cancer of the breast do not appear to be at any more risk than those without a family history (De Gregorio and Taras 1998), and some state the opposite. However, the patient can be encouraged to discuss any risk with her GP. The community and breast care nurses play a significant role in teaching women on HRT to be breast aware and to attend for screening. Women on HRT are usually of a higher social status and at greater risk anyway, and also may self-examine more often. They are more likely to accept screening invitations. Any risks must be balanced against the benefits.

Also women who are diagnosed whilst on HRT have lower grade tumours and no greater risk of disease recurrence (Harding et al. 1996). Studies have shown an improved survival rate from breast cancer in women who have had long-term HRT. This would suggest that cancers are diagnosed early as women are more breast aware and therefore treatment will be more successful. They are also more likely to be ER+ and PR+ and not have involved lymph nodes; therefore, hormone treatment may be more successful (Baum et al. 1994).

The increasing numbers of women who survive breast cancer face a dilemma over the use of HRT. Many of them undergo an early menopause as a result of breast cancer treatment. Usually HRT is not used for women with a history of breast cancer as oestrogen is a growth factor for most breast cancer cells. A holistic intervention, which includes counselling, education and non-hormonal drug therapy, has been shown to reduce menopausal symptoms in breast cancer survivors (Ganz et al. 2000).

The Royal Marsden and the Institute Of Cancer Research are co-ordinating a trial into whether HRT is safe for women with a history of breast cancer. The study aims to discover if taking HRT does increase the risk of breast cancer recurrence. It will also examine how effective it is in relieving menopausal symptoms, with half of the participants receiving HRT and half receiving advice on complementary therapies. Although it may not be advisable to prescribe oestrogen-only HRT for a woman treated for breast cancer, the same may not apply to combined HRT. This can be effective in managing severe symptoms of the menopause in women who have had breast cancer treatment. However other methods of symptom control should be tried first (Stoll 1990).

Women who have undergone an artificially early menopause are also not at any greater risk of recurrence than if their ovaries were still functioning (Cancer Bacup online 2000).

The Imperial Cancer Research Fund, now Cancer Research UK, funded the 'million women study' in 1997 to investigate HRT use in post-menopausal women. It aimed to answer how HRT affects the breast, if the risk of breast cancer is greater, if the type of HRT makes a difference, if HRT affects the mammogram and if it protects against heart disease (Marsden and Sacks 1997).

A study in the US (Writing group for the Women's Health Initiative Investigators 2002) was undertaken to find out whether HRT can prevent heart disease in healthy post-menopausal women. It was stopped when it was found that their risk of breast cancer was increased beyond an acceptable level. The drug is not available in the UK although a similar one is. The results of American and British studies on HRT to date are to be reviewed by an independent international committee of advisers. Advice to women remains the same – to keep the increased risk of breast cancer in perspective and to discuss concerns with their GP who will help weigh up the risks and benefits of HRT (Breast Cancer Care online 2002b).

Breast cancer and the Pill

Despite many very large-scale studies the issue of whether or not the Pill is linked to breast cancer is still unclear. There is, however, concern about a small increase in risk after long-term use – this applies to the combined Pill, which contains oestrogen and progesterone. The synthetic oestrogen in the combined Pill and its effect on breast tissue needs to be considered. The monthly growth and proliferation of breast tissue occurs at a higher rate and lasts longer than that of women not on the Pill. It is, however, unlikely that the Pill could initiate the changes leading to breast cancer but it may be a promoter of existing disease (Baum et al. 1994).There is, as yet, no clear research to prove that exogenous hormones may stimulate breast cancer.

Some recent studies have shown no association between the Pill and the development of breast cancer whereas others have shown a slightly increased risk especially in women with a family history of breast cancer. It has also been suggested that women who take the Pill from a very young age for more than five years before their first pregnancy have an increased risk. The risk also continues for 10 years after the woman has come off the Pill but the risk is very small (Dixon 2000).

Current opinion does not feel that the oral contraceptive pill is contraindicated in women with a history of benign breast disease (Cancer Bacup online 2000).

The small risk must be set against the patient's personal and family history. If a woman is on the Pill and develops breast cancer she will probably be advised to stop taking it and other methods of contraception would be discussed. A breast cancer would then be treated the same as it would if she had not taken the Pill. Breast cancer in women using the Pill tends to be less advanced then cancers in women who have never used the Pill – this may be because women taking the pill are more likely to self-examine (Collaborative Group on Hormonal Factors in Breast Cancer 1996). As with HRT the benefits of using the Pill must be weighed against the very small risk (Baum et al. 1994).

A woman who has been diagnosed with breast cancer would be advised to use non-hormonal contraception to avoid becoming pregnant for up to three years when the risk of recurrence is at its highest. She would also be advised not to become pregnant whilst taking Tamoxifen. Consequently if the Pill is the only suitable method for the patient, its use may be acceptable. In a contraceptive emergency the morning after pill may be used as a single exposure to hormones is unlikely to cause harm (Cancer Bacup online 2000).

References

Baum M, Saunders C, Meredith S (1994) Breast Cancer: A Guide For Every Woman. New York: Oxford University Press.

Breast Cancer Care (2002) Factsheet – Coping with menopausal symptoms. London: Breast Cancer Care.

Breast Cancer Care online (2002a) www.breastcancercare.org.uk/Breastcancer/DrugTherapy/Zoladex (accessed April 2002).

Breast Cancer Care online (2002b) Breast Cancer Care responds to American study on HRT. www.breastcancercare.org.uk/News/Statements&Releases (accessed April 2002).

Cancer Bacup online (2000) Health Professionals: Breast Cancer, the Pill and HRT. www.cancerbacup.org.uk/reports/breast_hormones_mac.htm (accessed April 2002).

Cancer Bacup online (2001) Cancer Treatments: Individual Hormonal Drugs: Anastrazole (Arimidex). www.cancerbacup.org.uk/info/anastrazole.htm (accessed March 2002).

Cancernet.co.uk online (2002) Hormone Therapy. www.cancernet.co.uk (accessed 2002).

Cancer Research UK online (2002) Hormone Therapies: Types of Hormone Therapies. www.cancerhelp.org.uk (accessed March 2002).

Colditz C, Egan KM, Stampfer MJ (1993) Hormone replacement therapy and the risk of breast cancer in results from epidemiological studies. American Journal of Obstetrics and Gynaecology 168(5): 1473–80.

Colditz C, Hankinson SE, Hunter DJ, et al. (1995) The use of estrogens and progestins and the risk of breast cancer in post menopausal women. New England Journal of Medicine 332(24): 1589–93.

Collaborative Group on Hormonal Factors in Breast Cancer (1996) Breast cancer and hormonal contraception: Collaboroative reanalysis of individual data on 53,297 women with breast cancer and 100,239 women without breast cancer from 54 epidemiological studies. The Lancet 347: 1713–27.

De Gregorio MW, Taras TL (1998) HRT and breast cancer: Revisiting the issues. Journal of the American Pharmaceutical Association 38(6): 738–46.

Dixon M (2000) Facts about Breast Cancer. www.netdoctor.co.uk (accessed March 2002).

Early Breast Cancer Triallists' Collaborative Group (1992) Systemic treatment of early breast cancer by hormonal, cytotoxic or immune therapy. Lancet 339: 1–15, 71–85.

Early Breast Cancer Triallists' Collaborative Group (1998) Tamoxifen for early breast cancer: an overview of the randomised trials. Lancet 351(9114): 1451–67.

Fenlon D (1996) Endocrine therapies for breast cancer. In Denton S (Ed.) Breast Cancer Nursing. London: Chapman & Hall.

Ganz PA, Greendale GA, Petersen L, et al. (2000) Managing menopausal symptoms in breast cancer survivors: Results of a randomised controlled trial. Journal of the National Cancer Institute 92(13):1054–64.

Harding C, Knox WF, Faragher EB, et al. (1996) Hormone replacement therapy and tumour grade in breast cancer: Prospective study in screening unit. British Journal of Medicine 312: 1646–7.

Loprinzi C, Sloan JA, Perez EA, et al. (2002) Phase 3 evaluation of Fluoxetine for treatment of hot flashes. Journal of Clinical Oncology 20(6): 1578–83.

Marsden J, Sacks NPM (1997) HRT and breast cancer. Endocrine Related Cancer 4(3): 269–79.

Mera S (1997) Pathology and Understanding Disease Prevention. Cheltenham: Stanley Thornes.

National Cancer Institute online (2002a) Aromatase Inhibitors Show Promise for Early Breast Cancer. www.cancer.gov/clinicaltrials/results/aromatase-in (accessed April 2002).

National Cancer Institute online (2002b) Tamoxifen and chemotherapy. www.nci.nih.gov/cancerinfo/pdq/treatment/breast/healthprofessional/#section_258 (accessed April 2002).

National Surgical Adjuvant Breast & Bowel Project (NSABP) (1998). A Clinical Trial to Determine the Worth of Tamoxifen for Preventing Breast Cancer. www.nsabp.pitt.edu/BCPT_Information.htm (accessed April 2002).

Osborne CK (1985) Heterogenity in hormone receptor status in primary and metastatic breast cancer. Seminars in Oncology 12(1) (Suppl 1): 12–16.

Stoll B (1990) HRT for women with a past history of breast cancer. Clinical Oncology 12: 309–12.

Tan-Chui E, Wang J, Constantino JP, et al. (2003) Effects of Tamoxifen on benign breast disease in women at high risk for breast cancer. Journal of the National Cancer Institute 95(4): 302–7.

Writing group for the Women's Health Initiative Investigators (2002) Risks and benefits of estrogen plus progestin in healthy post-menopausal women. Journal of the American Medical Association 288: 321–33.

CHAPTER TEN

Prosthetics and clothing

Introduction

There are several ways for a woman to restore her appearance after breast surgery and also to regain her body balance. Choices include breast reconstruction and also external breast forms or prostheses. The decision is a very personal one and is ultimately up to the woman herself. Providing a well fitting prosthesis is essential in helping the patient feel confident in resuming her normal life and to feel that no one will know that she has lost a breast. It may also help her adjust and come to terms with her altered body image.

Breast care nurses, prosthetic fitters and some support groups as well as the actual companies manufacturing breast forms are all sources of advice and information. It is very important that the prosthetic fitting service is carried out by a skilled practitioner who can also advise on clothing. Often this is a trained nurse with a special interest and experience in breast care who is recognized as part of the breast care team. This ensures continuity of care and allows another opportunity to observe how the patient is coping after surgery.

When mastectomies were first performed in the early 1900s there were no prostheses (breast forms) available. Women had to make their own out of limited available materials or go without. The results were unsatisfactory and usually unflattering. Through years of research and design the manufacturers have improved the technology of their products and determined the needs of women who require breast forms.

Temporary breast forms

Following surgery the patient will be given a temporary prosthesis to wear. This is a very light, soft polyester fibre-filled prosthesis (a 'Cumfie' or 'Softie') to wear until she has healed enough for a permanent prosthesis, usually around 6–8 weeks. These are provided by the ward nurse or breast care nurse, generally following removal of the wound drains to ensure a correct fit. The Cumfie can be worn next to the scar in a soft bra or crop top and should not cause any irritation. It can also be pinned into a night-dress or camisole. Time should be taken when fitting the temporary prosthesis. With the wound drains removed this may be the first time that the patient can really see how she looks. It may be an opportunity to allow her to look at the scar if she has been reluctant to do so before and to assess how she is coping. The fitting should be carried out in privacy and the pro-cedure explained thoroughly to the patient.

It may be necessary to try on a few different sizes to obtain the correct one. Some hospitals may stock a choice of different makes of temporary prostheses. The patient may be encouraged that she can leave the hospital looking 'equal'. All patients should be offered a temporary prosthesis prior to discharge. Some women may feel that their scar area is too tender to wear one immediately, or may refuse one altogether. The patient's choice should be respected.

The nurse should show the patient how to position the temporary pros-thesis either in the bra or nightdress. Looser clothes can be worn until the permanent prosthesis is fitted. The lack of weight of the Cumfie needs to be taken into account – the bra strap will need adjusting. It can then be pinned into the bra to avoid movement. The cover and filling can be hand washed and allowed to dry before reshaping. Extra filling can be added or some removed to suit each individual patient (Parker 1996).

Following the fitting the nurse may feel it appropriate to discuss perma-nent prostheses with the patient and arrange an appointment for the fitting in 6–8 weeks.

Types of breast prostheses

Manufacturers are constantly striving to improve the technology and designs of breast forms. The most common shapes tend to be triangular, heart shaped, pear shaped, teardrop and round to correspond with the most common breast shapes. Some breast prostheses have a tapered upper chest and underarm extension to fill in where tissue has been removed extensively. Breast forms are available with the nipple built in or the patient can use stick-on silicone nipples if she prefers.

Breast forms come in various densities to suit the needs of all women in all age ranges. As women get older their breast tissue becomes less dense so the prosthesis needs to be softer. Young women require a breast form that creates a more youthful appearance. The patient's breast shape, body type and lifestyle should all be considered.

High-grade prostheses are made from silicone. The companies may manufacture their own silicone to be sure of high quality. Silicone will drape like natural tissue and manufacturers hope that their product will pass the 'hug test' so that only the wearer knows that she has a prosthesis. Silicone feels very lifelike under clothing. It can be whipped with air to create a lighter prosthesis whilst still holding the natural shape and appearance. It can also be used in different densities in the same prosthesis to create a soft drape in front and a firm back.

The breast forms are covered in a polyurethane skin which is inert and hypoallergenic, flexible and wears well although silicone can also be used as a skin (Amoena US 2001).

Some women may develop complications following a mastectomy if they have a prosthesis that is too heavy. This can lead to neck and back pain and shoulder droop. Through data collection the mass to weight ratio was developed to recreate the weight of a natural breast. The lighter weight prostheses were created for women who cannot tolerate the weight of a prosthesis that would otherwise be the right size. The lightweight breast forms are made with a special silicone that reduces the weight; they can be about 12–15 per cent lighter than ordinary breast forms. Some have a soft back that fits over excess tissue and uneven chest walls. Others have a firm back layer to simulate muscle tissue and a soft front layer that moves like a natural breast (Amoena US 2001). Often the back is moulded to allow air to circulate for coolness and a more comfortable feel. This reduces fatigue but provides enough weight to restore balance. Lightweight breast forms are suitable for elderly patients or women who have back problems, osteoporosis or lymphoedema. Leisure breast forms, which are lightweight, are available with weights to give a more natural feel.

Some breast forms are attachable to the body so that they look and feel more like a natural breast. They are attached to the chest wall with a special gel adhesive. The backing on the attachable form must be scrubbed as directed with the special gel and air dried to reactivate its adhesive qualities (Amoena US 2001). Some breast prostheses are attached to the chest wall by a system of strips applied to the skin to which the prosthesis attaches. The strips can be changed every seven days. Smaller breasted women will be able to go without a bra whilst using these attachable breast forms and they can also be used whilst swimming. Women with an active lifestyle may choose an attachable breast form.

Partial breast forms are available for filling out missing tissue and evening out the patient's figure following breast reconstruction or breast conservation surgery. They can be used whilst the patient is undergoing inflations if she has had a reconstruction with an implant. (The breast care nurse needs to be aware of the surgeon's preferences, some do not like any prosthesis to be used whilst undergoing inflations.) Even when the reconstruction is complete the new breast may differ from the other so the patient may still choose to wear a partial prosthesis. The same may apply to women who have had a lumpectomy or after radiotherapy where one breast is smaller, to balance the figure. Partial prostheses or shells can also be used to balance underdeveloped breasts.

A silicone breast form is now available that can be used soon after breast surgery, very lightweight with a two-part back in a soft breathable fabric. This can be used post-operatively to ease the transition from surgery to wearing a silicone prosthesis, during breast reconstruction, during radiotherapy and chemotherapy or as a leisure breast form (Trulife online 2002).

Swimsuits can still be worn following breast surgery. Swimming forms are available which can be worn on either side of the body. These have a concave, hollow back to minimize weight in and out of the water. A temporary or foam prosthesis can be used but needs to be discreetly squeezed on leaving the water as otherwise it will be visible as it will retain water (Parker 1996). Adhesive breast forms can be worn for swimming as can the silicone prostheses as long as they are rinsed properly. The woman's swimsuit would need to be pocketed to hold the silicone prosthesis.

Prostheses are available in a limited number of colours although a patient could order a custom-made one to get an exact skin colour match if the standard ones are not satisfactory.

Fitting the permanent prosthesis

Breast forms are available in various shapes, colours and sizes to accommodate women's various body types, breast shapes and types of surgery. When the breast form is fitted the woman will hopefully feel more balanced, both physically and psychologically.

The prosthesis is worn externally to closely simulate a natural breast both in looks and in the body's balance. This is a non-surgical option that many women choose following a mastectomy. External breast prostheses can be made from silicone, foam or fibrefill. The prosthesis can be worn in an ordinary bra or a post-mastectomy bra with a pocket to hold the breast form securely in place. If the patient wants a pocket one can usually be sewn onto an ordinary bra either by the hospital or by the patient herself. A weighted silicone breast form helps the body maintain its balance and helps to prevent back, neck and posture problems.

The timing of the fitting for a breast prosthesis is important. The patient must be able to wear a bra comfortably, the wound and chest wall need to be healed and the swelling to have reduced. The patient also needs to be prepared psychologically – a fitting too early may cause the woman to hate the prosthesis and too late may cause her to be upset about the light temporary prosthesis making clothes ill-fitting (Thomson 1996).

The fitting session may last a few minutes or an hour or more. It is the woman's time and gives her a chance to find the most suitable breast form. The fitter needs to take a sensitive approach, listen carefully to the woman's wishes and needs, then offer a variety of choices. She can try on a number of breast forms in order to find the right one for her.

The fitting area should be a comfortable private room with a lockable door. It should have a full-length mirror, comfortable seating, adequate lighting and a wide selection of breast prostheses and bras to try. The selection of bras should be samples only but the patient can try them on and the fitter can advise where they can be purchased locally. The fitter can measure the woman if necessary to gain the best fit as many women wear the wrong size bra (measuring will be covered below). It is generally advised that the woman is measured when being fitted for a breast form so that the breast form is the correct one. The bra needs to adequately support the weight of the prosthesis and hold it securely against the body.

To fit the breast form, the top one or two of the bra hooks should be unhooked, the shoulder strap slipped off and the breast form slipped into the bra cup. The bra is then fastened and the breast form and the remaining breast settled into place. This ensures that all the breast form and breast tissue is contained within the bra. The bra should be comfortable and contain the breast and prosthesis without bulges or wrinkles in the fabric (Trulife online 2002). The fitter should warn the patient that the breast form will feel cold at first but reaches body temperature very quickly.

It is advisable for the patient to wear or bring a plain, light coloured top which is not too loose so that the shape can be determined. A favourite bra, swimsuit or other clothing such as a favourite dress or top can be brought along to see how it will look. It is important to emphasize that the woman can still wear eveningwear, swimsuits and close fitting clothes if she wishes.

A soft cover is usually included with each breast form as some women do not like the feel of the silicone and find a covered one more comfortable.

If the patient is very large or there is no suitable breast form available the fitter can order one specially from the manufacturer. The representatives from the various companies are very willing to visit breast units and give advice on breast forms and fitting. Often special sessions can be arranged where the representative will fit women who are finding it difficult to find the correct breast form for their needs. They will also give advice and guidance on bras and swimwear, and will usually bring samples to try.

Underwired bras can be worn with a breast form and many women prefer this style. The wires need to be flat against the body, if the bra or cup size is wrong the wires may protrude and damage the prosthesis. The shape of the breast form is important. Forms with an underarm piece will not fit.

If the form is too big the unnatural shape it is forced into will cause the silicone to eventually break down. Symmetrical shapes with a rounded base are best, for example a heart shape, but other shapes can be rotated to fit within the wire (Trulife online 2002).

A patient who has had a double mastectomy will need extra time for the fitting. She can choose to have prostheses in her original size or any size providing that she looks equal and balanced. It is important that the new breast size is in keeping with her body shape and size. It may be useful to have her partner or a close friend at the fitting for an extra opinion.

Care of the breast form

Breast forms can be washed with soap and water, except for the attachable forms which require the special gel. Powder, perfume or lotion should not come into contact with the breast form. It can be stored in the foam cradle of the box to maintain its shape when not being worn. It should not be placed on a radiator but left to dry naturally away from direct heat or with a towel. Breast prostheses are replaced every 2–3 years. The breast form can be replaced in the meantime if the patient has lost or gained weight, or if the prosthesis is damaged. The breast care nurse should ensure that a system is in place so that the patient can obtain a replacement as soon as possible if accidental damage occurs (Thomson 1996). If a prosthesis splits the split can be covered with Elastoplast until a new one is obtained.

Breast forms are free to women who have had their surgery on the NHS. Private health insurance may cover them or they can be bought through mail order suppliers. Breast forms vary in price but, at the time of writing, start at about £85.

Measuring for a bra

There has been some research undertaken in the past which claimed that wearing a bra can cause breast cancer. It was claimed that bras impact on the lymphatic system, which rids the body of toxins. According to this research, the bra constricts the lymph nodes in the axilla and the lymphatics causing lymph to build up in the tissues. This build up results in toxins accumulating and therefore causes tissue degeneration. This is, therefore, claimed to be a breast cancer trigger (Singer and Grismaijer 1995). However, this theory is flawed as family history, reproductive history or use of hormones were not taken into account, and this was carried out before the discovery of the BRCA1 and BRCA2 genes so these also were not taken into account. Therefore, this cannot be considered to be evidence and women will continue to be advised to carry on wearing supportive, well-fitting bras.

Special mastectomy bras may be preferred by some patients and can be obtained via mail order. They look like ordinary bras but include special features such as wider shoulder straps, additional back closures, extended underbands, higher necklines in some styles and elasticated cups. They are generally pocketed (Trulife online 2002). The fitter will have a range of leaflets and brochures from various companies and the patient can choose at her leisure.

The patient can choose to be measured by the fitter or by the lingerie department of most major stores. These are very aware of the needs of women who have had breast surgery and usually offer a sympathetic fitting service by specially trained staff. Women should be measured yearly to allow for changes in body weight and shape. Women who have had breast surgery need to be measured as drug therapy such as Tamoxifen can cause weight gain. Most bras need to be replaced every 3–6 months. Different brands will vary in size so the tape measurement is only a starting point. Hospital sewing departments will generally sew pockets onto ordinary bras and swimsuits if required as some patients feel more secure with a pocket.

The bra should fit close to the chest wall between the cups and the cups should be of sufficient fabric to cover the prosthesis.

- If the underband feels tight on breathing then the bra size is too small.
- If the breast form or bra bulges visibly at the front or underarm the cup size is too small. A larger cup size or deeper style is required.
- If there are wrinkles or excess fabric or if the breast form moves around loosely the cup size is too big. A smaller cup size or different breast form should be tried.
- If the underband rides up or the size feels loose the bra size is too big and a smaller one can be fitted (Trulife online 2002).

To find the bra size measure all around the body underneath the bust. If this measurement is an even number add 4 inches. If it is an odd number add 5 inches. For example, underbust 27ins/28ins = 32ins bra size; underbust 29ins/30ins = 34ins bra size. To find a cup size measure over the fullest part of the remaining breast from the centre of the sternum to the centre of the spine. This measurement is then doubled. The cup size is decided by the difference between the bra measurement and the cup measurement.

Difference in bra/ cup measurement	Cup fitting	Difference in bra/ cup measurement	Cup fitting
–1 inch	AA	3 inches	D
0 inches	A	4 inches	DD
1 inch	B	5 inches	E
2 inches	C		

The patient may be worried how her partner and children will feel at seeing her with a breast prosthesis. Some women find it hard to come to terms with 'putting the breast on' each day. It may be useful for her to discuss her feelings with the breast care nurse, a support group or an organization such as Breast Cancer Care who have helplines available.

References

Amoena US (2001) Breast Form Options. www.us.amoena.com (accessed May 2002).

Parker J (1996) Prosthetics. In Denton S (Ed.) Breast Care Nursing. London: Chapman & Hall.

Singer SR, Grismaijer S (1995) Dressed to Kill: The Link between Breast Cancer and Bras. New York: Avery Press.

Thomson L (1996) Breast cancer. In Tschudin V (Ed.) Nursing the Patient with Cancer. 2nd edn. London: Prentice Hall.

Trulife online (2002) Breast Care. www.trulife.com (accessed May 2002).

CHAPTER ELEVEN

Psychological and psychosocial aspects

Introduction

A breast cancer diagnosis can have a huge impact on a woman's self-esteem and quality of life. Women especially who have been diagnosed through the screening programme have to cope with the concept of going from being well to having a potentially life-threatening illness within a short space of time. They may feel that they are now dependent on medical specialists. The outcome is uncertain – the patient may feel that treatment may not be successful and will result in recurrence and death.

Treatments for breast cancer are complex. All have possible side effects and all can have a huge impact on a woman's self-esteem and body image. Chemotherapy and radiotherapy can cause fatigue, nausea, hair loss, skin problems and isolation. Some women may experience side effects whilst taking Tamoxifen and face five years of coping strategies. The severity of side effects and coping with them can increase emotional distress.

A breast cancer diagnosis has social consequences – the whole family is affected. The majority of patients rely on partners and family members for support but some may feel stigmatized and isolated. Repeated hospital attendance can have financial implications if the patient has far to travel and she may feel that she is a burden to the family. Family, sexual and employment relationships may change. Women with a family history will be concerned about the potential risk to daughters.

Spiritual well-being may suffer – some women may undergo a crisis of faith, loss of hope and constant uncertainty over their future (Hassey Dow 2000).

In fact, many of the psychological and psychosocial effects of breast cancer can be understood in terms of reaction to multiple losses:

- of physical well-being/physical loss, for example loss of breast, loss of body image, fatigue, weight gain, lymphoedema
- of independence
- of role

- of interpersonal relationships – communication problems
- of sexual function and fertility
- of life expectancy
- of control
- of mental integrity – experiencing unfamiliar emotions (Barraclough 1994).

The prevalence of psychosocial problems that have been reported in cancer patients underlines the need for comprehensive psychosocial support for these patients and their families. Psychosocial support should preserve, restore or enhance the patient's quality of life, which includes the management of cancer symptoms and treatment side effects. The rehabilitation of the patient through psychosocial support should ideally begin at diagnosis. Quality of life concerns should be considered throughout and include the patient's physical, psychological, social and spiritual well-being (Hassey Dow 2000). Psychosocial intervention can be divided into five categories:

1 Prevention – designed to avoid the development of predictable morbidity secondary to disease and treatment.
2 Early detection – early intervention could have effective therapeutic results superior to those of delayed support.
3 Restoration – restore to optimum functional status when a cure appears likely, the aim is the control or elimination of any remaining cancer disability.
4 Support – supportive rehabilitation is planned to maximize function and prevent possible secondary disabilities where the disease persists.
5 Palliation – required when curative treatments are ineffective and comfort is the main aim (Razavi and Steifel 1994).

Psychosocial interventions therefore tend to take many different forms and be multidisciplinary. The NHS Cancer Plan (Department of Health 2000) states that patients with cancer and their families commonly experience psychological problems, some experience severe levels of anxiety and depression. Nurse specialists and other health professionals provide essential support for patients with mild psychological distress.

All women diagnosed with breast cancer will suffer but some will experience sufficient distress to warrant formal psychological treatment. It is important that the breast care or community nurse can identify those who are more at risk for psychological difficulties. Some variables that predict which women will be at risk include age, previous stressful life events and social support (McCaul et al. 1999).

Coping responses

There are many possible coping responses to a cancer diagnosis which vary between people and the situation:

- Fighting spirit – the patient regards the illness as a challenge and aims towards practical goals. This attitude does not suit everyone and some patients may feel guilty that they weren't positive enough (Barraclough 1994). The idea is about taking control of the controllable aspects rather than being constantly optimistic and positive. However, optimism based on reality is different to false hope.
- Helplessness/hopelessness – the patient feels unable to do anything about the impact of cancer and feels at a loss. May abandon work/hobbies long before being forced to do so. (It is important to rule out a depressive illness, which could be treated.)
- Fatalism – the patient accepts things and does not attempt to take control.
- Anxious preoccupation – the patient allows the disease to dominate everything else.
- Avoidance (denial) – the patient chooses to avoid thinking about the illness or blocks worrying thoughts, 'playing it down'. Real denial is uncommon. This may be used as a strategy to cope with the side effects of treatment. It may prevent the patient making considered decisions (McCall et al 1999).

It is important to note the coping response in order to facilitate effective communication (Watson 2000). Good communication between the patient and health professional is essential for the delivery of high-quality care. Patients consider health professionals to be willing to listen and explain, honest, sensitive, approachable and respectful (Department of Health 2000).

Anxiety

Anxiety is often seen in individuals at various stages of the cancer journey, during screening, diagnosis, treatment, recurrence or when terminally ill. Anxiety can also increase when primary treatment ends and the patient is responsible for checking symptoms. As a symptom without relation to a psychiatric disorder it is very common in cancer patients. Anxiety can seriously interfere with the quality of life of cancer patients and their families and should be evaluated and treated.

Anxiety occurs in varying degrees and can be part of the normal adaptation to cancer. Breast cancer is a stressful life event and it is natural that it may cause anxiety. This reaction may motivate patients and their families to take steps to reduce anxiety, for example by seeking information which may help them to adjust. However, anxiety reactions that are prolonged or of an unusual intensity that interfere with the patient's ability to function or with her social activities are classified as adjustment disorders and require intervention (Razavi and Steifel 1994).

The stress of a breast cancer diagnosis and its subsequent treatment may cause a relapse of a pre-existing anxiety disorder. These disorders can be disabling and require treatment. Many factors can increase the likelihood of developing anxiety disorders during cancer treatment including:

- a history of anxiety disorders
- anxiety at the time of diagnosis (Nordin and Glimelius 1999)
- severe pain
- lack of social support
- functional limitations
- history of trauma (Green et al. 2000)
- inability to accept changed body image
- no social life/hobbies/interests
- low expectations of the effectiveness of treatment (Watson 2000).

Medical conditions and interventions can cause anxiety disorders, including lung metastases, central nervous system metastases and treatment with corticosteroids and other medications. Previous experiences or associations with cancer may reactivate memories and contribute to anxiety. Certain factors such as being female and developing cancer at a young age are associated with increased anxiety in medical situations. Patients who have problems communicating with their families, friends and health professionals are also more at risk (Friedman et al. 1994).

Symptoms

Symptoms include intense fear, inability to co-operate with procedures or absorb information, shortness of breath, dizziness, light-headedness, palpitations and sweating. These may be because the patient is experiencing a specific anxiety disorder which was present before and which recurs because of the stress of the cancer diagnosis and treatment.

Cancer patients can present with adjustment disorder phobias, panic disorder, obsessive-compulsive disorder, post-traumatic stress disorder or generalized anxiety disorder. These are distressing for the patient who generally wishes to co-operate with intervention.

The following questions may be asked when trying to assess for anxiety disorders:

- Have the symptoms been present since the cancer diagnosis or treatment?

- When do they occur?
- How long do they last?
- Does the patient feel jittery, shaky or nervous?
- Does the patient feel tense or apprehensive?
- Does the patient have a fear of certain places, fear of sleeping in case they die, fear of dying, fear of losing control, fear of pain?
- Does the patient have palpitations, sweating, breathlessness, trembling?
- Does the patient pace around?
- Does the patient worry about the next appointment weeks in advance?
- Is the patient confused or disorientated? (National Cancer Institute online 2002).

Adjustment disorder

Adjustment disorder is diagnosed in patients who display maladaptive behaviour and moods in response to a stressor and include worry, jitteriness, severe nervousness and impairment in normal functioning. These are usually in excess of normal reactions to cancer and occur within six months of the stressor, although in cancer patients the stressor is ongoing. There is not usually a history of psychiatric disorder. However patients with other chronic disorders are likely to have experienced adjustment disorder before and this may recur at a cancer diagnosis. It is prevalent among cancer patients especially at critical points such as diagnostic tests, diagnosis or relapse. Most will respond to reassurance, relaxation techniques, low doses of short-acting benzodiazepines and patient support, counselling and education (National Cancer Institute online 2002).

Panic disorder

Intense anxiety is the overriding symptom. Breathlessness, dizziness, nausea, tingling and trembling can also be experienced. Attacks of periods of discomfort can last from minutes to hours. It can be difficult to differentiate from other medical disorders although the patient may have a known history. The patient may be referred for cognitive behavioural therapy, which is useful but may not offer an immediate solution. Antidepressants and benzodiazepines can help.

Phobias

Intense anxiety is experienced and the feared situation avoided. Cancer patients may fear needles, scan machines (claustrophobia) or blood for example. This can complicate medical procedures. Counselling, hypnotherapy and cognitive behavioural therapy can help.

Obsessive-compulsive disorder

The patient experiences persistent ideas, images or thoughts and performs repetitive behaviours to alleviate their distress. This must be severe enough to affect the patient's ability to function to be classed as obsessive-compulsive. Patients with a history of this may be affected so badly that they cannot comply with treatment. Antidepressants and cognitive behavioural therapy can help. The patient may be referred for psychotherapy if the previous treatments are ineffective. Obsessive-compulsive disorder is rare in patients without a previous history.

Post-traumatic stress disorder

The diagnosis of a life-threatening illness now qualifies as a traumatic stressor. Cancer patients suffering from this can become extremely anxious before procedures, surgery, chemotherapy or dressing changes. Cognitive behavioural therapy and psychotherapy are used to overcome long-term anxiety and anxiolytic medications are given prior to any treatments. The experience of previous hospitalization or traumatic treatment can reactivate this.

General anxiety disorder

General anxiety disorder is characterized by ongoing, excessive and unrealistic worry about two or more life circumstances, for example finance or social support, even if there is no problem with these. It is often preceded by a major depressive episode. The patient experiences muscle tension, restlessness, fatigue, shortness of breath, palpitations, sweating, feeling on edge and irritability. Uncontrolled pain may also cause anxiety and anxiety can potentiate pain. Anxiety must be treated to manage the pain in this case (Velikova et al. 1995). Anxiety management measures include medication, cognitive behavioural therapy, relaxation techniques and hypnotherapy.

Treatment and psychological support

Assessment of the patient must be carried out and an accurate diagnosis made. The normal fears and anxieties associated with cancer must be taken into account before reaching a diagnosis of anxiety disorder. Even following treatment, cancer patients may develop anxiety regarding follow-up, further tests, recurrence, returning to work and finances. Fear of screening procedures, body image changes, sexual problems and reproductive issues can also cause anxiety (National Cancer Institute online 2002).

It must be decided how the patient's quality of life and activities of daily living are affected. A method used to screen patients for anxiety and depression may be a self-administered questionnaire as in-depth interviews are time consuming and require training. The HAD Scale (Hospital Anxiety and Depression Scale) may be used (Zigmond and Snaith 1983). If anxiety is caused by another medical condition, for example pain or a hormone secreting tumour, treatment of this will control the symptoms of anxiety (Breithart 1995).

Benzodiazapines, for example diazepam or lorazepam, may be prescribed – the dosage depends on the patient's tolerance. Diazepam is short-acting and can be useful for patients who are severely distressed as it reduces insomnia and daytime anxiety. Long-term use should be avoided due to the risk of dependence. The lowest dose for the shortest possible time is prescribed. Side effects must be discussed as they include drowsiness and light-headedness. Any medication will be monitored and discontinued when symptoms improve.

Health professionals need to understand the ways in which people cope with cancer in order to offer holistic care (Watson 2000). Coping strategies can be suggested to improve quality of life. These may include:

- encouraging the patient to view the situation as a challenge
- encouraging fearful patients to confront the problem
- encouraging the patient to seek information
- encouraging the patient to be flexible
- encouraging the patient to use resources and support
- encouraging the patient to talk through issues – provide information, answer questions truthfully and avoid the use of jargon
- encouraging the patient to decide her priorities
- helping the patient to set some goals
- helping the patient to become aware of which activities give a feeling of control and to avoid those that make her feel helpless.

The patient can also be helped to schedule a 'normal' life by asking questions such as:

- Can you think of some ways to get over this?
- What do you think you can do to get back to normal?
- What is the main thing stopping you from living normally at the moment?
- What have you stopped doing that you used to enjoy? (Watson 2000).

Psychological support may range from information from the GP to the use of sophisticated techniques employed by oncologists and psychiatrists. It is important that all these health professionals assist adjustment by employing listening skills, using eye contact, allowing discussion by using open-ended questions and ensuring privacy and time when talking to patients and families. The patient's way of coping must be accepted and understood. The health care professional needs to be open to the patient's feelings and give permission for them to acknowledge their feelings. The patient's courage can be acknowledged and permission given to be frightened in a safe environment.

These are all measures that the breast care team can provide. If the patient does not respond to these, she can be referred for specialist therapy, for example counselling, psychotherapy or psychoanalysis. It is important that the nurse realizes her own limitations and knows the correct channels of referral to the appropriate therapist in order to obtain help as soon as possible.

Cognitive behavioural therapy

Behavioural therapies include relaxation, hypnosis and imagery. Behavioural therapies are based on conditioning theories and are effective in anticipatory nausea and vomiting relating to chemotherapy, controlling psychological reactions to painful procedures and adverse reactions to radiotherapy and surgery. They are often used for anxiety and depression in patients with early breast cancer (Bridge et al. 1988).

Cognitive behavioural therapy (CBT) is used increasingly as it is focused, brief, problem-oriented and worked through with the patient (Watson 2000). CBT is a practical treatment which centres on the understanding that thoughts, ideas and beliefs affect the way that people feel about themselves and each other in daily life.

CBT is based on the fact that many problems are caused and maintained by unhelpful beliefs and deeply held assumptions by the individual about themselves and others. These assumptions and beliefs are usually learned through past experiences and interactions. At the time these were probably helpful and assisted the individual to cope with the experience. However, now these beliefs may not be helpful and may hinder the individual's effective functioning. Common themes tend to be low self-esteem, self-criticism and self-blame. Depressed clients may be unable to escape thinking negatively.

The aim of CBT is for the client and therapist to work together to identify the beliefs and assumptions that are no longer helpful and affect their feelings, functioning and behaviours. Depending on the nature of the problem, the client and therapist work together to identify goals and form a treatment plan (Oxford Development Centre online 2002). Goals may include changing behaviour to become more assertive, changing feelings, learning how to cope with panic (Townend 2002).

The focus of therapy is on the here and now rather than the on past, and to find solutions to the client's problems that will help day-to-day functioning and well-being. A client may work through past negative experiences and explore how she wants to live her life now. Therapy aims to reduce unhelpful emotions by altering thinking patterns and behaviour. CBT achieves this by analyzing negative thinking patterns, implementing new behaviours and coping strategies, and teaching adaptive and rational self-talk skills (Townend 2002).

CBT can be used alone or in conjunction with medication. About 10–15 sessions are generally enough but this depends on individual problems and goals. An assessment session is undergone first so that the therapist can predict how many sessions will be needed. The client is then followed up at regular intervals to check progress. CBT appears to be particularly effective for patients with anxiety and depression.

Depression

Depression is a disabling condition which affects approximately 15–25 per cent of cancer patients (Bodurka-Bevers et al. 2000). Cancer patients in general will experience fear of death, changes in self-esteem and body image, changes in lifestyle and financial concerns, yet not all people with cancer experience severe depression. As sadness is common it is important to be able to differentiate between 'normal' degrees of sadness and depressive disorders. Major depression has recognizable symptoms, which should be diagnosed and treated; otherwise they will have an impact on the patient's quality of life (Lynch 1995).

Depression is associated with a chemical imbalance in the brain. Neurotransmitters (chemicals in the brain) carry messages from one cell to another. When there are imbalances in the neurotransmitters, diseases such as depression result. Antidepressants mainly alter the effective levels of the chemicals serotonin and norepinephrine but others such as dopamine may be affected.

When a cell releases a neurotransmitter, the chemical only has a short time to relay the message to the next cell before it is destroyed by the body or taken back up into the cell (re-uptake), ending its effects (Altruis Biomedical Network 2000).

Normally a person's response to a cancer diagnosis is relatively brief but a depressive state can last for more than two years. The emotional response to a cancer diagnosis may include anxiety, fears about the future and sleep disturbance. People who can maintain an active involvement in daily life, minimize the disruption to life caused by the illness and manage their feelings and emotions will successfully adapt. Early indicators, which may suggest a need for intervention, may include a history of depression, no social support, evidence of irrational beliefs about the diagnosis or a more serious prognosis.

Symptoms need to be assessed by the health professionals involved. Counselling or a self-help group may help mild depression. However, when symptoms are long lasting or more intense treatment is essential.

Assessment and diagnosis

Symptoms of major depression are:

- a depressed mood for most of the day on most days
- no interest in any activities
- loss of libido
- appetite and sleep disturbances
- fatigue
- agitation or lethargy
- feeling worthless
- feeling guilty
- recurring thoughts of suicide/death
- poor concentration
- weight loss.

Symptoms will have lasted a minimum of two weeks in order for a diagnosis to be made. Diagnosis can be difficult in cancer patients as it is necessary to distinguish depressive symptoms from symptoms of the disease or toxic treatments especially in those with advanced disease (National Cancer Institute online 2002). Feelings of guilt, hopelessness, suicide and loss of interest in activities are probably the most useful in diagnosing depression.

Evaluating depression in cancer patients should include:

- an assessment of the patient's perception of her illness
- any personal/family history of depression
- any suicidal thoughts
- current mental and physical status
- current life stressors
- social support
- any history of alcohol abuse.

Any patient with suicidal thoughts should be referred to a psychiatrist or psychologist immediately and attention given to the patient's safety (National Cancer Institute online 2002).

Reactive depression is the most common type of depression in cancer patients. This is an adjustment disorder with depressed mood, which prevents the person carrying out normal activities. When this affects normal functioning it should be treated in the same way as a major depression; that is, with crisis intervention, supportive psychotherapy and medication.

Specific assessment methods are necessary as are simple accurate tools for early screening of psychological disturbances in cancer patients. Early detection by the breast care nurse who sees the patient at diagnosis may identify patients who require help. Early treatment obviously has an effect on quality of life.

Screening for depression usually involves the same methods as screening for anxiety, generally the use of a questionnaire such as the Hospital Anxiety and Depression or HAD scale, which is widely used (Zigmond and Snaith 1983). The Psychological Distress Inventory (Morasso et al. 1996) or the Zung Self-Rating Depression scale may also be used (Dugan et al. 1998). These tools can be used in conjunction with a diagnostic interview and can prompt further assessment (Passik et al. 1998). Some patients may talk freely about their feelings, others will not. Some cases may go undiagnosed, as doctors may not be comfortable asking patients about their feelings (Razavi and Steifel 1994). A precise and accurate assessment and an understanding of the patient's social situation are very important for the effect of therapeutic intervention.

Depression caused by medical factors is best treated with medication rather than psychotherapy alone especially if the causative drug cannot be discontinued. Uncontrolled pain, electrolyte imbalances and endocrine abnormalities can also cause depression. Possible interactions with cytotoxic drugs, morphine, steroids and anticoagulants must be considered when prescribing antidepressants (Razavi and Steifel 1994).

Treatment

Treatment depends on the patient's degree of functioning, whether she may improve spontaneously and how severe the depressive symptoms are. Counselling can be used to help the patient express and understand her feelings about cancer and encourage her to cope. Breast care nurses, community nurses, volunteers, oncologists and GPs can all be said to use counselling skills in talking to breast cancer patients but counselling is a specialist role. Each discipline will require specific training in counselling skills (Razavi et al. 1993).

Major depression is best treated by medication and psychotherapy. Psychotherapy should aim to enhance coping skills, lower distress, enhance problem-solving skills and reshape negative thoughts. Dynamic psychotherapy can be used for patients who wish to explore their feelings and reactions to promote personality changes. It has a long duration so is indicated in cancer patients with a good prognosis (Razavi and Steifel 1994).

If the patient is suicidal, if medication is not helping, if the patient's symptoms are worsening and she is unable to co-operate a psychiatric opinion must be sought (National Cancer Institute online 2002).

Antidepressants

A study found the response rate for treatment with the newer antidepressants to be around 54 per cent (Williams et al. 2000). Choice depends on the patient's medical history and current problems, and any prior experience of antidepressants and their side effects. It may be necessary to try different combinations until the right treatment is identified. Treatment should be continued for two weeks before any difference in symptoms is experienced, then maintained at the optimum dose for 4–6 months after the depression has resolved. Antidepressants should be stopped gradually to give the body time to adjust as they can produce withdrawal symptoms if discontinued suddenly (Altruis Biomedical Network 2000).

- Tricyclic antidepressants such as amitriptyline, imipramine – these have many potential side effects including a sedative effect and cardiac effects and should be prescribed with care after full discussion with the patient. These affect the uptake of dopamine, serotonin and norepinephrin to different degrees.
- Selective serotonin re-uptake inhibitors, for example fluoxetine (Prozac) – side effects include possible blood sugar changes and hypersensitivity reactions. Selective serotonin re-uptake inhibitors (SSRIs) inhibit the re-uptake of serotonin although they may inhibit the re-uptake of other neurotransmitters in some individuals (Altruis Biomedical Network 2000).
- Monoamine oxidase inhibitors, for example phenelzine (Nardil) – these are used infrequently but may be prescribed if tricyclic antidepressants have been ineffective.
- Atypical antidepressants – these are new drugs and are classified as atypical as their action is not clearly understood. They include trazadone, nefazadone and buproprion (Zyban).

Side effects

Various antidepressants have different side effects, although the most common tend to be sedation, constipation, dry mouth, low blood pressure, dizziness and blurred vision. SSRIs tend to cause difficulty sleeping, sweating, headache, loss of appetite and sexual dysfunction.

The ongoing role of the breast care nurse

The specialist nurse is becoming increasingly important as an educator. The breast care nurse has been shown in several studies since the 1980s to reduce psychological morbidity in breast cancer patients by giving information, practical help and emotional support (Wilkinson et al. 1988; Speigel 1992; McArdle et al. 1996).

The nurse and other members of the breast care team can assist the patient by answering questions and giving reassurance. The patient should be given the opportunity to explore the present situation and how it relates to her previous experiences of cancer (National Cancer Institute online 2002). Often benefit is gained through acknowledgement of distress. A long talk with the breast care nurse, for example, where the patient can cry and express her feelings may be sufficient for some patients. Reiterating information about diagnosis, treatment and prognosis can also be helpful.

Providing the patient with information is the first step to helping the patient cope with cancer. Information is given by the consultant and reinforced by other health professionals, for example the breast care nurse or self-help groups. Information can be given to the family members as well as to the patient. Successful information giving may prevent or reduce the impact of expected disabilities and is the first step in the rehabilitation of the patient. Problems may arise where the patient cannot or will not absorb the information for whatever reason.

The role of the breast care nurse at diagnosis has already been discussed in Chapter 4. However, the supportive role is ongoing throughout treatment and includes the giving of appropriate information at different stages of the cancer journey. The patient with breast cancer will have a contact name and number and will come into contact with the nurse at various stages of her treatment – the breast care nurse may be the only health professional to have contact with the patient at every stage (Poole 1996). The breast care nurse ensures that she has the appropriate training and knowledge in order to fulfil the information giving part of her role. (The required qualifications are also discussed in Chapter 4.) This also enables her to assess the patient and family's need for psychological support. Any onward referrals are made with the agreement of the patient and family.

A study by Luker et al. (1996) examined the information needs of women at diagnosis and a mean of 21 months from diagnosis. At diagnosis the priority concern was survival. Further from diagnosis information about family members getting breast cancer showed an increase in importance. This study showed that women at follow-up tended to be concerned about the genetic transmission of breast cancer, which suggested an earlier deficit in information giving. This may have been due to a lack of knowledge or it may have been that this information was given at an inappropriate time and not recalled.

Women tended to use the breast care nurse for information at diagnosis whereas further along women tended to use media sources rather than a professional or volunteer. Adequate information regarding voluntary self-help groups could be useful as this resource is often seen as negative by patients (support groups are discussed further in Chapter 15). The breast care nurse was rated highly as a source of information but less so as time went on, patients felt that they would only contact her if they had a specific question.

It is therefore important to consider the timing of specific information as well as the right amount. The woman's information needs change over time and the imparting of information should be an ongoing process.

The primary health care team are in an ideal position to provide women with breast cancer with information and support. However, the PHCT often defer responsibility for information given to the hospital team. More information could perhaps be given to the PHCT for them to increase their knowledge base and play an important role in improving breast cancer services (Luker et al. 1996). District nurses who visit the patient postoperatively and community psychiatric nurses who regularly see clients with anxiety and depression are in a strong position to provide support to breast cancer patients. Some breast cancer units may have a social worker attached whose role is psychological support of the patient and family. These health care professionals play an important role as the breast care nurse is not always able to provide follow-up due to limited resources. Although the district nurse who visits for wound care is not a specialist, there is potential for further training so that they can undertake information provision as required by the patient (Luker and Beaver 2000). This may even take the form of an alternative name and contact number other than that of the breast care nurse.

The study by Luker and Beaver (2000) found that women did not utilize the primary care team as they perceived them as lacking knowledge. Women who are to be supported in this way need to be actively directed towards this resource. Alternatively, there may be a case for breast care nurses to be provided with more resources to follow-up women with breast cancer.

Cultural issues

Increasingly there will be patient populations of many different ethnic, cultural and religious groups. It is important to be aware of cultural and religious differences when considering how people adjust to having cancer.

It may be difficult to detect distress in patients from some cultural/
ethnic/religious groups because:

- expressions of distress may vary
- it may be difficult to judge how the patient is feeling
- behaviour, which seems abnormal in one culture but normal in another
  may be misunderstood
- the needs of different ethnic groups may vary
- it is necessary to understand different religious and spiritual beliefs of
  people coping with cancer (Watson 2000).

Impact on families

Changes in the formation of families over recent years have resulted in
complex patterns. Many women are lone parents and take on the stresses
of childcare, decision making and finances. Women may return to education later in life as mature students and a breast cancer diagnosis at this
time can be devastating with the loss of aspirations for the future and a
longer financial investment to continue following treatment. Many women
remain at home to care for children and many work part-time, resulting in
financial disadvantage. A high proportion depends on the benefits system.
Age, culture and personality affect the response to the diagnosis and the
initial period following diagnosis is vital to how the patient copes with the
ongoing disease and treatment (Radcliffe 2000).

It is important to understand the needs of family members and significant others so that support can be extended to those who are finding it
difficult to adjust. Many feel that they are not entitled to disclose problems
because the patient has priority. Some patients may be elderly and have
only one or two close relatives. The partner may be elderly and frail.
Spouses are often very distressed and cannot be considered to be the natural provider of support for the patient as they may require support
themselves. Also, family relationships, which were poor prior to the cancer
diagnosis, may have further stress placed on them by the illness. However,
a positive relationship with a partner provides a secure base for the patient
to face her illness.

When families are coping they can be enlisted to help the patients to
cope. Most studies agree that patients who maintain close relationships
with family and friends cope more effectively than those who cannot maintain relationships.

It is important for the health care professional to assess the family situation and to elicit any other support available, for example a neighbour, so
that there is someone to offer help. This also means that there will be

someone present at times such as breaking bad news (Faulkner and Maguire 1998).

The assessment should be ongoing and areas could include:

- the family's perception of the illness
- the family's perception of health care
- the family's perception of the patient's quality of life and response to treatment
- the family's functioning before and during the illness
- the marital relationship
- the patient's system of social support
- the impact of the disease on healthy family members – genetic risks
- the family's coping with previous family deaths
- intra-family issues
- the level of psychological distress in family members
- work and financial issues
- how much information the family require
- the family's commitment to the support of the patient (Baider 2000).

Families respond in different ways. It may be that they gain new coping skills and become closer or that relationships regress and disintegrate.

Techniques to support a family:

- Provide coping skills and a means of social support – as previously mentioned a social worker or counsellor attached to the unit could assist greatly by working with families.
- Provide effective problem-solving techniques to patients and family members to assist them to take control of the situation and support each other (Baider 2000).

A study by Harrison et al. (1995) found that there was a high level of concern among the relatives of cancer patients in the first weeks following diagnosis. The relatives reported more concerns than the patients, possibly due to feelings of helplessness and the provision of help given by health care professionals. However, the lower levels of concern showed by the patients could have been due to denial as a defence mechanism. These different levels of concern could indicate the need to talk separately to patients and relatives so each can talk freely about concerns. This raises questions as to how much support relatives should receive – should they also be screened and monitored for psychiatric disorders and who will manage their distress?

Health care professionals can help by offering information about the illness and providing support – a referral back to their GP may be appropriate if the relative develops serious emotional distress. Information on locally available support services should be offered where appropriate (Harrison et al. 1995).

The breast care nurse can also help by being aware of social trends affecting women and information regarding the benefits system. It is also helpful to be aware of self-help and voluntary groups available.

Men's responses to partners with breast cancer

The breast care nurse is well positioned to observe the responses of the patient's partner to the breast cancer diagnosis. Partners tend to express concerns about the patient rather than focus on themselves. Studies confirm that a woman's adjustment to breast cancer is improved by a partner's support.

However, the woman may feel that the partner is suffering and wishes to support him, but he will not express his concerns to protect her leading to a problem in communication. The breast care nurse needs to assess the communication process between couples by encouraging them to discuss concerns and feelings. It needs to be established whether to talk to the couple together or separately. Sensitive communication skills are required (Foy and Rose 2001).

The partner may feel overwhelmed and powerless to help the patient – it must not be automatically assumed that he is the main supporter. Men may find the periods when the patient is undergoing surgery particularly stressful as they are required to undertake household and childcare tasks as well as their usual role. Many adapt to this willingly but others feel threatened by change.

It is important not to deprive the patient of all her roles. However, after discharge the woman may still be trying to comprehend the impact of the diagnosis and treatment whilst the partner feels that things are getting back to normal. Sexual relations may be a problem – the man may be wary of hurting her or of looking at the scar. He may reassure the patient but avoid any discussion of worries or concerns.

Nurses might need to create opportunities to interact with the man if they are aware of problems. It may be that the woman wishes to discuss her cancer but her partner does not. This may lead to the patient receiving information about her disease and treatment alone as the partner does not wish to be present. Partners of breast cancer patients may need separate information but problems may arise when needs do not match (Faulkner and Maguire 1998). However, not all men will wish to confide in the nurse and each person should be assessed individually (Foy and Rose 2001).

The partner's response to the cancer diagnosis may be complicated by guilt or anger if there has been a past conflict in the relationship.

Sometimes a marriage in trouble can break down completely under the strain (Barraclough 1994).

Anger

Some patients can express their anger at a breast cancer diagnosis and move towards acceptance whereas in others anger becomes ingrained and destructive. Anger can sometimes be more marked in relatives. The anger can be directed at the illness, Fate, God or the health care professionals. It can also sometimes be justified, for example if there has been a delay in making a diagnosis or a problem with treatment.

It is difficult for members of the breast care team to have anger directed at them. It is best to listen to the patient and offer consistent professional concern. The breast care nurse can provide time and space and offer counselling if necessary. A counsellor can also be valuable where a couple appear to be consistently arguing. Any genuine problems can be acknowledged but it is important not to blame colleagues – listening without judging is best (Barraclough 1994).

Sexuality

Sexuality is complex, incorporating physical, psychological, interpersonal and behavioural dimensions. Sexuality is defined by each patient and her partner within a context of factors such as age, gender, personal attitudes and cultural and religious values.

Many types of cancer treatments are associated with sexual dysfunction. Around 50 per cent of women who have had breast cancer experience long-term sexual dysfunction (Ganz et al. 1998). Causes can be physical and psychological. Sexual problems can continue for longer than two years following treatment and can interfere with the patient's quality of life. Assessment for intervention and follow-up are important for maximizing quality of life.

Sexual function following breast conservation surgery has been the subject of much research. Several studies concur that breast conservation or reconstruction has only a small impact in preserving sexual function compared to mastectomy alone (Schover et al. 1995).

Chemotherapy is associated with loss of sexual function due to side effects of nausea, vomiting, diarrhoea and hair loss, which can leave patients feeling asexual. Alopecia also causes changes in body image and can lead to much distress. Cytotoxic drugs can cause vaginal dryness and dyspareunia. Premature menopausal symptoms caused by chemotherapy or radiotherapy associated with oestrogen loss include vaginal atrophy, vaginal dryness, hot flushes, mood swings, irritability and fatigue. Radiotherapy can cause nausea and sore skin. Hormonal therapies such as Tamoxifen can cause menopausal symptoms but the impact of Tamoxifen itself on sexual function is not clearly understood. In young women with breast cancer who are menopausal, concern about oestrogen replacement causing recurrence leads to high rates of sexual problems (Ganz et al. 1998).

Loss of sexual desire can be a symptom of depression; therefore, assessment to rule this out is very important. The stress of the diagnosis can have an effect on the sexual aspect of a couple's relationship.

The patient who is not in a relationship may worry about being rejected by a new partner when they have learnt about the cancer. Sexuality should be addressed as seriously even if there is no partner at the time. One of the most important factors in adjusting is how the patient felt about her sexuality prior to the cancer (Schover 1997).

Health care professionals can assist patients and their partners by asking open-ended specific questions to elicit health concerns, thus providing a safe environment in which the couple are encouraged to express concerns. The breast care nurse should be comfortable addressing sexuality or should refer on. The patient's concerns must not be ignored. Patients may not wish to discuss this but should be offered the option, giving the idea that it is fine to discuss this at a later date.

The patient can be monitored at follow-up by including a question on sexual problems in the routine quality of life questionnaire often given at clinics. A member of the multidisciplinary team can give immediate advice or refer on for specialist help, especially for younger women with fertility issues.

The partner must be taken into consideration – how they feel about the illness and the patient's concern about the partner. The breast care nurse should recognize that most couples have difficulty discussing sexual issues and this difficulty increases with the threat of a life-threatening illness.

Any previous anxiety and depression, mental illness, previous psychotherapy or medication should be noted (Schover 1997).

Cancer treatment produces change in body image and self-esteem. Patients have problems seeing themselves as sexually attractive during and after treatment. If a partner has to provide physical care, this can impact on sexuality. The change of roles and stressors such as financial concerns can also contribute.

It needs to be remembered that not all women will consider sexual attractiveness to be of high priority. This emphasizes the need to establish priority information for each patient rather than assuming that sexual attractiveness is a major issue for all women diagnosed with breast cancer (Luker et al. 1996).

Lesbian relationships

Some patients may have a significant other excluded by the family, for example lesbian partners or partners not accepted by the rest of the family. The patient and person concerned must take responsibility to avoid health care professionals becoming involved in family problems (Faulkner and Maguire 1998). Again sensitive communication skills are required.

Breast Cancer Care run a telephone support group for lesbian and bisexual women with breast cancer, it may be appropriate for the breast care nurse to suggest contacting this group. Many lesbian relationships involve a varied and flexible sex life, which can be helpful when trying to cope with changes due to cancer (Cancer Bacup online 2002). However, great value may be placed on physical appearance, which may be altered by breast surgery. Fertility can be just as much of an issue as for heterosexual couples.

Health care staff may be ignorant about the health care needs of lesbians and lesbians who have encountered discrimination may delay in seeking help for a health problem. Nurses need to convey to patients from the beginning that they will be treated with respect and their life is a normal variation in lifestyle.

Lesbian women may also be concerned about the labels used to identify them and may not always wish the word lesbian to be used. Nurses need to facilitate good communication by:

- avoiding the use of questions that assume that all patients are heterosexual and ensuring privacy and comfort before asking personal questions
- becoming informed about the specific health care needs of lesbian women – for example, ensure that the patient is comfortable undergoing breast examination and that this is carried out correctly. Homophobia can lead to rough treatment of lesbian women by health care professionals and nurses must recognize if this is the case and report misconduct
- using language that the patient can relate to
- displaying information in clinics and waiting areas in the unit which shows that staff are non-judgemental towards patient with same-sex orientation
- respecting the concerns of patients about confidentiality – they may fear discrimination if confidentiality is broken (Royal College of Nursing 2000).

Children

Many breast cancer patients have young children or teenagers. Telling children the cancer diagnosis is difficult and painful but children are aware when something is wrong within a family and may imagine far worse things than the situation if nothing is discussed. Talking about cancer also suggests that this is a subject that can be talked about. Children may otherwise develop an abnormal fear of illness. They need to be reassured that it is not their fault and will not feel isolated (Cancer Bacup online 1999).

Children under seven years may have difficulty understanding, although some show a matter of fact interest and acceptance. Teenagers may be more difficult to talk to due to existing communication problems but will have greater intellectual understanding.

Children may exhibit physical or behavioural symptoms of distress and may feel guilty or abandoned. Older teenage girls may worry about contracting breast cancer. Some children may exhibit:

- clinginess
- crying
- sleep disturbances
- bed wetting
- exacerbation of asthma/eczema
- headaches
- abdominal pain
- vomiting
- problems at school
- aggressive behaviour (Barraclough 1994).

Children need to be supported by relatives, friends and a consistent routine to provide a sense of security. Questions should be encouraged and answered honestly. They should be told about the diagnosis, treatment side effects and how the patient will feel, although too many frightening medical details should be avoided. Boundaries and discipline should be kept up and the children's feelings acknowledged. It is important to reassure them that they will still be cared for. Some clinical nurse specialists specialize in talking to children, also teachers, social workers or a parish priest are other individuals who can be involved.

Body image

Body image develops in childhood and is refined during adult years. Maintaining a satisfactory body image means retaining a sense of balance when illness or injury challenge the person's satisfaction with their body (Price 1998). The balance is generally easier to maintain when the patient has social support to help with the adjustment to physical change.

In a seminal work on body image, Price (1990) observes that body image is how we think and feel about our body's appearance and that it is a complex and abstract way in which we picture it. Three components are necessary for the formation and maintenance of a person's normal body image:

1 Body reality – the way in which the body is constructed, the way it really is.
2 Body ideal – how we think the body should look – constantly changing.
3 Body presentation – how we present our body to the world using dress, poise, actions – can be controlled within certain limits.

Each person holds an idealized image of their physical self. Once their perception of this body image is altered, emotional and psychosocial reactions can result. Altered body image exists when the patient's social and individual coping strategies to deal with changes in their body reality, ideal or presentation are overwhelmed by disease or disability (Price 1995). As body image is so important to the sense of self, this can have a profound effect on a person's well-being.

Threats to body image include pain and fatigue, loss of physical control, treatment affecting the face or sexual organs, conditions such as breast cancer requiring the use of a prosthesis, use of catheters and Hickman lines, and alopecia (Price 1998). Nausea and vomiting, mucositis and anorexia due to chemotherapy can cause much distress. Loss of libido is also a threat to body image and younger women may be trying to deal with fertility issues as well. Skin reactions caused by radiotherapy, especially if the skin breaks down, cause distress and some patients may find the marks of radiotherapy treatment are a constant reminder of the cancer (Salter 1997).

The female breast is seen as the symbol of femininity, sexual desirability and maternal comfort. It is central to many people's views about 'being a woman' and therefore any threat to the breast is potentially very stressful.

Patients who have had a mastectomy might be expected to regard this as a disaster but as women hold vastly differing views about their breasts this may not necessarily be the case. Many patients are also relieved to have the cancer removed without being particularly affected by the loss of the breast. The fear of pain and death may mean that body image is not immediately considered. This all depends on the woman's circumstances after surgery, her attitudes towards her breasts and the degree of social support available to her. Baseline questions to assess how much body image mattered prior to surgery should be part of the assessment by health care professionals.

Women who have undergone mastectomy or even breast reconstruction will have already undergone procedures affecting body image, such as clinical examination and biopsy. These may cause her to feel a loss of control over her body. The patient who has had a mastectomy following the menopause may feel that her feelings of femininity have suffered a double blow with the cancer diagnosis and treatment. Younger women may mourn the loss of a breast as breastfeeding will be affected, as well as dealing with a life-threatening illness (Price 1990). Assumptions are often made that elderly or sexually inactive women do not mind losing a breast so mastectomy will be performed. This may not be the case, all patients should be treated as individuals and these women may well opt for lumpectomy (Fallowfield 1994).

Each individual has different worries. The breast care nurse can play an important role in helping the patient to come to terms with the surgery and change in her body image. The loss of a breast and axillary lymph glands is major surgery and poses immediate body image problems. All three components for a normal body image are affected at once. Some women have a very pronounced sense of body image and develop great self-consciousness after mastectomy. Some may feel that they can cope when dressed but experience distress when unclothed.

Some women may show signs of becoming socially phobic. They become sure that everyone can tell that they have only one breast and start to wear baggy clothing. Attending social events can become a frequently avoided behaviour. The patient may feel that she is being stared at and talked about or even avoided. This can result in the displaying of considerable psychological difficulties, especially in social situations (Newell 2002a). Cognitive behaviour therapy to promote positive thinking may be useful. Some examples are:

- Exposure therapy – the patient enters a feared situation and remains until her anxiety reduces – the sooner and more frequently the better. The anxiety, although uncomfortable, will fade. Avoiding situations leads to the patient being restricted in the number of things she can do.
- Leaflets and information aids containing a cognitive behavioural element such as emphasis that confronting feared situations can help to contribute to psychological well-being.
- Advice when preparing the patients for surgery that confronting their fears will help them to cope with their disfigurement by increasing their sense of self-worth and confidence.
- Specialist intervention – some patients will require more intensive help due to the extent of their difficulties (Newell 2002b).

Breast reconstruction may play a vital role in the rehabilitation of women who are devastated by losing a breast. Women should be asked about their preference and offered the option if at all possible. Reconstruction should be offered as an important part of treatment, not as an afterthought if resources permit. All women should be offered this, it should not be assumed that an elderly woman would not want it or that a young woman would always want reconstruction (Fallowfield 1994).

The ways in which the patient can be helped post-operatively include:

- ensuring that all runs smoothly on the patient's return from theatre, for example drains remain patent, dressings do not become dislodged until the wound is due to be inspected
- maintaining comfort – ensure that drainage tubes do not block or drag on the wound, ensure adequate analgesia so that the patient can perform arm exercises properly
- assistance with personal hygiene if the patient is unable to do this herself
- providing a soft temporary prosthesis once the dressings are removed
- enabling the patient to look at the wound in her own time (Price 1990).

Removing the theatre dressing can be traumatic. Nurses can assist the patient by helping her to bath and dress. The presence of an empathetic nurse can be helpful. The patient should be gently encouraged, rather than forced, to view her wound. She should be given permission to show emotion. Sensitive care will facilitate adjustment to a significantly altered body image (Salter 1997).

Early mobilization of the affected arm and educating the patient about the risk of lymphoedema is also vitally important to minimize the risk of occurrence. Lymphoedema can be a chronic wearying condition and an added threat to the woman's feelings about her body image. A heavy, large arm can be an impediment to normal functioning. Some items of clothing will be impossible to wear and mobility is often impaired (Salter 1997). (Lymphoedema will be discussed in Chapter 12.)

Nursing staff may find that the patient seems to be relieved at first when the affected breast is removed but becomes more distressed when near to being discharged. The breast care nurse and ward staff can note certain factors that would indicate that the patient's perception of her body image is altering:

- observation of how she behaves towards the operation site
- listening to how she talks about her body
- observing for social withdrawal
- taking note of relatives' concerns and reports of how the patient is coping
- listening to how she feels she will cope outside hospital.

Some actions can be undertaken prior to discharge:

- planning care to minimize problems, for example suitable temporary prosthesis, appointment for permanent prosthesis along with appropriate information about fitting, etc., provision of a contact number, assurance that she will receive a visit from the community nurse shortly after discharge
- rehearsing with the patient coping strategies for when she is out in the outside world, for example trying the cognitive behavioural strategies
- encouraging relatives to give support and encourage coping strategies – hospital stays are often too short (Price 1998).

The recovery process may take time. The patient needs to regain trust in her body, which will never be quite 'back to normal' – she will have had a life-threatening disease and will always have to live with the fact. It may take time for the patient to recover her self-confidence and deal with the outside world. Some patients may feel abandoned when treatment comes to an end – after months of intensive treatment she may feel extremely insecure when she is not being monitored as often by health care professionals. Again, provision of a contact number may provide security and the breast care nurse may explore the possibility of the patient joining the local support group if appropriate.

Employment

Past studies have shown that women returning to work after treatment for breast cancer face various problems. Difficulties reported in the study ranged from other workers' reactions to their cancer history, wanting to work less hours or wanting more fulfilling work. However, the main problem was discrimination caused by their cancer history. Hostile attitudes of co-workers, confrontations regarding altered body image, dismissal, demotion and denial of promotion were all experienced (Feldman 1987). Breast cancer survivors may suffer increased fatigue and reduced stamina, which could be the cause of discrimination but further studies are needed (Rendle 1997).

New employers may feel that a cancer history is a reason not to employ someone. Employers feel that the employee will only be able to work for a short time, not taking into account ever improving survival rates and employment potential. This may be due to a public misunderstanding of cancer and how this attitude affects survivors' lives (Rendle 1997). Cancer survivors are as reliable and productive as their fellow workers and do not have higher levels of absenteeism (Brown and Tai-Seale 1992). More education of the public regarding their understanding of cancer is required, and more research is needed to ascertain the impact of breast cancer on employment.

Delay in reporting a breast lump

Some women may delay reporting a breast lump. Delayed presentation of a breast lump is associated with lower survival (Richards et al. 1999). More than 50 per cent of patients present to a GP within one month but 20–30 per cent delay more than three months (Ramirez et al. 1999).

They convince themselves that it is a minor condition until the symptoms of advanced cancer cannot be ignored any longer. Characteristics of this group of women include:

- older age groups
- lower social class and education
- clinically depressed and anxious patients
- fear of cancer
- fear of surgery
- those less likely to report any illness
- those constantly in denial
- women who are very inhibited about their bodies (Fallowfield 2000).

Marital status appears to be unrelated to delay in presenting with symptoms. Younger age can be a risk factor for delay by providers when presenting with symptoms other than a lump (Ramirez et al. 1999).

Although it is important that women report their breast lumps, health care professionals should emphasize that it is an emotional emergency rather than a medical one to allow the woman time to assimilate information and make choices.

Refusing treatment

There are many situations where the patient and/or doctor may decide that the side effects and trauma of the treatment outweigh the benefits. Even if the patient and doctor do not agree the doctor will generally respect the wishes of the patient. Occasionally the treatment, which would have been beneficial, is refused. The patient's wishes are given priority but it is worth the breast care nurse or doctor trying to elicit reasons:

- the patient may be misinformed about the treatment
- she may not appreciate the consequences of not undergoing treatment, for example the breast may become a fungating, ulcerated mass

- passive suicide – refusing treatment will lead to an early death in depressed patients or patients with an unhappy life
- the patient's way of exerting some control over the situation.

Relatives who hold a different view may try to dictate treatment for their family member.

Repeated information, advice and support may be effective, either from the breast care team or specialist counsellors. If the patient still refuses treatment, the breast care nurse can be available for psychological support and information. The patient will continue to be seen by the medical and nursing staff at the clinic. Referral can be made to the community nurses for additional support, practical help and management of a fungating wound. Social services may be involved. Referral to palliative care nurse specialists at the appropriate time can also be made.

References

Altruis Biomedical Network (2000) www.anti-depressants.net (accessed May 2002).

Baider L (2000) Update 5 – Family stress. Psycho-Social Impact of Breast Cancer. First series of updates for health professionals. Information about 2nd Psycho-Social Impact of Breast Cancer Meeting, Helsinki, June, www.cope.uicc.org

Barraclough J (1994) Cancer and Emotion: A Practical Guide to Psycho-Oncology. 2nd edn. Chicago, IL: John Wiley & Sons.

Bodurka-Bevers D, Basen-Endquist K, Carmack CL, et al. (2000) Depression, anxiety and quality of life in patients with epithelial ovarian cancer. Gynaecologic Oncology 78(3): 302–8.

Breithart W (1995) Identifying patients at risk for and treatment of major psychiatric complications of cancer. Supportive Care in Cancer 3(1): 45–60.

Bridge L, Benson P, Pietroni P, et al. (1988) Relaxation and imagery in the treatment of breast cancer. British Medical Journal 297: 1169–72.

Brown HG, Tai-Seale M (1992) Vocational rehabilitation of cancer patients. Seminars in Oncology Nursing 8(3): 202–11.

Cancer Bacup online (1999) www.cancerbacup.org.uk/info/talk-children.htm (accessed May 2002).

Cancer Bacup online (2002) www.cancerbacup.org.uk/info/sexuality.htm (accessed June 2002).

Department of Health (2000) The NHS Cancer Plan. A Plan for Investment, a Plan for Reform. London: DoH.

Dugan W, McDonald MV, Passik SD, et al. (1998) Use of the Zung self-rating depression scale in cancer patients: feasibility as a screening tool. Psycho-Oncology 7(6): 483–93.

Fallowfield L with Clark A (1994) Breast Cancer (The experience of illness). London: Tavistock/Routledge.

Fallowfield L (2000) Update 4 – Women's perspective on the psychological impact of breast cancer. Psycho-Social Impact of Breast Cancer. First series of updates for professionals. Information about 2nd Psycho-Social Impact of Breast Cancer meeting, Helsinki, June, www.cope.uicc.org

Faulkner A, Maguire P (1998) Talking to Cancer Patients and their Relatives. Oxford: Oxford Medical Publications.

Feldman FL (1987) Female cancer patients and caregivers: experiences in the workplace. Women and Health 12: 137–53.

Foy S, Rose K (2001) Men's experiences of their partner's primary and recurrent breast cancer. European Journal of Oncology Nursing 5(1): 42–8.

Friedman LC, Lehane D, Webb JA, et al. (1994) Anxiety in medical situations and chemo-related problems among cancer patients. Journal of Cancer Education 9(1): 37–41.

Ganz PA, Rowland JH, Desmond K, et al. (1998) Life after breast cancer: understanding women's health related quality of life and sexual functioning. Journal of Clinical Oncology 16(2): 5011–14.

Green BL, Krupnick JL, Rowland JH, et al. (2000) Trauma history as a predictor of psychological symptoms in women with breast cancer. Journal of Clinical Oncology 18(5): 1084–93.

Harrison J, Haddad P, Maguire P (1995) The impact of cancer on key relatives: a comparison of relative and patient concerns. European Journal of Cancer 31A(11): 1736–40.

Hassey Dow K (2000) Update 3 – Rehabilitation and Follow Up. Psycho-Social Impact of Breast Cancer. First series of updates for professionals. Information about 2nd Psycho-Social Impact of Breast Cancer Meeting, Helsinki, June, www.cope.uicc.org

Luker K, Beaver K (2000) An evaluation of information cards as a means of improving communication between hospital and primary care for women with breast cancer. Journal of Advanced Nursing 31(5): 1174–82.

Luker K, Beaver K, Leinster SJ, et al. (1996) Information needs and sources of information for women with breast cancer: a follow-up study. Journal of Advanced Nursing 23(3): 487–95.

Lynch ME (1995) The assessment and prevalence of affective disorders in advanced cancer. Journal of Palliative Care 11(1): 10–18.

McArdle JMC, George WD, McArdle CS, et al. (1996) Psychological support for patients undergoing breast surgery: a randomised study. British Medical Journal 312(7034): 813–16.

McCaul KD, Sandgren AK, King B, et al. (1999) Coping and adjustment to breast cancer. Psycho-Oncology 8(3): 230–6.

Morasso G, Constantini M, Barraco G, et al (1996) Assessing psychological distress in cancer patients – validation of a self-administered questionnaire. Oncology 53(4): 295–302.

National Cancer Institute online (2002) Emotional Concerns. Anxiety Disorder/Depression. www.nci.nih.gov/cancerinfo/coping (accessed May 2002).

Newell R (2002a) Living with disfigurement. Nursing Times 98(15): 34–5.

Newell R (2002b) The fear-avoidance model: helping patients to cope with disfigurement. Nursing Times 98(16): 38–9.

Nordin K, Glimelius B (1999) Predicting delayed anxiety and depression in patients with gastro-intestinal cancer. British Journal of Cancer 79(3/4): 525–9.

Oxford Development Centre online (2002) Cognitive Behavioural Therapy, www.oxdev.co.uk

Passik SD, Dugan W, McDonald MV, et al. (1998) Oncologists' recognition of depression in their patients with cancer. Journal of Clinical Oncology 16(4): 1594–6000.

Poole K (1996) The evolving role of the Clinical Nurse Specialist within the comprehensive breast cancer centre. Journal of Clinical Nursing 5: 341–9.

Price B (1990) Body Image: Nursing Concepts and Care. Hemel Hempstead: Prentice Hall.

Price B (1995) Assessing altered body image. Journal of Psychiatric and Mental Health Nursing 2: 169–75.

Price B (1998) Cancer: altered body image. Nursing Standard 12(21): 49–55.

Radcliffe P (2000) The psychological and financial support. Presentation to RCN Breast Care Nursing Conference, December.

Ramirez AJ, Westcombe AM, Burgess CC, et al. (1999) Factors predicting delayed presentation of symptomatic breast cancer: a systematic review. Lancet 353(9159): 1127–31.

Razavi D, Steifel F (1994) Common psychiatric disorders in cancer patients: 1. Adjustment disorders and depressive disorders. Supportive Care in Cancer 2(4): 223–32.

Razavi D, Delvaux N, et al. (1993) The effects of a 24 hour psychological training programme on attitudes, communication skills and occupational stress in oncology: a randomised study. European Journal of Cancer 29: 1858–63.

Rendle K (1997) Survivorship and breast cancer: the psychosocial issues. Journal of Clinical Nursing 6(5): 403–410.

Richards MA, Westcombe AM, Love SB, et al. (1999) The influence of delay on survival in patients with breast cancer: a systematic review. Lancet 353(9159): 1119–26.

Royal College of Nursing (2000) Issues in Nursing and Health. Aspects in the Nursing Care of Lesbians. London: RCN.

Salter M (1997) Altered Body Image: The Nurses' Role. 2nd edn. London: Balliere Tindall.

Schover LR (1997) Sexuality and Fertility after Cancer. New York: John Wiley & Sons.

Schover LR, Yetman RJ, Tuason LJ, et al. (1995) Partial mastectomy and breast reconstruction: a comparison of their effects on psychosocial adjustment, body image and sexuality. Cancer 75(1): 54–64.

Speigel D (1992) Effects of psychosocial support on patients with metastatic breast cancer. Journal of Psychosocial Oncology 10: 113–20.

Townend M (2002) Cognitive Behavioural Psychotherapy. www.townendm.freeserve.co.uk/index.html/cognitiv.htm (accessed May 2002).

Velikova G, Selby PJ, Snaith PR, Kirby PG (1995) The relationship of cancer pain to anxiety. Psychotherapy and Psychosomatics 63(3–4): 181–4.

Watson M (2000) Update 7 – Psychological adjustment over time. Psychosocial Impact of Breast Cancer. First series of updates for health professionals. Information about 2nd Psycho-Social Impact of Breast Cancer Meeting, Helsinki, June. www.cope.uicc.org

Wilkinson S, Maguire P, Tait A (1988) Life after breast cancer. Nursing Times 84(40): 34–7.

Williams JW Jr, Mulrow CD, Chiquette E, et al. (2000) A systematic review of newer pharmacotherapies for depression in adults: evidence report summary. Clinical guidelines part 2. Annals of Internal Medicine 132(9): 743–56.

Zigmond AS, Snaith RP (1983) The Hospital Anxiety and Depression Scale. Acta Psychiatrica Scandinavia 67: 361–70.

Chapter twelve
Lymphoedema

Introduction

Lymphoedema is a swelling of a limb and/or part of the body due to failure of the lymphatic system to drain lymph. Chronic lymphoedema is difficult to reverse. The deficient lymphatic system of the limb cannot compensate for the increased demand for fluid drainage. Lymphoedema can be primary, usually present at birth or occurring at puberty or midlife. In patients with breast cancer it is classed as secondary lymphoedema and causes include the following:

1 the tumour itself pressing on the lymphatic system
2 removal of the axillary lymph nodes during surgery. Removing the nodes provides valuable information on the staging of the cancer but puts women at risk of acquiring swelling of the affected arm and/or the adjacent truncal quadrant. Sentinel node biopsy is now being used in some centres to avoid axillary dissection and associated morbidity
3 radiotherapy – by affecting the inner walls of the lymphatic vessels therefore slowing the movement of the lymph fluid. Radiotherapy can also cause general scarring of the skin and soft tissues, leading to lymphoedema
4 infection – a major problem for patients with delayed wound healing or compromised immunity, caused by repeated aspiration of seromas or from sustaining cuts or insect bites Infection is a major cause of lymphoedema and will be discussed later in detail.

Lymphoedema can occur weeks, months or years after surgical treatment for breast cancer. Chronic lymphoedema cannot be cured but the swelling and discomfort can be relieved. It is often seen as a minor condition but can have a huge impact on quality of life. Daily lifestyle can be limited and the capacity to work is reduced. The onset of swelling and the realization that there is no cure can lead to depression (Lymphoedema Support Network 2002).

Although it is not life threatening it can take a strong psychological toll on the patient. Psychosocial maladjustment is more likely than in patients with breast cancer who do not have lymphoedema (Tobin et al. 1993).

Even with surgery reduced from radical mastectomy to lumpectomy and in some cases chemotherapy instead of radiotherapy, about 22 per cent of patients develop lymphoedema (Mortimer et al. 1996).

The lymphatic system

Anatomy

The lymphatic system includes superficial or primary lymphatic vessels that form a complex dermal network of capillary-like channels that drain into larger or secondary lymph vessels in the sub-dermal space. They are the most peripheral vessels and are blind-ended tubes consisting of endothelium (Board and Harlow 2002a). There are as many lymphatic vessels as blood vessels but the lymphatic system differs from the blood system in that blood continually circulates through the body but the lymphatics just drain from each part. Eventually lymph (see below) is filtered via the lymph nodes before emptying back into the bloodstream, mostly in the lower neck. The lymph vessels of the left arm drain into the left subclavian lymphatic trunk and then into the left subclavian vein. The right arm lymph vessels drain into the right subclavian lymphatic trunk and then into the right subclavian vein. On its way along the lymph is filtered into lymph nodes which remove foreign matter and start any necessary immune reaction. There are about 30–50 lymph nodes in the axilla, made of lymphoid tissue. The nodes filter out unwanted bacteria, infectious organisms or cancer cells. Lymphocytes within the nodes attack unwanted material and try to break it down before it is carried away in the bloodstream.

Physiology

Normally all tissues in the body are kept alive by a supply of oxygen, nutrients and water and by the removal of waste products. As blood does not reach all parts of the body a blood filtrate provides these supplies to each cell. This colourless fluid of water and protein (interstitial fluid) seeps out of the circulation and bathes all body tissues, providing nourishment to every cell and picking up waste. Approximately 16–18 litres of interstitial fluid is formed daily and 14–16 litres returns to the bloodstream. The remaining fluid, lymph, drains back from the tissues through the lymph vessels or lymphatics.

The exchange of fluid between interstitial fluid and blood plasma centres around the forces of filtration and reabsorption. The mechanism controlling it is known as Starling's Law of the Capillaries. The equilibrium of fluid exchange is maintained by the hydrostatic pressure of water in the fluid and by the osmotic pressure (the force exerted by plasma proteins).

The lymphatic drainage process occurs by changes in the pressure of the interstitial fluid through breathing and general muscle movement. The movement of adjacent muscles pumps lymph into and along the lymphatic vessels and the large lymphatic vessels' walls also contract. This pumping is aided by valves inside the vessels. The pulsation of arteries also compresses adjacent lymphatic vessels assisting the flow of lymph.

This muscle pump activity is crucial for the propulsion of lymph through the lymphatic vessels. Lymphatic vessels have a smooth muscle wall. Lymphatic return from the limbs is influenced by the extrinsic and intrinsic muscle pump. In relation to the extrinsic pump, the pressure applied to the venous system by movement, muscle contractions, respiration and arterial pulsation push fluid from the limb in the direction of the heart (Casley-Smith and Casley-Smith 1997). For the extrinsic pump to be effective the initial lymphatics must open when pressure on the tissues is low during rest and close when pressure is high during exercise. Alternating pressures cause lymph to be propelled towards the collecting vessels.

Lymphatics also possess an intrinsic muscle pump. When lymphatics contract and move fluid towards the heart a negative pressure is produced in the initial lymphatics which pulls lymph in through the tissues. The pressure is lower in the initial lymphatics than that in the tissues over a substantial part of the contraction cycle. During muscle contraction the frequency of pulsation can increase. In patients with lymphoedema these spontaneous contractions can be absent and passive movements will increase contractions of the intrinsic pump. It is also essential that muscle activity produces skin movement as movement between the skin and underlying tissues is essential for the filling of the initial lymphatics (Hughes 2000).

If the lymph nodes trap a cancer or infection they swell. With cancer the swelling is painless and does not cause any discomfort. The cancer cells are trapped by the 'filter system' and continue to divide and produce new cells within the node.

If a lymph channel blocks due to tumour or damage caused by surgery or radiotherapy the lymph fluid cannot pass along the lymph vessel. Protein still continues to enter the blood capillaries. Excess tissue fluid builds up in the tissues the lymphatics should be draining and causes swelling (lymphoedema). However lymph drainage never falls to zero and collateral routes are always established. In lymphoedema these fail to work properly. Continual lymphostasis causes dilation of the lymph vessels and

backflow of fluid to the tissue beds. The swelling decreases the oxygena-
tion of tissues and interferes with normal functioning. The protein is also
removed by cells such as macrophages in the tissues. These can partly take
over the role of the lymphatic system if it is blocked; however, in lymphoedema the chronic excess protein causes these cells to cease
functioning.

If the patient is immobile the use of the muscle is prevented and congestion of blood occurs in the veins causing venous hypertension. Fluid
accumulates due to the increase in capillary filtration rate caused by the
backwards pressure. Local tissue movement propels lymph through the
lymphatic vessels in subcutaneous tissues and when this movement is
absent lymph accumulates in interstitial spaces already congested by
venous hypertension (Board and Harlow 2002b).

Diagnosis

Lymphoedema differs from other oedema being not solely due to water
accumulation but also a solid component comprising fat, fibrosis and
inflammation exists. A lymphoedematous limb will be cool to the touch.
However, collagen proteins can accumulate and inflammation occur as the
body attempts to degrade the excess proteins. More blood capillaries are
formed and dilated leading to heat in the limb. This heat plus the stagnant
protein can cause acute inflammation and the patient may be very ill.
These infections worsen the lymphoedema as greater loads are placed on
the lymphatics.

If the swelling is rapid it can cause pain and adjacent areas such as the
shoulder, which are receiving excess lymph from the blocked region, also
ache. Fibrosis of the interstitial connective tissue causes the stiff non-
pitting oedema that does not respond to elevation, gentle exercise or elastic compression garments making treatment difficult (British Lymphology
Society 1999b).

Early diagnosis and therapy is vital to improve lymph flow, reduce
swelling, improve tissue structure and reduce the risk of further debility. A
swollen arm can be reduced to near normal size and can be maintained
with the appropriate treatment. Patient compliance needs to be 100 per
cent for daily therapies. The patient who does not adhere to the recommended regime may not fully understand the condition, may be unable to
take part, may not wish to take part or may not have a supportive network.

Research is ongoing to challenge the view that removal of the lymph
glands results in the obstruction of lymphatic drainage from the arm. A
more complex mechanism may involve regional differences in lymphatic
function within the limb, possibly arising from local failure of lymphatic
vessels and re-routing of lymph through skin and sub-cutaneous tissues.

Research will focus on what happens deep in the muscle of the forearm following treatment for breast cancer as well as whether fluid can escape via other routes such as the bloodstream, and prevent swelling (Lymphoedema Support Network 2002).

Symptoms of lymphoedema

Diagnosis of lymphoedema in breast cancer is made on the basis of the medical history and clinical examination. Other causes of oedema must be eliminated such as renal, hepatic or cardiac disease or deep venous thrombosis. Symptoms and clinical features include:

- changes in skin texture and/or tight, stretched skin
- increase in the thickness of the skin folds in the arm/axilla
- swelling of the arm and/or trunk (Keeley 2000)
- dull ache
- burning/pins and needles (due to nerve damage)
- pressure in joints and reduced joint movement
- muscle wasting
- soft, pitting oedema
- heat and irritation (only if cellulitis present).

With a recurrence of breast cancer the remaining axillary lymph nodes may enlarge and lymphoedema will be exacerbated (Keeley 2000). The brachial plexus may be involved causing neuropathic pain and weakness of the arm. Metastatic skin nodules on the chest wall or upper arm can reduce lymphatic drainage and the resulting severe lymphoedema is difficult to manage. Lymphoedema may be the first sign of a recurrence of breast cancer. The patient requires a full examination if any major swelling occurs.

Prevention

Patients who have undergone surgery for breast cancer that involves axillary node dissection are always given advice on reducing the risk of lymphoedema. The main advice is to undertake regular gentle active exercise and to prevent trauma because injury and infection are major avoidable causes.

- Do not have blood taken, blood pressure readings, injections or acupuncture from or on the affected arm. If the patient has had a bilateral mastectomy the leg can be used for venepuncture and blood pressure readings.

- Prevent scratches and cuts by wearing rubber gloves in the kitchen and gardening gloves when working outside.
- Use a thimble when sewing.
- Use oven gloves to avoid burns.
- Try to avoid sports injuries.
- Try to avoid being scratched or bitten by pets.
- Do not wear tight cuffs or tight fitting jewellery.
- Apply antiseptic to any cuts and go to the GP if any signs of infection occur.
- Use a high protection sun cream or cover up in the sun.
- Use an insect repellent to avoid being bitten especially when travelling abroad – it may be advisable to obtain prophylactic antibiotics.
- Use an electric razor or depilatory cream for removing hair. Waxing is not recommended.
- Do not carry heavy bags/packages.
- Care must be taken when manicuring nails.
- Avoid extremes of temperature, for example hot baths, saunas.
- Prophylactic antibiotics may be required for major dental work/general surgery.
- Deodorant can be used but avoid antiperspirants as the chemical can block the drainage system.
- Keep weight stable within normal limits (Todd 1996).

Following a mastectomy the patient should wear a well-fitting bra. The straps should not cut into the shoulders and any underwires should not cause red marks or indentations – lymphatic drainage will be restricted. The opposite breast is also at risk of swelling due to overload of the natural collateral drainage. The opposite breast is also at risk following a lumpectomy and radiotherapy and should be correctly supported.

Breast lymphoedema presents as swelling of part or all of the breast and is the result of the disruption of lymphatic drainage of the breast and axilla. The breast may feel tight and heavy, with the swelling primarily in the lower part of the breast. Tenderness and skin changes may be present. Breast cancer can spread through the superficial vessels that drain the skin of the breast on the affected side and presents as cutaneous nodules (Kirschbaum 2000).

Management of lymphoedema

Diuretics will have little or no effect and can exacerbate long-term problems of fibrosis and possibly increase swelling. Surgery is never recommended except as a last resort in few extreme cases (Lymphoedema Support Network 2002).

Management consists of skin care and prevention of infection. Physiotherapy to increase shoulder function and prevent scarring from surgery and radiotherapy, which could block lymph flow, is advisable. The massage used in manual and simple lymphatic drainage (see later) helps to increase lymphatic drainage, softens breast tissue and disrupts scarring.

Treatment for lymphoedema takes into account diagnosis, the patient's medical history, clinical findings and any factors that may affect the outcome. There are four cornerstones of treatment for lymphoedema:

1 skin care
2 exercise
3 manual lymphatic drainage (massage)
4 compression bandaging and/or hosiery.

Treatment falls into three categories each comprising all the four cornerstones – maintenance, intensive and palliative. The overall goal is to reduce and control the symptoms and allow patients to manage their condition independently (Todd 1999). It is crucial that the patient complies as this is a lifelong, chronic condition. The patient needs to thoroughly understand the principles of treatment and care. The lymphoedema therapist spends much time explaining the treatment, outcome and potential problems. Written information is usually given to back up discussion and a contact number provided. Treatment is generally realistic and short- and long-term goals are set, tailored to the individual needs of the patient.

The aim of maintenance treatment is long-term control of the oedema, which is generally mild and uncomplicated. The limb volume is no greater than 20 per cent when measured against the other unaffected limb. The formula used is:

$$\frac{circumference^2}{\pi}$$

The shape remains normal and there is no active malignancy. The skin is intact and the subcutaneous tissue pits. Treatment involves skin care, compression hosiery, exercise and massage. Advice and education are given to enable the patient to perform the treatment daily. Regular appointments are given to monitor and support, usually about four monthly. The majority of breast cancer patients with lymphoedema are in the maintenance phase.

The aim of intensive treatment is to reduce the amount of oedema and improve the skin so that the patient can enter the maintenance programme. Intensive treatment would be undertaken if the swelling is uncontrolled with the maintainance treatment or if the patient presented primarily with a large, distorted limb. The excess limb volume is greater than 20 per cent of the contralateral limb with some oedema extending to the trunk. The limb is distorted with fragile, damaged skin and tissue changes. Lymph may be leaking through the skin (lymphorrhoea). Treatment involves skin care, multi-layer bandaging, exercise, support and manual lymphatic drainage for 2–3 weeks with compression hosiery being applied at the end. The intensive phase is also known as Decongestive Lymphatic Therapy.

The aim of palliative treatment is to palliate the oedema and assess symptoms as the patient approaches the terminal stage of the illness. Patients who have active cancer causing oedema require this category of treatment. Symptoms vary depending on the nature and speed of the disease. There is often gross oedema involving the root of the limb and adjacent body trunk. The skin is often compromised with lymphorrhoea (fluid oozing from the skin), pain, heaviness and restricted use. Treatment is flexible and involves skin care, multi-layer bandaging and/or compression hosiery, exercises, support and manual lymphatic drainage (Board and Harlow 2002c).

Acute inflammatory episode (cellulitis)

All the advice regarding prevention of lymphoedema, that is, avoiding the risk of injury or infection, applies to patients with a lymphoedematous arm. This should be emphasized to the patient along with the need for meticulous skin care (see below). A break in the skin can lead to an acute inflammatory episode, which can start rapidly and the patient can quickly become unwell. Fever, rigors, vomiting and delirium can result, with redness and swelling of the arm, and the patient may be admitted to hospital. Acute inflammatory episodes (AIEs) can recur, and intervals between attacks may be short leading to severe debility. Infection elsewhere, such as a dental infection can also result in an attack as bacteria are a causal agent (Mortimer 2000).

Treatment consists of rest and antibiotics. Penicillin V 500mg qds orally for two weeks is the treatment of choice. Erythromycin may be prescribed if the patient is allergic to penicillin or Augmentin 625mg three times daily orally for two weeks. If there is marked systemic upset and patient debility the patient will be admitted to hospital and treated with Benzylpenicillin intravenously. The infection is usually streptococcal but *Staphylococcus aureus* may be present and Flucloxacillin added as cover. Community GPs are often advised of treatment regimes by lymphoedema therapists so a patient presenting with an AIE can be commenced on treatment without delay.

For recurrent AIE long-term prophylactic penicillin 500mg daily or 500mg twice daily for a large patient is recommended. If penicillin is ineffective Clindamycin 150–300mg twice daily can be used, reducing the dose to a minimum to prevent recurrence. Long-term treatment must be monitored by regular blood tests for kidney and liver function.

The patient is always advised to take a supply of antibiotics when travelling abroad even if an AIE has not yet been experienced.

Rest is very important during an attack of cellulitis and should be enforced. Resuming daily regular exercise and the wearing of compression garments is a matter of judgement.

The four cornerstones of treatment

Skin care

The recommended skin care regime for patients who have lymphoedema is designed to keep the skin supple and hydrated. It also reduces the risk of infection and the possibility of skin complications (Linnitt 2000). Aqueous cream or another soap substitute is used for washing and the skin is moisturized daily using aqueous cream or equivalent to prevent water loss and dry skin (Williams 1995). Unperfumed bath oils can also be used.

It is important that the patient maintains daily skin care at home as part of lymphoedema management. It is recommended that the skin is washed and dried carefully morning and night and that moisturizing is carried out at night before bed. This is to prevent the skin from becoming dry and cracked. The cream should be applied using an upward stroke, from elbow to shoulder and from hand to shoulder (Todd 1996). Extra care should be taken with skin folds as cream can collect and the skin can become macerated.

Skin should be washed and dried carefully especially between the fingers to prevent fungal infections, and all precautions (as above) against infection and injury taken. Cool or slightly warm showers and baths are beneficial and the application of a cool damp towel to the arm can relieve burning or tightness (Todd 1996).

The lymphoedema therapist checks the skin at each appointment and provides support and encouragement to the patient to maintain the daily regime. Preventive measures against infection are emphasized.

Exercise

Exercise is vital for the maintenance of lymphatic drainage as the lymphatic system relies partly on factors like muscle pump activity for the propulsion of lymph (Mortimer 1995). (The extrinsic and intrinsic muscle pump is discussed above.) Forty per cent of lymph is formed within skeletal muscle. Venous return must be maximized, although this will not fully compensate for poor lymphatic drainage. Venous return is increased by muscle activity and movement. Slow rhythmical movement is beneficial as it drives blood out of the limb reducing the load on the lymphatic system (Hughes 2000).

Exercise is part of both the intensive and maintenance programmes for lymphoedema. The exercise programme is tailored to the individual and taught by the lymphoedema therapist. The therapist carries out a thorough assessment of the patient's range of movement taking into account age, physical fitness, previous musculo-skeletal problems and degree of oedema. Referral may be made to a physiotherapist if necessary to improve the range of movement. Following breast cancer surgery some patients may find the arm exercises difficult and may experience adhesive capsulitis or 'frozen shoulder' as a result. 'Cording' may also occur. This is the development of cord-like structures down the inner aspect of the arm, axilla or on the chest wall. These two conditions both cause restriction of movement and pain, and the patient can benefit greatly from physiotherapy (Twycross 2000).

An exercise programme should incorporate flexibility, aerobic and strengthening exercises. It is important that the patient understands the importance of maintaining normal muscle tone. The exercises should not cause pain, which would cause trauma and increase swelling. The patient is encouraged to wear compression hosiery or support bandaging to prevent excess filtration of fluid into the tissues and increase the efficiency of the muscle pump. Exercises are performed daily and are fit into the patient's routine, they should be easy to do and not time consuming to maintain motivation. Ill or immobile patients can have passive exercises performed by carers where possible (Board and Harlow 2002c).

Advice to patients

- Rest with the arm in elevation with the hand above the level of the heart to maximize venous and lymphatic return. The arm should be well-supported along its length with the shoulder at approximately 90°, no higher or venous return is obstructed. A pillow on a chair arm when sitting is acceptable. The arm must not hang down for long periods. The hand can be tucked in a pocket or supported with the other arm.
- Good posture should be maintained whilst exercising. Move normally and carry out deep breathing exercises to promote thoracic venous and lymphatic return.
- Avoid static exercise such as carrying heavy bags. It may be easier to load shopping into smaller bags.
- Maintain a range of movements in day to day life, for example if using a computer keyboard support the arm and remember to move the arm several times a day.
- When static exercise cannot be avoided grip and relax the hand and elevate the arm at rest for a period.

- Discuss work and lifestyle so activities can be managed to prevent swelling, for example intersperse heavy activities in the house and garden with gentler ones.
- Resume sporting activities slowly as increased activity can increase swelling. A higher grade of compression sleeve may be required. There is an increased risk of trauma and infection if sports are undertaken, especially contact sports.
- Swimming is ideal. Muscle tone is helped and the water provides a degree of external compression.
- Prevent or reduce obesity (Hughes 2000).

Some tasks carried out by women need to be performed with care as they may increase swelling. A rest period may be necessary each hour, during which the hand can be pumped and the arm and wrist bent and stretched for 10 minutes. Activities that involve stretching at the shoulder, pushing, lifting, movements such as ironing, vacuuming, dusting, driving for instance need to be attempted cautiously. Very heavy activities that put an extra strain on the lymphatics should be avoided if possible; these include moving heavy objects, heavy DIY tasks, decorating, hanging curtains, weight training (Todd 1996). The condition of the patient's arm is generally a guide as to how much activity can be undertaken.

Examples of some of the exercise techniques for patients with lymphoedema are given below. These exercises should be done slowly and rhythmically twice a day. The arm sleeve should be worn when exercising to aid with the pumping away of fluid. Each session should be commenced with five deep breaths with relaxed abdominal muscles.

- Shrug shoulders up and down, then backwards and forwards.
- Straighten the arm and then bend at the elbow 20 times.
- Turn the palm of the hand to face the ceiling then the floor.
- Place the hands at the back of the neck, then slowly bring them forward and down to behind the waist 10 times.
- Bend and stretch the fingers 10 times (Todd 1996).

Other exercises can be recommended by the lymphoedema therapist to help with posture. The patient and therapist agree a programme together taking into account the ability of the patient. Leaflets are generally provided with diagrams and written instructions to follow and include a contact number in case the patient has any problems.

Massage

Massage is used within an intensive regime for lymphoedema to control swelling, or as part of a maintenance regime to maintain comfort, reduce pain and fibrosis, and enhance feelings of well-being. The aim is to stimulate lymphatic fluid to move away from the swollen quadrant so that it can drain away to the unaffected quadrant.

The therapist carries out a full physical and psychosocial assessment. Contra-indications include: cardiac insufficiency, asthma, superior vena cava obstruction, chronic inflammation, history of thrombosis, thyroid dysfunction, recent abdominal surgery. It is used very carefully in patients with advanced cancer.

There are two types of massage used for lymphoedema, manual lymphatic drainage and simple lymphatic drainage

Manual lymphatic drainage

This is very specialized and is only carried out by trained therapists. The technique depends on where the therapist trained but all have the same aim. The aim is to enhance the removal of proteins from the tissues and to increase the flow of lymph. Excess interstitial fluid will be reabsorbed without increasing capillary filtration (British Lymphology Society 1999c).

Massage commences at the neck working towards the trunk adjacent to the swollen arm. The collateral routes are then prepared for an increased workload and fluid is encouraged to drain away from the limb (British Lymphology Society 1999c). A variety of manual techniques are used, for example:

• The therapist starts at the neck and unaffected lymphatics and works towards the quadrant adjacent to the affected area before treating the swollen part. This ensures the movement of lymph towards the functioning lymphatics.
• Hand movements work across divisions between the superficial lymphatic drainage system (watersheds) so that collateral drainage is stimulated.
• Very light pressures are used.

It is not recommended to use deep or strong massage because of potential tissue damage and increase in oedema. It is necessary for the therapist to undergo approved training as the pressure used needs to be demonstrated in practice. The level of pressure applied should not exceed 40mm Hg. Each therapist will have an individual technique. Sessions last around 30–60 minutes depending on symptoms. Oils and creams are not used as the therapist needs to be in direct contact with the skin (Board and Harlow 2002c).

The massage is carried out daily for three or more weeks and may be repeated at intervals of three months to a year.

Simple lymphatic drainage

This is taught by the lymphoedema therapist and carried out by the patient or carer as part of the daily regime. The aim is to provide a technique of simplified manual drainage that the patient can perform independently. The patient needs to be dextrous and motivated. It incorporates simplified hand movements in a set sequence taught by the therapist. The patient is carefully assessed and time is allowed for teaching and ensuring competence, often over several sessions. It is advised to carry out this massage for 20 minutes a day to maintain lymph flow and softening of tissue. Patients are advised to set aside a regular time period to ensure continuity of treatment and establish a routine (Board and Harlow 2002c).

It may take a while for the patient to learn the technique. The therapist can teach by demonstrating on the patient and then letting the patient practise themselves. If teaching is successful the patient will feel more comfortable with their condition (Bellhouse 2000).

The movements work across the lymphatic watersheds towards the functioning lymphatics. Treatment is mainly to the neck and trunk area and again no oils or creams are used as the massage is done directly on the skin. The patient is advised to carry out the massage lying down, and that it is important to be relaxed. Compression hosiery should be worn. The carer can be taught the technique if this is acceptable to the patient.

Massage should be done in a quiet, warm room. No jewellery or clothes should be worn on the affected side. The patient can sit or lie with the arm well supported.

The massage starts with deep breathing as for exercising.

- Using the flats of the fingers and a circular motion press enough to make the skin move but not hard enough to cause redness. Place the fingers on each side of the neck with little fingers touching the earlobes and fingertips pointing backwards. Move the fingers in a circle to take the skin down and back five times. The skin's elasticity should take the hand back.
- The above movement is repeated a finger width down the neck and so on until the index fingers touch the collar bone.
- The whole neck massage is repeated three times.
- Cross the arms so that the hands rest above the collar bone and move fingers in a stationary circle (circular pressure made with the hands remaining in one spot) directing them forward and in. This is repeated five times.
- Place one hand with the fingers resting in the unaffected armpit. Move the hand in a stationary circle directing the movement in and up.
- Repeat the above four finger widths down the side of the chest wall. The skin is moved up and in towards the unaffected armpit.

- Place the hand on the front of the chest near to the unaffected armpit.
- Move the hand in three stationary circles to gently push the fluid towards the armpit. Repeat the circles moving towards the affected side gradually. Repeat two or three times.
- Place the hand on the affected shoulder towards the back. Direct the movement back and up away from the affected armpit. Repeat all around the shoulder and upper arm above the compression sleeve.
- Finish with abdominal breathing (Todd 1996).

Lymphoedema therapists provide the patient with written information as well as verbal in the form of leaflets with easy-to-follow diagrams and instructions. A video may be available to borrow. A contact number should be included.

Compression

Graduated compression sleeves allow the muscles to work more effectively to pump fluid away. Pressure is exerted on the tissues by forces within the material acting compressively (Badger et al. 2000). A firm resistance is provided against which the lymphatic vessels are squeezed by the muscle during activity promoting lymphatic and venous drainage. Lymph is moved up the arm more effectively and lymphatic drainage away from the affected arm is promoted (Breast Cancer Care 1999). Interstitial pressure is raised, capillary filtration is limited and support for tissues is provided.

Sleeves are used when the lymphoedema is mild or in the maintenance phase to maintain the size and shape of the arm. The pressure is sustained over a longer time period. Sleeves are not used on very swollen arms or where the skin is folded, pitting or leaking. In these cases multi-layer bandaging is carried out (see below).

Indications include:

- limb is a normal shape
- there is less than 20 per cent excess limb volume
- skin is healthy and intact
- oedema is soft and pitting
- oedema is confined to the limb.

Contraindications include:

- distorted limb shape
- arterial disease
- skinfolds
- cellulitis
- loss of skin integrity
- thrombosis
- neuropathic pain
- allergy to the hosiery (British Lymphology Society 1999a).

There are three classes of graduated compression hosiery each identified by the level of compression in mm Hg measured at the wrist. Sleeves contain elastomer and the degree of compression is dictated by the weave and type of material used. Compression sleeves are a higher compression class than those used for venous disorders. Both sleeves and mittens are used for hand and arm oedema. If ready-made sleeves are inappropriate made-to-measure can be obtained. Regular sleeves are made for regularly shaped limbs. Arm sleeves are generally not available in different colours.

Class 1 – Light   –   14–17mmHg at wrist circumference.
Class 2 – Medium   –   18–24mmHg at wrist circumference.
Class 3 – Strong   –   25–35mmHg at wrist circumference
(British Lymphology Society 1999b).

The strongest pressure is exerted at the distal part of the arm. The pressure is inversely proportional to the limb circumference. A lower class sleeve is used for limbs of smaller proportion as the pressure exerted by the garment will be greatest over a limb with a smaller circumference (Todd 2000).

The sleeve is provided on prescription by the lymphoedema therapist who carries out a thorough assessment and selects the most appropriate garment for the patient's needs:

- An accurate medical history is taken. Other causes of oedema must be eliminated, for example cardiac, renal or hepatic disease or DVT.
- Details of onset, duration and pre-disposing factors are noted.
- Contraindications to compression such as arterial insufficiency are eliminated.
- All clinical features are noted.
- A physical examination is carried out.
- Psychosocial factors are assessed – the patient's competence, motivation, ability and movement (Badger 1993).

The sleeve must be properly measured and fitted and should feel firm but not uncomfortable. The unaffected arm is used as a baseline measurement. The site and extent of the oedema and the appearance of the underlying skin and tissues are examined. Both arms are measured to identify the total excess volume, the fluid distribution and the degree of distortion. (Badger 1993). Circumferential measurements are recorded at 4cm intervals along the arm using the cylinder formula:

$$\frac{\text{circumference}^2}{\pi}$$

If one arm is swollen the percentage volume difference can be calculated by comparing the measurements taken from both arms using:

$$\frac{100 \times \text{excess limb volume}}{\text{normal limb volume}}$$

The degree of distortion in shape can be calculated by dividing the measurements of the upper segment of the arm by the lower segment. This ratio is then compared for both arms. The difference is established by subtracting the swollen ratio from the normal ratio. In bilateral oedema the calculations cannot be done and the degree of percentage volume and distortion is subjective. If misshapen or excess percentage volume is over 20 per cent the arm is bandaged with compression bandaging (Board and Harlow 2002b).

If the patient has required multi-layer bandaging the sleeve should be ordered and ready to fit at the end of this treatment. Measurements should be taken when volume reduction appears to be static.

The patient wears the sleeve all day and removes it at night following massage and exercises. Sleeves are not used on very swollen arms or where the skin is folded or pitted. The patient must report any pain, tingling, pins and needles or change in skin colour as the sleeve is too tight. Management should be safe and effective. An increase in weight can alter the sleeve's effectiveness (Todd 2000).

Full explanation and instructions should be given. The patient is advised to keep nails short and remove jewellery to avoid damage to sleeve. It is put on first thing in a morning following washing and drying of the skin. Moisturizing is done at night with aqueous cream as the sleeve would be very difficult to put on. To put a sleeve on it is turned inside out as far as the wrist, pulled over the hand and eased up a bit at a time. It should not be pulled up by the top. The top should not be turned over as this restricts blood flow. A little unperfumed talc to the arm may help with application. The fabric should be smooth with no creases or wrinkles. An overlapping mitten may be supplied if the hand is swollen. Rubber gloves can be worn to prevent damage. Two sleeves are supplied, one to wear and one to wash and these are replaced 4–6 monthly as they become less elastic over time. Measurements may be rechecked at this point to ascertain whether a different size is required.

Patient compliance is paramount when prescribing compression hosiery as the patient needs to be motivated. The wearing of the sleeve and the skin care is a lifelong routine and success depends on the patient's perseverance and motivation. Education is very important and the therapist spends a long time on this. If the patient is frail or has problems with dexterity a carer or spouse will need to be educated (British Lymphology Society 1999b).

Some patients find the sleeve difficult to cope with. They can be advised to wear it at active times and it can be removed when activity is lower. The sleeve will be least useful during rest and most useful when muscles are active. However, the constant use of a sleeve can have a negative effect on the patient's body image, being seen as an additional stigma causing embarrassment and reducing self-esteem. The patient needs time to express her feelings; more emotional support may be required prior to the sleeve fitting. If the patient understands the sleeve's role in management she may accept it more readily. Patient information should include clear verbal/written information and the establishment of achievable goals. Once the swelling reduces and self-management is undertaken confidence and motivation may improve.

Multi-layer bandaging

If compression garments are contraindicated multi-layer bandaging can be used. This reduces symptoms and allows the patient to enter the maintenance phase. Short stretch bandages are used to create a graduated pressure – greatest at the wrist and gradually decreasing up the arm. The pressure of fluid in lymphatic and venous vessels of limbs is greatest distally and gradually reduces towards the proximal end of the limb. Fluid is encouraged upwards towards the root of the arm. The efficiency of the muscle pump and joints are improved. Voluntary muscle contraction and relaxation within the inelastic bandage cause variations in tissue pressure and stimulate the flow of lymph (Todd 2000). Graduated compression reduces the tourniquet effect. The bandaging helps to prevent the arm refilling with lymph and helps to break down deposits of scar and connective tissue, and minimizes inflammatory changes.

The short stretch bandages are 100 per cent cotton and are applied at 90 per cent stretch. The bandage is inelastic and provides a rigid support around the arm, which expands when the muscle contracts. This creates a high pressure beneath the bandage (sub-bandage pressure) when the muscle contracts as it meets the resistance of the bandage. The increase in pressure within the bandage is brought about by skeletal muscle activity and causes changes in the circumference of the limb. Graded pressure is achieved by selecting the correct width of the bandage, bandage overlap and the use of layers. All are held in place by tape.

A low sub-bandage pressure is created when the patient is still and the muscle is inactive.

This high-working, low-resting pressure provided by the short stretch bandage is comfortable for the patient. The bandages are inelastic and are reapplied daily as they will not fit the limb as it shrinks. The therapist must have a sound knowledge of the principles of bandaging in order that the procedure is safe and effective (Board and Harlow 2002c). This is a specialist technique and must be carried out by a trained, skilled therapist.

As with the other cornerstones of lymphoedema treatment a full medical history is taken by the therapist prior to bandaging.

Method

Each bandage is started distally, with more layers used at the distal end of the limb, and taken proximally. The fingers should be relaxed and are spread apart when applying the hand bandage. The patient is asked to make a fist during arm bandaging to achieve the tension required for a comfortable degree of exercise pressure.

1 The arm is washed and dried, and a non-perfumed moisturiser applied.
2 Stockinette is applied from the base of the fingers to the axilla with a hole cut out for the thumb.
3 Elastic gauze bandage is secured by a turn at the base of the hand with minimal tension and taken across to the dorsum of the hand to wrap each finger in turn. The wrist is not covered. Coming from the dorsum the first turn is taken at the base of the fingernail followed by circular turns around each finger. Slight tension is maintained. The thumb and fingertips may be left free as this does not adversely affect the reduction in swelling of the fingers (Todd 2000).
4 Padding is applied to the hand, wrist and arm to achieve a cylindrical shape and for protection. If a double layer of padding is required the bandage overlaps the prior turn by 50 per cent. The padding can be increased to protect the inside of the elbow (cubital crease). A second padding bandage can be used if one is not sufficient.
5 A 6cm bandage is secured by a turn at the wrist with minimal tension and taken across to the dorsum to wrap twice around the hand adjacent to the base of the fingers. All the hand is covered in successive wraps including the knuckles. The circles overlap and a number of circles are used to build up pressure. The fingers are kept open and extended. The remaining bandage is around the forearm in a spiral (Klose 1998).
6 An 8cm bandage starts at the wrist and covers the forearm. Each turn should overlap the previous one by two-thirds. After reaching the slightly flexed elbow the bandage runs across the cubital crease, once around the distal aspect of the upper arm and back down to the forearm, proceeding in a spiral to cover the elbow.
7 The 10cm bandage starts at the distal end of the forearm applied in the reverse direction to the previous bandage. This extends to the top of the arm and is secured by tape (Todd 2000). A moderately strong tension is kept on the bandage.
8 The bandage is checked for proper compression – the muscles of the limb are tightened and the degree of compression can be felt with one or both hands.

9 The arm should be easy to move with the bandages in place, it may, however, feel heavy. If the patient complains of pain, pins and needles, numbness or altered colour in the fingers the bandages must be removed (Klose 1998).

Padding and short stretch bandages are available on prescription. The procedure is done daily for 2–3 weeks and is very time-consuming. The patient or carer may be trained in the procedure; this should be encouraged and monitored carefully.

Compression pumps

Compression pumps can be used to move more fluid out when manual lymphatic drainage has been performed to trunk and arm. The pump consists of a power unit and various sizes of inflatable sleeve. These have a lining for easy cleaning and can be multi-chambered. The chambers inflate in a sequential pattern of compression up the arm. This ripple effect is more effective at moving fluid than a squeezing effect of a single chamber.

Usually lymphoedema which is mild responds best, very fibrotic lymphoedemas do not. There should be no truncal oedema present. Compression pumps tend to force fluid into the adjacent area and do not necessarily improve drainage in the long term. The trunk and the affected limb need to be cleared by manual or simple lymphatic drainage prior to the use of the pump. This may not always be done adequately. Small lymphatic vessels are fragile and easily damaged when a pressure of more than 60mm Hg is applied. Slightly deeper vessels may also be damaged. Scar tissue can form and block drainage in adjacent channels. The region of the arm above the sleeve can become overloaded, the lymphatics rupture and fibrous tissue can be formed in a band around the upper arm, making the lymphoedema worse (Casley-Smith and Casley-Smith 1998).

Low pressures are used, not more than 40mm Hg. Higher pressures can cause the lymphoedema to worsen. Compression pumps are not used if the arm is inflamed or infected. The arm is generally supported on the arm of a chair during treatment.

Compression pumps should not be used if the patient has an active cancer as there is a potential risk of spread.

Complications of lymphoedema

Acute inflammatory episode or cellulitis is the most serious complication experienced by patients with lymphoedema. A primary immune response cannot develop without lymphatics. In breast cancer related lymphoedema cutaneous responses are significantly impaired in the affected arm (Mallon et al. 1997).

Pain in lymphoedema can manifest in different ways, for example aching, throbbing, burning. The pain can increase as the day progresses and use of the limb can exacerbate it. Patients may have difficulty sleeping. Analgesia is not always effective but supporting the arm can give relief. Once treatment for swelling commences the ache generally eases (Twycross 2000). A patient with recurrent disease may experience brachial plexopathy causing neuropathic pain and a nerve block may be necessary.

High protein oedema can over time create fibrotic changes to the tissues. Thickness of the skin will occur with hyperkeratosis and papillamatosis (nodules protruding from the skin's surface). This generally occurs in the palliative stage of breast cancer.

Large amounts of lymph can leak through the skin and weep down the limb. This is known as lymphorrhoea and also generally occurs in the palliative stage of the disease. Non-adherent dressings and multi-layer bandaging are used. An emollient to act as a barrier is applied (Shankar et al. 2000).

Hyperkeratosis is scaly, warty changes to the skin. Fifty per cent white soft paraffin and 50 per cent liquid paraffin daily can be used to soften. Five per cent salycilic acid ointment is used in severe cases to ease the scales. Hydrocolloid dressings can be applied and left for 3–5 days to soften the hyperkeratosis and enable the scales to be lifted without damaging the underlying skin (Linnitt 2000).

Deep vein thrombosis can be caused by lymphoedema. This may be due to immobility of the limb, reduced venous flow or venous compression by a tumour in a patient with active malignant diseases (Keeley 2000).

Psychosocial aspects

Lymphoedema can become a social and physical handicap. It can affect quality of life and make everyday tasks difficult. Skilled psychosocial care is required to maintain motivation and encourage the patient to adapt.

The therapist empowers patients with lymphoedema and encourages them to achieve personal goals. The therapist develops a relationship that allows the patient to express her needs and ensures that she feels supported. Confidence and motivation may be very low and the patient may have a negative self-image and low self-esteem.

The visible change in the size and shape of a limb is a problem. It can be difficult to cover up with clothes and is a constant reminder of the cancer. The woman may dress differently than before, using baggy clothes to cover the arm where formerly she wore fitted clothes. However, even baggy clothes may not fit well if the swelling increases and buying clothes can be very depressing.

The patient may also find that wearing a compression sleeve has a negative effect on her body image. It may be difficult to put on and be a constant reminder of a chronic condition. Support and encouragement to wear the sleeve are very important.

Functional impairment can occur as the result of the weight of a swollen arm which becomes more difficult to move. The patient may have to remove rings and jewellery due to swollen fingers and fine movements used in writing, dressing and personal hygiene are difficult. Continuing to work may be problematic especially if computers are involved – lengthy periods at a computer can make swelling worse especially if the arm is unsupported.

Loss of self-esteem may lead to difficulties in family and sexual relationships as the strain of coping with lymphoedema takes its toll. The use of compression garments can cause the woman to feel less attractive with resulting problems with intimacy.

It is vital that the therapist is aware of potential psychosocial problems and her attitude can be very influential. The patient should feel able to discuss concerns and feel supported whilst aiming for a normal life. Good communication skills are vital (Woods 2000).

References

Badger C (1993) Guidelines for the calculation of limb volume based on surface measurements. British Lymphology Interest Group Newsletter 7: 3–7.
Badger CMA, Peacock JL, Mortimer PS (2000) A randomised, controlled, parallel-group clinical trial comparing multi-layer bandaging followed by hosiery v hosiery alone in the treatment of patients with lymphoedema of the limb. Cancer 88(12): 2832–7.
Bellhouse S (2000) Simple lymphatic drainage. In Twycross R, Jenns K, Todd J (eds) Lymphoedema. Oxford: Radcliffe Medical Press.
Board J, Harlow W (2002a) Lymphoedema 1: Components and functions of the lymphatic system. British Journal of Nursing 11(5): 304–9.
Board J, Harlow W (2002b) Lymphoedema 2: Classification, signs, symptoms and diagnosis. British Journal of Nursing 11(6): 389–95.
Board J, Harlow W (2002c) Lymphoedema 3: The available treatments for lymphoedema. British Journal of Nursing 11(7): 438–50.
Breast Cancer Care (1999) Living with Lymphoedema after Breast Cancer Treatment. London: Breast Cancer Care.
British Lymphology Society (1999a) Chronic Oedema: Population and Needs. Sevenoaks: BLS. www.lymphoedema.org/bls/blsd0010.htm

British Lymphology Society (1999b) Strategy for Lymphoedema care. Sevenoaks: BLS. www.lymphoedema.org/bls/blss0010.htm

British Lymphology Society (1999c) Guidelines for the Use of Manual Lymphatic Drainage (MLD) and Simple Lymphatic Drainage (SLD) in Lymphoedema. Sevenoaks: BLS. www.lymphoedema.org/bls/blsm0030.htm

Casley-Smith JR, Casley-Smith JR (1997) Modern Treatment for Lymphoedema. Adelaide: Terrace Printing.

Casley-Smith JR, Casley-Smith JR (1998) Other treatments for lymphoedema. Lymphoedema Association of Australia online. www.lymphoedema.org.au/tret_oth.htm

Hughes K (2000) Exercise and lymphoedema. In Twycross R, Jenns K, Todd J (eds) Lymphoedema. Oxford: Radcliffe Medical Press.

Keeley V (2000) Clinical features of lymphoedema. In Twycross R, Jenns K, Todd J (eds) Lymphoedema. Oxford: Radcliffe Medical Press.

Kirschbaum M (2000) Breast lymphoedema. In Twycross R, Jenns K, Todd J (eds) Lymphoedema. Oxford: Radcliffe Medical Press.

Klose G (1998) Lymphedema bandaging: Practical Bandaging Instructions for Lymphedema Patients and Therapists. Neuwied : Lohmann & Rauscher GMBH & Co.

Linnitt N (2000) Skin management in lymphoedema. In Twycross R, Jenns K, Todd J (eds) Lymphoedema. Oxford: Radcliffe Medical Press.

Lymphoedema Support Network (2002) www.lymphoedema.org. (accessed June 2002).

Mallon E, Posell S, Mortimer P, et al. (1997) Evidence for altered cell mediated immunity in post-mastectomy lymhoedema. British Journal of Dermatology 137: 928–33.

Mortimer PS (1995) Managing lymphoedema: clinical and experimental. Dermatology 20: 98–106.

Mortimer P (2000) Acute inflammatory episodes. In Twycross R, Jenns K, Todd J (eds) Lymphoedema. Oxford: Radcliffe Medical Press.

Mortimer PS, Bates DO, Brassington HD, et al. (1996) The prevalence of arm oedema following treatment for breast cancer. Quarterly Journal of Medicine. 89: 377–80.

Shankar S, Marshall K, Mortimer P (2000) Skin care in lymphoedema. British Lymphology Society Newsletter 28: 5–8.

Tobin MB, Lacey HJ, Meyer L, Mortimer P (1993) The psychological morbidity of breast cancer related arm swelling. Cancer 72: 3248–52.

Todd J (1996) Living with Lymphoedema. Your Guide to Treatment. London: Marie Curie Cancer Care.

Todd J (1999) A study of lymphoedema patients over their first 6 months of treatment. Physiotherapy 85(2): 65–76.

Todd J (2000) Containment in the management of lymphoedema. In Twycross R, Jenns K, Todd J (eds) Lymphoedema. Oxford: Radcliffe Medical Press.

Twycross R (2000). Pain in lymphoedema. In Twycross R, Jenns K, Todd J (eds) Lymphoedema. Oxford: Radcliffe Medical Press.

Williams A (1995) Skin care in patients with uncomplicated lymphoedema. Journal of Wound Care 5(5): 223–6.

Woods M (2000) Psychosocial aspects of lymphoedema. In Twycross R, Jenns K, Todd J (eds) Lymphoedema. Oxford: Radcliffe Medical Press.

CHAPTER THIRTEEN

Diet and complementary therapies

Diet and breast cancer

The area of research into diet is difficult as people eat a wide range of foods in varying amounts. Researchers recently have suggested that about 35 of every 100 cases of cancer can be prevented by altering the diet (CancerHelp UK 2001).

There is widespread professional and public interest in the possible link between diet and breast cancer. Much research is ongoing, and it appears to suggest that the risk of breast cancer can be reduced by making dietary changes. However, reports tend to be conflicting. For example, some research shows that high fat diets link with a higher incidence of breast cancer; other research does not. Women in South East Asia eat a diet much lower in fat and higher in soy and have few menopausal symptoms and a lower rate of breast cancer and this is often cited. Some studies have found a link with alcohol consumption; others have not. Other factors such as environmental, cultural and lifestyle must be considered (Breakthrough Breast Cancer online 2002).

A large-scale project, European Prospective Investigation into Cancer started in 1992 and will be producing reports on various types of cancer over 10–20 years commencing with breast and colon cancer. The research concentrates on the main food groups – fats, starchy carbohydrates and sugars, fibre, fruit and vegetables and proteins. Other research looks at the effects of obesity, alcohol, food additives and pesticides (CancerHelp UK 2001).

Women are generally advised to follow healthy eating guidelines. Women with a strong family history of breast cancer may be advised to eat a diet including foods that are thought to cut the risk of cancer. A woman who is taking Tamoxifen may be worried about weight gain and will be advised on healthy eating. Maintaining a normal body weight is an important consideration. There is strong evidence that obesity and breast cancer are linked.

As with all other aspects of breast cancer treatment the patient is assessed individually. Breast care units can usually involve the services of the dietitian if required.

Fruit and vegetables

All nutritional advice includes the recommendation that people eat five or more portions of fruit and vegetables per day. This is important as fruit and vegetables contain antioxidants, which protect cells from damage. Cell damage may start the process of a healthy cell becoming a cancer cell. Molecules of oxygen within cells known as free radicals are produced naturally by the cell as a by-product of activity or in response to harmful contact with something. These antioxidants absorb free radicals.

Fruit and vegetables also enhance the immune system. Oestrogen levels may also be altered as some parts of vegetables and fruit cause the breakdown of oestrogen to weaker levels. Some chemicals, for example dithiolthiones found in broccoli increase the action of detoxifying enzymes in the body – these enzymes detoxify carcinogens (Naieralski and Devine 1999).

Important antioxidants in vegetables and fruit are vitamin C and beta-carotene, a carotenoid. Carotenoids are chemicals that are found in dark green leafy vegetables such as spinach and brightly coloured vegetables such as carrots. Carotenoids may contain vitamin A, which has a possible activity against breast cancer. However, the conversion of beta-carotenes to vitamin A by the body weakens the antioxidant effect. Lycopene is a carotenoid found in tomatoes and tomato products although some can be found in canned apricots, watermelon and pink grapefruit. It is a more powerful antioxidant than beta-carotene as it is not converted to vitamin A when ingested. The availability of lycopene increases with food processing so there is more in canned tomatoes than fresh. It has been suggested that lycopene can reduce the risk of breast cancer (British Nutrition Foundation online 1999). However, there have been no placebo controlled clinical intervention trials in humans yet so advice is generally given to consume a wide variety of fruit and vegetables including ones containing lycopene.

Sweet potatoes and carrots are especially high in beta-carotenes, some of which are converted to vitamin A by the body. A compound such as carotenoid derived vitamin A encourages a cell to differentiate (develop) and interferes with the process of uncontrolled division typical of a cancer cell (Naieralski and Devine 1999). Vitamin A can be obtained from animal sources such as dairy products and oily fish.

Increasing vitamin A from fruit and vegetables can be beneficial for healthy breast development, teenage girls can be encouraged to help prevent breast cancer in the future by increasing vitamin A in the diet. It does not have to be eaten every day and a varied, balanced diet should be sufficient.

However, all beta-carotenes should be obtained from the diet. Caution should be used in the use of high doses of purified supplements of micronutrients such as vitamins C and E as they cannot be assumed to be without risk. Beta-carotene supplements should be avoided as high doses of vitamin A are toxic and may be carcinogenic in high risk patients. A healthy, balanced diet should provide all vitamins and minerals necessary (Food Standards Agency online 2002).

Other antioxidants include some substances that colour and flavour fruit and vegetables. Some also contain vitamin E, another antioxidant – nuts, seeds, vegetable oils and some cereals (British Nutrition Foundation online 1999).

Other valuable vitamins include:

- Vitamin C (ascorbic acid) – found in citrus juices and fruits, for example oranges, grapefruits. Also found in green peppers, cauliflower, tomatoes, strawberries and leafy green vegetables.
- Folic acid – a vitamin found in leafy green vegetables, asparagus, broccoli, beets and some types of beans.
- Selenium – a mineral obtained by plants from the soil. Can be taken as a supplement.

Fruit, vegetables, wholegrains and cereals are also high in fibre, important in healthy eating. Wheat bran fibre has been found to lower oestrogen levels in pre-menopausal women but it is not clear how.

Phytoestrogens

Phytoestrogens are found in plant foods especially soya beans. Most phytoestrogens come from one of three chemical classes – isoflavanoids, lignans or coumestans. Isoflavanoids are found in beans from the legume family, soy beans and soy products. Some epidemiological evidence and evidence from animal studies suggests that soya beans may reduce the risk of breast cancer developing. Isoflavanoids include genistein and daidzen, which have been shown to act as weak oestrogens (British Nutrition Foundation online 1999). Genistein has been shown in a recent study to kill one type of breast cancer cell (American Institute of Cancer Research 2002).

Lignan phytoestrogens are found in brans and flaxseeds. Coumestan phytoestrogens are found in split peas, lima beans, alfafa and clover sprouts. Many fruits and vegetables including apples, pears, carrots, onions, corn as well as garlic and olive oil contain phytoestrogens. Phytoestrogens can either act like oestrogen or block its effects. Oestrogen receptors can be activated by phytoestrogens depending on the dose (Warren and Devine 2001). Phytoestrogens compete with oestradiol by trying to bind to the oestrogen receptor complex but fail to stimulate a full oestrogenic response on binding.

Early research showed that women who have a diet high in phytoestrogens have a lower risk of breast cancer. In the late 1990s, women were often advised to eat foods and supplements containing isoflavones to reduce menopausal symptoms as women in cultures whose diet is high in soy products rarely experience these symptoms.

However, it is currently unclear whether soy foods affect breast cancer risk. Some studies show that potentially soy phytoestrogens can behave like oestrogen and increase risk. Caution should be exercised over eating large amounts. Moderate consumption of these foods is probably advisable. As phytoestrogens are naturally present in many fruit and vegetables, a broad-based diet will almost certainly contain some (Lawson and Lawson 1999).

There would also appear to be a possible increased risk from genetically modified soya from the US but the link is unclear. Also as phytoestrogens have a weak oestrogenic effect it is uncertain how this affects the growth of oestrogen sensitive breast tumours. Women with oestrogen receptor positive tumours or women who are taking Tamoxifen should avoid eating large amounts of soy until research is concluded (American Cancer Society 2000). The role of phytoestrogens is currently the subject of much research. Soy foods have been used for a very long time with safety but it appears that any expectations with respect to prevention of breast cancer should be treated with caution.

A study reported in July 2002 by Cancer Research UK, the National Cancer Institute in America and the National University of Singapore found that women who eat a soya rich diet had breast tissue that was less dense than women on low soya diets (BBC News Health online 2002). Higher breast density has been linked with an increased risk of breast cancer. This is the first study to link soya with an effect on breast density.

Alcohol

The link between alcohol intake and breast cancer is also the focus of much research. Information regarding this association may offer a practical way for women to reduce the risk of developing breast cancer.

Studies involving several different populations of women in several countries have shown a weak association between drinking low levels of alcohol and breast cancer risk, the risk increasing as the amount of alcohol consumed increases. However, other risk factors should be taken into account, for example age, family history, early menarche, all of which are established risks. Many studies have taken these into account and have also looked at factors such as diet and smoking. The results of many of these have suggested a direct link. Other researchers continue to study all aspects of behaviour and lifestyle as they are not convinced of the direct link.

There is a weak association between breast cancer and alcohol consumption in women who have one drink per day. Between two and five drinks per day may be associated with a rate that is 40 per cent higher than the rate for non-drinkers. This risk is around the same proportion to that of other risk factors (Naieralski and Devine 1998). The highest risk category therefore appears to be those women who 'binge' drink on more than five drinks per day.

The way in which alcohol influences breast cancer risk is being studied. The influence of alcohol on oestrogen may be significant, in some studies oestrogen levels have been shown to rise when alcohol has been consumed. However, results are not conclusive.

Low Vitamin B intake may increase the risk of breast cancer as DNA does not have the same capacity to repair. Alcohol intake increases the risk – evidence has been found from prospective studies of an interaction between alcohol and folate. The risk of a post-menopausal woman contracting breast cancer may be increased if she has a low folate intake and consumes alcohol (Sellers et al. 2001).

In all cases the woman needs to decide for herself but women with a strong family history of breast cancer may be advised to limit alcohol consumption.

Obesity and fat in the diet

Western nations where fat can make up 35-45 per cent of the diet have increased rates of breast cancer. In South East Asian nations, for example Japan, the diet is about 15 per cent fat and the incidence is lower (Oncolink online 2002). When Japanese women emigrate to the USA where the incidence is high their breast cancer risk goes up. This suggests that the difference must be due to the lifestyle or environment. The dietary change is the most obvious as Americans eat far more fatty foods. Populations currently at highest risk of breast cancer are North America and Europe where the risk is five times higher than in Asia according to the government document 'Nutritional Aspects of the Development of Cancer' (DoH 1998). This recommends that adults maintain a healthy body weight and do not increase it during adulthood. Studies in this area are contradictory but it may be that fats eaten in childhood and teenage years are increasing the risk of breast cancer (CancerHelp UK 2001).

There appears to be strong evidence of an increased risk of breast cancer in post-menopausal women who are obese. There is a positive association between Body Mass Index and post-menopausal breast cancer. Obese is more than 40 per cent overweight. The role that fat plays is unclear but the level of fat intake may influence oestrogen levels. An increased risk of breast cancer is associated with a higher serum concentration of oestrogen in post-menopausal women. Oestrogen is synthesized from the precursor hormone androstendione in adipose tissue. This becomes the main source after the menopause and therefore in women who lose weight serum concentrations fall. Post-menopausal overweight women have a two-fold greater risk of breast cancer. The effect of weight in pre-menopausal women does not seem to be consistent (Cummings and Bingham 1998). A high-fibre, low-fat diet may lower oestrogen levels in pre-menopausal women but it is not known whether it is the high fibre or low fat which is responsible.

There is moderate evidence that the consumption of red and fried meat may also increase the risk. The consumption of red and processed meat should be reduced. The World Cancer Research Fund recommends that red meat should provide less than 10 per cent of total energy on average. The Department of Health (1998) report recommends that people who consume more than 14 portions of red meat per week should consider reducing this.

Therefore, it is prudent for patients with breast cancer and high-risk women to cut back on dietary fat to about 20 per cent of calories from fat with about five per cent coming from animal sources such as milk, butter, yoghurt, meat and 10 per cent or more from fish or plant sources, for example vegetables, seeds, nuts and fruits. Too little fat can also be harmful and going under 15 per cent of total calories per day from fat will require a supplement of flaxseed oil for essential fatty acids. These are necessary for healthy skin and for brain and nervous function. Omega-3 fatty acids are found in oily fish, some seeds, nuts and vegetables. Evening primrose, borage and flaxseed are good sources of gamma linoleic acid (GLA), important for regulating hormones. Fish oil supplements can be taken instead of eating fish.

Different kinds of fat may have different effects on breast cancer risk. Studies have found that polyunsaturated fat found in many vegetable oils increased the risk but monounsaturates, for example olive oil, reduced it. This reflects another benefit of the 'Mediterranean' diet rich in fruit, grains, little meat and olive oil as the principal fat. The Bristol Cancer Help Centre also recommends healthy eating to strengthen emotionally, physically, mentally, spiritually and to promote healthy immune function. It is recommended that intake of fruit, vegetables, grains (for example wholewheat bread, brown rice), beans, lentils, seeds, nuts, sunflower/olive oils and water is increased. These foods have the added benefit of being rich in fibre, another important constituent of a healthy diet.

Psychological factors such as improvement of mood may influence adherence to dietary change. Besides the possible direct effects of a healthy diet, there are added psychological benefits – improved self-esteem, motivation and mood that may accompany a person's ability to change her behaviour and to maintain that change (Hebert et al. 2001).

Dairy foods

Studies are inconsistent and there is not enough information available for women to choose individual dairy foods or no dairy foods to reduce the risk of breast cancer. Emphasis has to be placed on optimum nutrition for healthy eating and factors such as eating for a healthy heart should be taken into consideration. Also calcium intake is an important issue for women and calcium taken within the first 30 years of life establishes bone density. Any studies linking high bone density with increased breast cancer risk are thought to be the result of raised oestrogen levels and not associated with diet (Warren 2000).

Milk and dairy products may also be supplemented with vitamins A and D, which both have a possible activity against breast cancer.

It has been claimed recently that a dairy free diet can prevent breast cancer but the charity Breakthrough Breast Cancer has challenged these claims (BBC News Health online 2000).

The general consensus for optimum health, therefore, appears to be to eat more healthily in general. Health care professionals can help patients by recommending that they eat:

- less fat
- more fruit and vegetables and fibre
- grilled/stewed meat
- more poultry, fish and vegetable protein instead of red meat
- more starchy foods
- less processed/sugary foods
- polyunsaturated or monounsaturated fats instead of animal fats
- less alcohol.

Complementary therapies

Most treatments in this country are based on Western medicine, which uses a scientific model to prove the benefits of the treatment. Some complementary therapies originate from Eastern traditions. Complementary therapies may be available on the NHS and are viewed as treatments that are given alongside conventional cancer treatments.

Complementary therapies share some common characteristics:

- Natural healing – the purpose of cancer treatment would be to restore the ability of the immune system to locate and destroy cancerous cells.
- Holistic medicine – seeks the root and treatment of disease in the individual's mind, body, family, community and environment. For example, the theory that a person's temperament, family and social links affect the onset and course of the disease.
- Non-invasive medicine – therapeutic procedures are gentle and can even be pleasurable, for example massage, which has a low risk of side effects. The therapeutic partnership between the patient and practitioner is particularly important.
- Patient participation – patients take an active role, for example making lifestyle and dietary changes, practising exercises mentally and physically and playing the central role in decision making about treatments (Vickers 1996).

However, many of these characteristics are also found in conventional medicine:

- Most doctors avoid intervention where possible.
- The holistic approach is increasingly common practice.
- Many conventional practices are non-invasive.
- Many practitioners recognize the importance of building a relationship and giving time to talk and listen.
- Many doctors are increasingly willing to share information and decision making with patients and are increasingly aware of the trend for self-help and lifestyle changes (Vickers 1996).

In the past, alternative and some complementary therapies have not been scientifically studied or validated. However, studies have now been undertaken in some therapies, for example hypnotherapy and relaxation, and some are ongoing.

Patients must not miss the conventional methods of cancer treatment and can be advised that complementary therapies can improve well-being and offer support. They should discuss their treatment with the breast cancer consultant who will be generally supportive but may advise against certain alternative therapies. Seeking alternative treatment instead of conventional may be because the patient is confused, lacks information or feels that she has not been listened to. She may feel that the medical team can do no more for her. It is important that the patient is encouraged to get all the information and support relevant to her cancer from her doctor and breast care team to avoid seeking help from alternative practitioners.

Alternative therapies are generally intended for use instead of conventional treatments. Some doctors are concerned as they believe that there is no scientific evidence that alternative therapies can cure or arrest cancer. They do not wish patients to be misled or given false hope. Alternative medicine is becoming increasingly popular throughout our culture. Some common forms of alternative nutrition therapy include herbs and enormous doses of minerals and vitamins (10 times the recommended daily allowance). These are potentially toxic and benefits have not been proven (Hannon and Silagyi-Rebovich 1999).

Dietary regimes and unconventional medicines are other alternative therapies and may be harmful. Herbal medicines may interact with conventional medication. Treatments such as Essiac and shark cartilage are unproven to have an effect on cancer.

Some patients may try unconventional therapies such as homeopathy. Homeopaths may use homeopathy to treat symptoms of the disease or the side effects of treatment such as chemotherapy or radiotherapy. It is important to ascertain whether patients are taking homeopathic remedies or indeed any other alternative therapies when planning treatment for breast cancer. It is important that the breast cancer team feel that it can do no harm and that the therapist is not trying to dissuade her from undergoing conventional treatment.

However, certain complementary therapies, for example counselling are recognized as having positive effects on patients' well-being. Often counselling is part of the conventional treatment. Others, for example massage and relaxation are accepted as they make patients feel better and cope better with the illness (Cancer Bacup UK 2001/2002). The patient's relatives or carers may also be offered the same service to help them to cope with the cancer diagnosis.

Patients must seek advice from the breast care team before consulting a complementary therapist. The therapist must be qualified and the cost of the therapy should be ascertained. However many cancer units now offer various complementary therapies as part of treatment. The therapy chosen must suit the patient's needs and if the therapist is not allied to the unit it should be checked that a cure is not being promised as no reputable therapist would offer this.

Some examples of conventional support offered by cancer treatment centres and hospices may include: psychotherapy, counselling, relaxation, massage, aromatherapy, hypnotherapy, healing, art therapy and self-help groups.

The concept that a change in attitude to having cancer may affect the outlook influences many complementary approaches. Although a positive attitude helps people to cope with cancer, it is not always possible to be positive and show a fighting spirit. This does not mean that the chances of a good outcome are lowered. Anything that helps the patient to cope is valuable but patients must not be made to feel guilty if they are too tired or are experiencing feelings of helplessness, which are common in cancer patients.

The effect of complementary approaches is difficult to evaluate but many people find them helpful in improving quality of life (Cancer Bacup UK 2001/2002). A study by Downer et al. (1994) found that patients using complementary therapies tended to be younger, female and of a higher social class. They tended to be anxious and found that the benefits of complementary therapies were mainly psychological – improved optimism and hope.

Psychological and self-help therapies

Counselling

Often counselling is not formal, it is undertaken by family and friends in the form of careful listening. However, it is easier sometimes to talk to an impartial person. The patient will be allowed to express her feelings in a safe environment and may be able to put a different perspective on things and make decisions. Counselling is usually available at GPs' surgeries or the cancer centre or patients can be advised to contact the British Association of Counselling. Cancer Bacup and Breast Cancer Care also do telephone counselling.

Relaxation

Relaxation techniques can be used to relieve many symptoms of tension such as tense muscles, racing heart, hyperventilating, persistent exhaustion, difficulty sleeping, aches and pains, loss of appetite and inability to concentrate. Simple breathing and relaxation self-help exercises are very useful and the technique is easily learned. Anxiety and muscle tension are relieved and patients and their relatives can learn to relax and be calm. A group or self-help cassette can be accessed. Motivation and practice are required for the use of a cassette, so a group may be better for some people. Exercises do not necessarily need to be done lying flat; sitting up is fine. Learning to physically relax muscle groups, meditation, mental relaxation and prayer are all possible approaches.

Visualization

This involves the use of imagination whilst in a state of meditation or relaxation. By imaging a peaceful scene the patient feels more relaxed. Therapists who use visualization in the treatment of cancer believe that the immune system can be stimulated to affect the growth of the cancer. Visualizing feeling better and stronger can help, and can assist mood improvement in breast cancer patients who are undergoing treatments.

Hypnotherapy

Hypnotherapy is the application of hypnotic techniques in order to bring about therapeutic changes. There is a variation in therapists' techniques. The mind and body are totally relaxed and nearly asleep but will remain aware and conscious of surroundings. The part of the mind on which the therapist is working will also be awake (National Council for Hypnotherapy 2001). Hypnosis can be useful in dealing with symptoms and side effects of treatments such as chemotherapy and radiotherapy, for example nausea and vomiting. Suggestion can then be used to benefit the patient by enabling them to gain control over symptoms or feel better.

Art therapy

Art therapy is used in many cancer centres to allow people to express them-selves through art. It is a non-verbal way of revealing deeper emotions that may not otherwise be clearly expressed. The therapist encourages the patient to communicate their feelings through drawing, painting or mod-elling. Reflecting on the images produced can help patients to understand and deal with the issues that arise. Patients may then become aware of pent-up feelings, which can be discussed if appropriate in their counselling sessions. It is not necessary to be able to paint well, patients are encouraged to be spontaneous. Sometimes the therapist will ask for something specif-ic, for example a picture of the cancer but generally it is a creative approach to dealing with a distressing experience (Cancer Bacup UK 2001/2002).

Self-help groups

Self-help groups are organized groups for patients and families. They can be helpful and are a source of information and support. Some are run by health care professionals; some by people with cancer. Coping strategies may be taught along with practical information and emotional support. In some areas there may be a separate support group set up for younger women who have specific issues such as bringing up a young family and career issues.

It is important to make new patients aware of the group so that they can attend if they wish. The group can be advertised in the breast care and oncology unit, and if the group is run by former patients they may leave a contact number in case there are any enquiries. An advertisement in the local newspaper may reach more people. It is important to hold meetings in a suitable venue. The room should be private and informal. If there is a centre for complementary therapies attached to the unit for example, meetings may be held there. Some areas may use a hospital conference room, local community centre or a volunteer's home for example. Refreshments should be provided. Groups often arrange a programme of speakers for the year so that the first part of the meeting is given over to a topic. This may be a talk from a health care professional or anyone with a special interest. The rest of the meeting should give members a chance to talk and share experiences.

The facilitation and running of the group are very important. Designated volunteers or health care professionals need to co-ordinate speakers, refreshments, finances and venues. A small charge per week may be made to cover costs and perhaps pay for trips out occasionally. All members need an opportunity to share feelings, anxieties and questions and the facilitator needs to control the group so that all who wish to do so speak and all feel valued. It may be especially difficult if a member has died. The remaining members need to feel supported and safe. It is important that the breast care nurse supports the group and facilitators if she does not run it herself and checks that the format is meeting members' needs, perhaps with a yearly audit in the form of a simple questionnaire.

The size and balance of the group will change over time as people move on and cease attending and new members arrive. It is important that the facilitator is flexible and moves the day and/or time of meetings each year if members wish it and the venue allows.

The charity Breast Cancer Care also run telephone support groups. Women with breast cancer can be linked together from their own homes and can discuss issues and feelings. This is facilitated by a breast care nurse and counsellor and run weekly for two months at a time. Various groups are running including young women, women with secondary breast cancer, lesbian and bisexual women with breast cancer and women who are Urdu speakers (Breast Cancer Care 2002).

Healing

Healers believe that they act as a channel through which healing energy flows into the patient. Healing can provide an important support for cancer patients and their families, but people seeking healing need to be aware that it cannot offer a miracle cure.

Meditation

Meditation is a deeper form of relaxation which clears all thoughts from the mind leaving the patient in a calm, peaceful state. This helps to reduce pain, fear, anxiety and depression. Meditation techniques do take practice but regular meditation can help people to feel in control. The patient's local cancer centre can probably provide contacts for people to learn how to meditate.

Physical therapies

Massage and aromatherapy

Almost all cultures throughout history have used massage as a form of health care. It is increasingly being accepted by the medical and nursing professions. Massage is a manual technique using a variety of strokes to move the soft tissue and muscles of the body. Fibrous tissue is broken up, stiff joints loosened and joints and tissues cleared of acids and deposits. Various techniques are used; a common one is the Swedish technique, which incorporates flowing, rhythmic movements. The key to massaging people with cancer is to be gentle and to make the massage enjoyable and calming (McNamara 1999).

Touch can relieve pain and distress and massage can be used to relieve muscle pain, tension, to relax and bring comfort. Massage may also improve vitality and aid sleep. It may also result in the release of fear and generate a feeling of being open to change (Vickers 1996). The use of touch can be useful in overcoming loneliness in patients with a cancer diagnosis. Patients who have difficulty expressing their feelings may find that the trust built up between them and the practitioner through touch provides the atmosphere for emotional expression. Massage can also help patients to improve their perception of their altered body image (Stevenson 1996). Practitioners provide emotional support just by their presence and by the time spent on massage.

It is also important to remember that some patients, for cultural or religious reasons will not want to be massaged or touched and differences must be understood and respected to prevent misunderstandings (McNamara 1999).

Aromatherapy oils are used to prevent friction and pain. These are highly concentrated essential oils. They are obtained from plants and aromatherapists use only whole essential oils from a single botanical source, for example rose, lavender, peppermint, lemongrass, camomile, bergamot. Benefits can also be gained from inhalation and adding to baths. The therapist will give the patient different oils to smell and let them choose. Different oils have different effects – care must be taken with some as they have oestrogenic properties. These are contraindicated in oestrogen dependent cancers. Some mood-altering oils may be used for depression. Massage and aromatherapy can also be stimulating and certain oils can be used to improve the lethargy and fatigue induced by radiotherapy (Stevenson 1996). If the patient does not want aromatherapy oils to be used, a carrier oil such as sweet almond oil can be used.

A full history is taken prior to a massage. The patient is usually referred by a health professional, often the breast care nurse, so will have been assessed prior to referral. Any allergies are noted. Practitioners should be fully trained and qualified.

The therapist working in a cancer unit will have understanding of anatomy and physiology but will also require some knowledge of cancer and knowledge of how the unit works so that the patient is reassured that she or he is part of their cancer team.

The whole body may be treated but often a massage is given to the head, hands, feet or back. For patients with breast cancer the affected arm will be avoided and also any areas undergoing radiotherapy. Any areas near a tumour or lymph nodes affected by cancer are avoided. Great care is taken when massaging a patient with bony metastases. Some other contraindications to giving a massage are:

- areas of skin infection because of the risk of spread
- recent scar tissue
- lesions, these should heal before being massaged
- bleeding
- thrombosis
- phlebitis
- hypertension
- hypotension (McNamara 1999).

The room is kept warm and quiet and the therapist may play soft music but not all do. It is important that the room is not too small to give the patient the feeling of maintaining some space. The room is designed to encourage relaxation as patients are generally very anxious on their initial visit. Explanation of the procedure and answering any questions the patient may have is done at the initial assessment prior to the actual massage.

It is important that the therapist bears in mind body image issues and takes time to put the patient at ease. A massage may last about 35–45 minutes, about 20 minutes for very ill patients (may be given in a hospice setting). A massage can be given with the patient lying down or sitting up – whatever is appropriate for the individual. The setting is tailored to the patient. The patient may appreciate the therapist checking verbally halfway through that she is comfortable and wishes the massage to continue.

An initial series of about six sessions may be planned, possibly more. The earlier the service is accessed the better the patient may cope. Massage sessions may be incorporated into a programme of therapies including relaxation and counselling, for example.

The therapist may work closely with the lymphoedema therapist who will undertake the bandaging and the therapist may undertake the specialized lymphoedema massage to assist her.

Yoga

Yoga is an ancient discipline concerned with developing a holistic and healthy lifestyle. It is a combination of mental and physical exercises to promote flexibility, increase stamina and reduce stress. Yoga classes work on suppleness, strength, stamina and concentration and aim to strengthen the body and calm the mind. Daily practice may increase strength, increase bone density and reduce the possible risk of osteoporosis (British Wheel of Yoga 2001).

Alexander technique

This is very helpful in cancer patients but some may find it too invasive as the therapist has to be close to the patient. It can help with tension and muscle problems, and with symptoms of stress. It can provide coping skills for the patient and improve movement and posture. The lessons are one-to-one and involve the patient's active participation. The teacher uses explanation and a guiding touch to help the patient rediscover their balance and poise. Co-ordination is improved and the patient learns how to relieve tension. The lessons involve some movement so are ideal for the newly diagnosed breast cancer patient who may be quite active, and also for carers.

Reflexology

Reflexology is a form of complementary medicine that uses massage to reflex areas in the feet. These reflex areas correspond to all parts of the body. Reflexologists work by applying pressure to the areas to release the blockages in energy channels running through the body and restore energy. This may not be offered at all cancer units as it is draining for the patient. It is also a diagnostic aid so may not be appropriate.

Acupuncture

Acupuncture is the placing of sterile needles to affect energy points below the skin. It is part of traditional Chinese medicine. In Chinese medicine chi is the life force. Acupuncture needles are placed along points in this system to help release the flow of chi and restore health and balance. Endorphins are released relieving pain and relaxing muscles. Acupuncture may be used to treat the side effects of chemotherapy such as nausea (Cancer Bacup UK 2001/2002). It may not be available on the NHS and may not always be advisable for breast cancer patients. The affected arm would need to be avoided when inserting the needles. Acupuncture is not widely available in cancer units.

Shiatsu

This is a Japanese form of massage. It is based on the concept that health depends on the balanced energy flow through channels in the body called meridians. Pressure is placed on these meridians to help the person's energy regain balance. Again, this may not be available in breast cancer units.

The NMC and complementary therapies

The Nursing and Midwifery Council (NMC; formerly the UKCC) states that complementary and alternative therapies are used increasingly in the treatment of patients. Nurses who practise these therapies must be competent in this area having undertaken thorough training. The patient must be aware of the therapy and give informed consent.

The Council does not have the responsibility for the standards of other bodies that offer training in complementary therapies. Therefore, it is the responsibility of individual practitioners to judge whether or not the qualification obtained in their chosen training has brought them up to a suitable level of competence.

Use of complementary therapies should be discussed within the health care team but individual practitioner is accountable for their practice. Employers may establish a framework of local policies for the use of complementary therapies to ensure that the practice falls within the scope of employment. Practitioners are still accountable to the NMC (NMC 2000).

References

American Cancer Society (2000) Soybean. www.cancer.org (accessed June 2002).
American Institute of Cancer Research (2002) www.aicr.org (accessed June 2002).
BBC News Health online (2000) Row over breast cancer diet claim. http://news.bbc.co.uk/1/hi/health/781089.stm (accessed June 2002).
BBC News Health online (2002) Soya reduces breast cancer risk. http://news.bbc.co.uk/1/hi/health/2097053.stm (accessed October 2002).
Breakthrough Breast Cancer online (2002) FAQ (Frequently Asked Questions) about breast cancer. www.breakthrough.org.uk (accessed June 2002).

Breast Cancer Care (2002) Telephone support groups 2002. Leaflet. London: Breast Cancer Care.

British Nutrition Foundation online (1999) www.nutrition.org.uk (accessed June 2002).

British Wheel of Yoga (2001) About Yoga. www.bwy.org.uk (accessed June 2002).

Cancer Bacup UK (2001/2002) Cancer and complementary therapies. www.cancer-bacup.org.uk (accessed June 2002).

CancerHelp UK (2001) Healthy Eating. www.cancerhelp.org.uk (accessed June 2002).

Cummings JH, Bingham SA (1998) Diet and the prevention of cancer. British Medical Journal 317: 1636–40.

Department of Health (1998) Nutritional Aspects of the Development of Cancer. Report on the Working Group on Diet and Cancer. Report on Health and Social Subjects No 48. London: The Stationery Office.

Downer SM, Cody MM, McCluskey P, et al. (1994) Pursuit and practice of complementary therapies by cancer patients receiving conventional treatment. British Medical Journal 309: 86–9.

Food Standards Agency online (2002) www.foodstandards.gov.uk/healthiereating/ (accessed June 2002).

Hannon HL, Silagyi-Rebovich EJ (1999) Alternative Nutrition Therapy and Breast Cancer. Nutrition Research Newsletter March: 1.

Hebert JR, Ebbeling CB, Olendzki BC, et al. (2001) Change in women's diet and body mass following intensive intervention for early stage breast cancer. Journal of the American Dietetic Association 101(4): 421–31.

Lawson A, Lawson J (1999) Breast Cancer – Can You Prevent It? Sydney: McGraw-Hill.

McNamara P (1999) Massage for People with Cancer. London: The Cancer Resource Centre.

Naieralski JA, Devine C (1998) Alcohol and the risk of breast cancer. Factsheet #13. Cornell University Programme on Breast Cancer and Environmental Risk Factors in New York State (BCERF). www.cfe.cornell.edu (accessed June 2002).

Naieralski JA, Devine C (1999) Fruits and vegetables and the risk of breast cancer. BCERF www.cfe.cornell.edu (accessed June 2002).

National Council for Hypnotherapy (2001) www.hypnotherapists.org.uk (accessed June 2002).

Nursing and Midwifery Council (2000) Complementary and Alternative Therapies. (Advice statement). London: NMC.

Oncolink online (2002) Risk factors and breast cancer. www.oncolink.com (accessed June 2002).

Sellers TA, Kushi LH, Cerhan JR et al. (2001) Dietary folate intake, alcohol and the risk of breast cancer in a prospective study of post menopausal women. Epidemiology 12(4): 420–8.

Stevenson C (1996) Cancer care. In Vickers A (Ed.) Massage and Aromatherapy: A Guide for Health Professionals. London: Chapman & Hall.

Vickers A (1996) Massage and Aromatherapy: A Guide for Health Professionals. London: Chapman & Hall.

Warren BS (2000). Dairy foods and the risk of breast cancer. Factsheet #33. BCERF www.cfe.cornell.edu (accessed June 2002).

Warren BS, Devine C (2001) Phytoestrogens and breast cancer. Factsheet #01. BCERF www.cfe.cornell.edu (accessed June 2002).

World Cancer Research Fund (1997) Food, nutrition and the prevention of cancer: a global perspective. Washington DC: WRCF. American Institute for Cancer Research.

CHAPTER FOURTEEN

Fungating malignant breast wounds

Introduction

The presentation of cutaneous skin metastases in breast cancer patients varies and can even be taken for benign skin changes. Lesions develop as hard, immobile nodules, plaque formations and ulcerating wounds. They are characterized by tumour invasion with rupture of capillaries, infection and necrosis, which results in a fungating, malodorous lesion. This is characterized by pain, bleeding and exudate, as well as by malodour. Cutaneous metastases occur in about 2.7–4.4 per cent of all cancer patients. A fungating wound may also develop from a primary tumour of the skin or from an underlying tumour. These wounds are associated with advanced systemic disease and in many cases expected survival is less than a year (National Cancer Institute 2000). However, some may be present (often unreported) for many years. The reasons why some women delay in reporting a breast lump are discussed in Chapter 11. The presence of an exuding, necrotic, malodorous skin lesion is a constant visible reminder that the cancer is incurable and progressive. Health professionals must not underestimate the seriousness of these distressing wounds for patients. These lesions present a major challenge to the multidisciplinary team. Their presence is a constant reminder that the patient is in the terminal stage of their cancer and that in most cases treatment is palliative. The goal is to improve or maintain quality of life through effective symptom control. The individual should be the focus of assessment and management and all subsequent care should be holistic (Bird 2000). Community nurses will manage fungating breast wounds for much of the time and will require support from the breast care team and also from the palliative care team. Women with fungating breast wounds require much help and support to ensure that their quality of life is as good as possible.

Prevalence

Fungating wounds tend to develop in more elderly patients (over 70 years) with metastatic cancer in the terminal stages of the disease (Ivetic and Lyne 1990). Approximately 62 per cent of fungating wounds will develop in the breast area (Thomas 1992). The incidence in recent times is unknown as these wounds are not recorded in population-based cancer registries and it is difficult to determine accurately the number of patients in the UK with fungating wounds. Sometimes a fungating wound is only discovered when the patient is admitted to hospital or onto the community nurse's caseload for another reason – the patient may have been dressing it herself for a long period of time informing no one of its presence.

The significance of fungating wounds should be considered in terms of the impact on the individual, family and community resources of a long period of managing an uncontrolled, malignant wound (Grocott 2000b). Patients may live for years with a fungating wound if it is localized but healing is unlikely.

The disease process

The term 'fungating' refers to a malignant process of proliferative and ulcerating growth (Grocott 1995). A cancerous tumour is an expanding mass of disorganized tissue produced by the replication of abnormal cells. It will invade and destroy adjacent tissue and can spread to other tissues within cells that break off and travel in the lymph or blood system. The tumour can develop its own blood supply, sometimes outgrowing it and causing the tumour to become necrotic in the middle. Fluctuations in local blood supply and cell perfusion lead to hypoxic regions within the tissue margins increasing the likelihood of necrosis.

Lesions with a predominantly proliferative growth pattern may develop into a nodular 'cauliflower' or 'fungus' shape, whereas an ulcerating lesion will present as a wound which appears to be crater-like (Grocott 1999). Some lesions may appear with a mixture of both characteristics. They may develop in different ways:

- from a primary skin tumour, for example malignant melanoma/squamous cell carcinoma
- through direct invasion of the skin structures by underlying tumour, for example in breast cancer
- from metastatic spread of a more distant tumour. Metastases can occur along lymph vessels, capillaries or tissue planes (Grocott 1999).

As the tumour extends, it causes capillaries to rupture leading to tissue breakdown. The cancerous infiltration of the skin's epithelium results in ulceration and the lesion presents as a fungating, malodorous mass, which is constantly enlarging and changing shape if untreated. Disruption of the epithelial layer, which supports the blood and lymph vessels, can affect the blood, lymph, cellular and interstitial environments causing bleeding and lymphoedema (Lisle 2001).

The skin may be massively damaged by proliferative growth, ulceration and loss of vascularity leading to necrosis. As the skin is the body's largest organ the physical and psychological impact on the patient of an uncontrolled tumour infiltration is overwhelming. It is important to be aware of the routes for metastases and loco-regional spread so that some insight is gained to be able to plan clinical needs (Grocott 2000b).

The smell from fungating wounds is caused by a mixture of volatile agents, including short-chain organic acids, produced by anaerobic bacteria, for example, clostridium and bacteroids. Aerobes such as Klebsiella, Proteus and Pseudomonas also produce foul odours. These organisms cause a secondary bacterial infection by colonizing areas of slough and necrosis, the end products of ischaemia which has led to cell death and a build-up of dead cells.

A mixture of diamines and amines such as putrescine and cadaverine, which other proteolytic bacteria produce via their metabolic processes, also contribute (Thomas et al. 1998). The exudate from a wound can also lead to odour problems, leading to wet dressings and soiled clothing. More exudate is produced as the infection increases.

The effects of fungating wounds

Physical, psychological and social problems are associated with fungating wounds. A fungating, ulcerating wound usually indicates that the patient is coming to the end of their life and the patient and family have to face many problems. Issues are complex and as well as facing impending death they have to deal with pain, malodour, exudate and bleeding which have a devastating effect on the patient's physical and emotional well-being. A multidisciplinary approach is necessary so professionals can pool resources and manage these wounds effectively (Williams 1998).

Healing of a fungating wound is unlikely although chemotherapy or radiotherapy may sometimes elicit a good response. However, most will continue to deteriorate causing the patient to feel distressed, embarrassed and isolated. A fungating breast cancer is a double threat as the woman is facing a life-threatening disease. The emotional suffering can be greater than the physical pain and the patient may fear disfigurement and discomfort.

A fungating breast wound will affect the woman's self-image and her sexuality. Altered body image is a major problem. The female breast is regarded as a symbol of sexual desirability and femininity and society places great importance on having an attractive body. Body image is linked to feelings of self-worth and self-esteem. A healthy body image is desirable so a woman with a fungating wound, feeling less than physically acceptable, may do things to improve her self-image such as covering up the wound and denying that it is there. Although these wounds are not confined to late presentation, there are patients who for complex social and psycho-logical reasons delay presentation until the tumour is advanced and fungating (Fairbairn 1993). Others feel that the alteration of the breast by a fungating tumour means that they are no longer whole and lose the moti-vation to look attractive as the breast is non-functional and unrecognizable.

The woman may feel a great sense of loss of physical well-being and sex-ual function and may fear rejection. Intimacy with a partner may be affected. Feeling out of control and fear of the future leads to anxiety and depression. Sexual dysfunction may result in a fear of being touched due to the woman's negative feelings about her body.

The fungating breast wound is a problem as it is in close proximity to the woman's face. She may experience nausea, loss of appetite and weight loss (Benbow 1999). The smell causes social stigma and leads to feelings of guilt, shame, withdrawal, loneliness and depression. It reminds the patient that her body is infected or 'rotting' (Moyle 1998). This can also be extremely unpleasant for the carers who may experience gagging and vom-iting reflexes (Collier 1997a). People can become accustomed to odours but not those produced by putrescine and cadaverine (Van Toller 1994). Nurses must display great empathy and sensitivity but may not always be able to mask their instinctive responses to a malodorous wound and may find it distressing to deal with. This adds to the embarrassment and disgust felt by the patient especially as the odour may linger and permeate the home or ward. The psychological effect on the patient is heightened through the reactions of others (Moyle 1998). She may be reluctant to engage in social activities and quality of life will be affected. It also height-ens the sense of stigma (Kelly 2002).

Patients feel stigmatized socially when body fluids are uncontrolled (Goffman 1963). Leakage, staining and wetness of clothes by exudate can be extremely distressing for the patient and carers, leading to loss of con-fidence and social isolation. Lives can be ruled by dressing changes and laundry. Effective management using a socially acceptable dressing increas-es comfort and improves self-confidence. It is important that the patient continues with a normal life as much as possible. A wound management system that controls odour and wetness, restores body symmetry and takes into account the patient's physical appearance is desirable (Naylor 2002).

A fungating breast wound may also affect the adjacent limb causing lym-phoedema, pain, inflammatory episodes and immobility of the arm.

Referral to the lymphoedema specialist will be necessary (Grocott 2000b).

The incidence of psychiatric problems increases with advanced disease. The health care professional needs to be aware of this and be vigilant for signs of psychological distress and psychiatric problems. This may particularly apply to patients with disfiguring complications and may lead to despair and avoidance (National Cancer Institute 2000).

Nurses managing these wounds must assess the patient holistically and take a calm and sensitive approach. When breast cancer presents in this form, death is the most frequent outcome. Knowledge of current treatments and communication with other members of the multidisciplinary team are vital to maintain good symptom control and meet all the needs of the patient with a fungating breast wound.

Wound assessment

Fungating wounds can be managed equally as well in the home as in hospital or hospice and carers should be part of the team. The nurse needs to develop an understanding of the effects of the disease, physically, psychologically, spiritually and emotionally and how it impacts on the patient and family. Much of the care is carried out by primary care nurses in the community and good channels of communication with the hospital staff are required.

Community nurses may find that the care of a patient with a fungating wound has a considerable impact on the caseload – a visit to undertake the dressing and support the patient may well be lengthy. The patient could require more than one visit per day. It may be necessary to request extra resources and assistance wherever possible. It is important that continuity of care is maintained due to the complex wound care.

The patient should be assessed holistically and it should be ensured that planned dressings or treatments do not interfere with other treatments such as radiotherapy. Assessment should include:

- relevant history
- cause and stage of the disease
- present treatment
- physical limitations of the patient
- nutritional status
- emotional and spiritual considerations
- the patient's understanding of the disease and self-perception
- the carer/family's understanding of the disease
- patient/carer influences
- environmental influences

- support systems
- condition of the wound and associated symptoms (Williams 1998).

A full wound assessment is also carried out:

- Location of wound – if the wound is extending to the axilla this could cause further problems related to lymphoedema.
- Size of wound – should be measured as accurately as possible and records kept of visual change. Photography can be used. This provides a two-dimensional view of the wound. It is important that the camera angle, the position of the patient and the focal length are consistent each time (Griffin et al. 1993). Digital photography is now increasingly being used and photographs can be stored within the computer. Written permission from the patient is necessary for these. A woman with breast cancer may find this intrusive so it is necessary to build a rapport with the patient before requesting consent for photographs. It is not always advisable to use wound tracing on fungating wounds as the contact can cause bleeding.
- Percentage of devitalized tissue within the wound margins. A wound classification tool can be used to note whether the wound is necrotic, sloughy or granulating (Collier 1997b).
- Depth of wound.
- Amount of exudate.
- Odour (an odour assessment tool can used – see below) – also the patient's reporting of the odour should be taken into account.
- Pain – pain in the wound, pain during the dressing procedure, pain in between (often related to the disease process) (Schulz 1999).
- Condition of the surrounding skin – whether red, inflamed, macerated, affected by radiotherapy or adhesive tape used for dressings.

The nurse should have an up-to-date knowledge of the disease process and of the principles of wound healing. Community nurses are often very knowledgeable about wound care and should ensure that they maintain clear channels of communication with the breast care or palliative care nurses regarding changes to the planned treatments. However, the nurse should bear in mind that the theory of moist wound healing accounts for epithelialization in a wound that is healing, not for the processes involved in managing chronic malignant wounds as these may deteriorate due to uncontrolled disease (Grocott 2000a).

Assessment of fungating wounds can be difficult as the assessment of factors such as malodour and exudate tend to be subjective. It is important that they are estimated accurately and consistently. A very heavily exuding wound requiring daily or more changes or a dry wound are easy to assess – less heavy and moderate levels present a difficulty (White 2001).

An appropriate documentation system should be in place. Regular wound assessments, measurements and photographs should be kept in the nursing notes. Nurses should ensure consistent care through the setting of goals and objectives and the formulation of a plan of care. This should take into account the holistic assessment of the patient's problems and needs, both physical, psychological and social.

Wound management

A histological assessment in the form of a wound swab can be carried out to confirm the presence of aerobic and anaerobic organisms. The metabolic by-products of these organisms can be identified by liquid gas chromatography, a process that can be undertaken in clinical laboratories (Collier 2000a). However, the bacteriology of fungating wounds is not fully established and the prescription of antibiotics may have a limited value (White 2001). The presence of slough or necrotic tissue could also mean that antibiotics may not be effective and the patient may also experience gastric side effects.

When selecting a dressing the nurse needs to consider such factors as:

- the level of exudate
- presence of infection
- stage of healing
- if the patient is to be treated at home or in hospital
- the position of the wound
- objectives for treatment of the wound
- any skin preparation to be used around the wound
- will the dressing be a primary dressing or a wound contact layer and secondary dressing
- how will a secondary dressing be secured to fragile skin
- the correct size of dressing (White 2001). The size and shape of the wound determines the size of the primary dressing, which should cover the wound and leave a margin of at least 2cm for adhesion.

Wound malodour

An odour assessment tool can be used, although it should be remembered that if the odour worries the patient it should be addressed even if the nurse feels that it is not a problem. Not all fungating wounds are necessarily malodorous.

Odour assessment tool:

- odour is classed as strong if the odour is evident on entering the room 6–10 feet (2–3 metres) from the patient with the dressing intact.
- odour is classed as moderate if the odour is evident on entering the room 6–10 feet (2–3 metres) from the patient with the dressing removed.
- odour is classed as slight if the odour is evident at close proximity to the patient with the dressing removed.
- no odour present if there is no odour evident even at the bedside with the dressing removed (Haughton and Young 1995).

The odour may be eradicated if the slough and necrotic tissue is removed by debridement. This should be autolytic or enzymatic, not surgical due to the risk of bleeding. The use of occlusive dressings such as hydrocolloids (for example, Tegasorb, Granuflex) will maintain the temperature and hydration of the wound and facilitate the autolysis of slough. Enzyme preparations (for example, Varidase) contain streptodornase to liquefy pus and streptokinase to activate fibrinolysis. These are effective for desloughing and removing dry eschars but are expensive.

Cadexomer iodine preparations (for example, Iodoflex) are also effective but may be uncomfortable for the patient and must not be used if the patient is allergic to iodine.

Hydrogels (for example, Intrasite) will also debride a wound, but more gently. They are insoluble hydrophilic polymers, which can retain and absorb fluid and also donate fluid to dead tissue to remove dry necrotic or sloughy wounds. It can be applied to a wound and covered with a secondary dressing – a hydrogel and a hydrocolloid will have a debriding effect.

Sugar paste and honey are old-fashioned remedies which both have debriding and antibacterial properties. The high sugar content produces a hyperosmotic wound environment, which inhibits bacterial growth. Some varieties of honey contain potent antimicrobial agents (Thomas et al. 1998). Frequent dressing changes are required and both honey and sugar paste are available in hospitals but not on prescription for patients in the community (Kelly 2002). However, some patients may wish to have a simple dressing that uses natural substances for the terminal stage of their life.

Larval therapy has also been investigated. If patients can tolerate it it may debride necrotic tissue and ingest the bacteria responsible for the odour (Thomas et al. 1996).

If the wound is infected and causing odour it should be appropriately treated. Topical antibiotics can be used if a wound swab indicates that they would be appropriate. Metronidazole is commonly prescribed, 400mg twice daily orally for 10 days. However, there may be side effects including nausea, vomiting, unpleasant taste, furred tongue and visual disturbances. The dose can be reduced to 200mg twice daily, which will reduce the side effects but still be effective (Young 1997). Metronidazole works by preventing bacterial replication through binding to aerobes' and anaerobes' DNA (Hampson 1996).

Metronidazole may be used topically for fungating wounds to treat odour. This is a clear transparent gel with a concentration of 0.8 per cent metronidazole and 0.02 per cent benzalkonium chloride solution and is available as Metrotop. Metronidazole is usually associated with anaerobic infection but in the concentration used topically it may have an effect on a range of aerobic organisms (Thomas et al. 1998). It is usually applied 1–2 times daily to the wound and covered by a secondary dressing. It can also assist in debridement of sloughy and necrotic wounds by facilitating autolysis. Care should be taken in pregnant or lactating women, as it can be systemically absorbed (Haughton and Young 1995).

Activated charcoal dressings are increasingly being used to control odour in the management of fungating lesions. A suitable cellulose fabric is carbonized by heating it under controlled conditions to produce activated charcoal cloth. The surface of the carbon then breaks down to form small pores. These increase the effective surface area of the fibres and therefore remove unpleasant odours – it is believed that the molecules responsible for the production of the odour are attracted to the surface of the carbon and adsorbed (held there) by electrical forces. These molecules are small and can be detected by smell in low concentrations in the air. A single dressing has a large surface area of carbon and can take up large numbers of molecules therefore removing odours over a long period (Thomas et al. 1998). Actisorb was the first produced commercially and is now obtained as Actisorb Silver (0.15 per cent silver chemically bound to the carbon) and is on nurse prescription for community nurses. The silver imparts extra anti-bacterial activity and kills the bacteria adhering to the cloth. It can be placed directly onto the wound and removes molecules causing odour and toxins and other materials in the wound fluid.

Many dressings are now available containing carbon. It is intended that some, like Actisorb Silver, be placed in direct contact with the wound. These vary in function and therefore in their ability to cope with wound exudates, another feature of fungating wounds. Carboflex is a multi-layered dressing that consists of a wound contact layer composed of both an alginate and Aquacel fibres. These are bonded to a plastic film that facilitates the passage of liquid in one direction only. Behind the film is a charcoal cloth and an absorbing layer. A sealed perforated plastic layer completes the dressing structure. It can be placed directly onto the wound (Thomas et al. 1998). Other primary charcoal dressings include Carbonet, Kaltocarb and Lyofoam C.

Other carbon dressings are designed to be used as a secondary dressing beneath a retaining dressing (for example, Clinisorb).

Miscellaneous measures for controlling odour include practical measures such as opening windows, having scented plants around and changing clothing and bed linen more frequently. Soiled dressings should be disposed of correctly. Aerosols or air fresheners may be used or the patient may prefer to use scented candles or aromatherapy oils in a burner. However, the patient and carers may come to associate the smell of scented products with the cancer.

A Prozone unit may be used in the hospital or hospice for the elimination of malodours. This is an ozone generator and is a fairly small and compact unit for commercial use. Ozone is a powerful oxidizer. Ozone is generated when a molecule of oxygen is illuminated by high-energy ultraviolet light. Ozone is formed when three atoms of oxygen are bound together instead of the normal two and it is this extra atom that makes ozone a highly energetic oxidizer. The unit eliminates unpleasant odours and creates a fresher atmosphere. Ozone also destroys bacteria with no harmful by-products, therefore levels of airborne micro-organisms are reduced and bacterial growth on surfaces are retarded.

Exudate

The amount of exudate produced by a fungating breast wound can be difficult to manage. High exudate levels are caused by increased permeability of blood vessels within the tumour and the secretion of vascular permeability factor by tumour cells (Haisfield-Wolf and Rund 1997).

If exudate is not effectively controlled maceration of the skin will occur. Maceration is the excoriation or stripping of the epidermis due to the prolonged presence of toxins on the skin (Collier 2000b). Excessive moisture is retained causing softening of tissue. Excessive wound exudate can cause maceration and delay healing. Peri-wound maceration and odour can be controlled by the control of exudate and is essential for the patient's quality of life. Maceration, or excoriation, often arises due to inappropriate dressings or too long a wear time. Judgement of a realistic wear time and careful dressing selection may avoid this (Nielsen 1999).

The size of a fungating wound and tissue necrosis present significant problems for the management of exudate. The problem is compounded by the site of the lesion and its shape, which affect the fit of the dressing selected. Exudate management depends critically on fitting conformable, high-quality materials that are suitable for the size of the wound.

Managing exudates therefore requires the maintenance of a moist environment for wound healing without excessive wetness. Certain factors need to be considered:

- the level and nature of the wound exudates
- the site and condition of the wound
- the fluid handling capacity of the dressing
- the specific needs of the patient
- the optimal wear time for the dressing
- the possibility of damage to surrounding skin by adhesives.

Partially occlusive dressings, which rely on absorbency and moisture vapour transmission rate (MVTR) for their ability to handle fluid, may reduce the risk of maceration. (Fluid handling is the method by which a dressing absorbs, retains and evaporates fluid from the wound bed and intact skin (Cutting and White 2002).)

Moisture vapour transmission rate is the ability of a dressing to absorb fluid from the wound and to permit a controlled loss by evaporation through the backing surface. This avoids a build-up of fluid in the dressing and the wound (Cutting and White 2002).

If a dressing has been designed for this purpose it will take up fluid from the wound and then lose it through its outer layer (MVTR). However dressings differ, from dry gauze dressings through to occlusive dressings. Occlusion may be appropriate providing that the dressing has sufficient absorptive capacity for the exudate as occlusive dressings have no effective MVTR. The ideal dressing would absorb exudate rapidly whilst still leaving an optimum moist wound healing environment. Then the absorbed exudate would pass through the dressing and into the atmosphere by MTVR (Cutting and White 2002). All exudates could then be coped with without maceration. A clear, aqueous exudate would be more likely to be absorbed and lost by MVTR than the viscous exudate from an infected fungating wound and dressings may need to be changed more frequently. The dressing's combined absorbency and MVTR would give as long a wear time as possible. This is the subject of much research and progress is being made.

Effective fixation of these dressings is critical. Training of nursing staff in their application may be necessary – for example, the stripping of the skin may be avoided by the 'patterned' application of adhesive (Grocott 1998). Dressings tend to be ineffective on irregular shaped, extensive fungating lesions on curved body sites. Dressings tend to be a standard size and shape and a patient with an uncontrolled lesion may experience severe pain and exudate leakage and soiling especially when moving about.

A study has been undertaken in collaboration with a dressings manufacturer to investigate new materials in a wide range of sizes. This has been trying to solve the problems of leakage, poor dressing fit and soiling of clothes, the need to repad dressings between changes and peri-wound maceration. Several different systems have been examined but the ideal system is not yet commercially available (Grocott 2000a).

A variety of dressings can be used to manage exudate. If the amount is low, dressings with a low absorbency can be used, for example semi-permeable film dressings or thin or regular hydrocolloids. Regular hydrocolloids come in a plain or bordered form. A gel is formed when exudate is absorbed into the hydrocolloid mass of the dressing (White 2001).

If exudate is moderate to high the dressing needs to be more absorbent and maintain a moist wound environment. A secondary dressing may be necessary irrespective of the type of primary dressing used. Hydrofibre dressings that are of a fibrous material but contain a hydrocolloid (for example Aquacel), or foam/hydropolymer dressings such as Tielle, Lyofoam, Biatain or Avance (which is impregnated with silver) may be suitable. Alginates can be used (for example Sorbsan); these will absorb fluid from the wound to form a gel and are effective in superficial or cavity wounds with moderate or high exudate. However, the alginate in available dressings tends to be insufficient for extensive exuding wounds (Grocott 2000a). Alternatively a non-adherent wound contact layer (N/A Ultra, Mepitel) with an absorbent pad, which allows venting of moisture through the back (e.g. Mesorb) can be tried (Grocott 1999). A heavily exuding wound may require more than one daily change – a stoma appliance can be used although care must be taken with the surrounding skin. A protective barrier product such as Cavilon can be used to reduce the macerating effects of the exudate on the skin.

A deep, full thickness wound or a cavity may require the insertion of an alginate ribbon. Cavity shaped foam dressings for very deep wounds such as Silastic foam can be used in hospital. This can be shaped to fit the wound and can be removed from the wound for cleaning. They help to restore body symmetry without the use of very bulky dressings. These dressings are not available on prescription for community nurses.

Cosmetic acceptability is vital even in the terminally ill patient, especially for a woman with a breast wound. A Netelast vest can be worn to hold dressings in place and reduce the need for tape on fragile skin. The nurse may be required to advise on suitable clothing so that the patient feels comfortable and confident enough to be with other people.

Pain

The pain of a fungating malignant wound can have various causes. The tumour can press on blood vessels and nerves. The exposure of the dermis means that the nerve endings are exposed leading to a stinging pain. Removal of the dressing or a poor dressing technique can cause a great deal of pain.

It is vital to assess pain properly to ascertain the appropriate treatment. Analgesia should be administered in accordance with the World Health Organisation (1996) guidelines for the control of cancer pain, and also local prescribing protocols. Analgesia should be administered so maximum benefit is gained during dressing changes, for example Oramorph can be given as a booster if the patient is taking slow-release morphine. If the dressing change is very painful the patient may be given Entonox during the procedure (Naylor 2002).

Non-adherent dressings are generally used to minimize the pain of dressing changes. Dressings that maintain a moist wound environment to reduce adherence and protect nerve endings should be selected. A product requiring fewer changes may be necessary. Irrigation with warm saline or water will be less traumatic than cleaning with a gauze swab. Assisting the patient into the most comfortable position and complementary therapies to aid relaxation may help.

Topical opioids can be used to reduce wound pain; 10mg of morphine or diamorphine to 15g of a hydrogel, for example Intrasite, can help the cutaneous stinging that is sometimes experienced (Back and Finlay 1995).

Palliative radiotherapy, chemotherapy or hormone therapy may also have an effect on pain. These may also help if the patient is experiencing pruritis – a creeping, itching sensation due to the activity of the tumour especially in inflammatory breast disease and cutaneous infiltration (Regnard and Tempest 1998). The side effects of these treatments should be carefully monitored as they may be unacceptable in a palliative care setting. Tamoxifen can be used to achieve tumour regression if the patient is not already taking it and may reduce the size and progression of the tumour.

Bleeding

Bleeding is common in fungating wounds. Malignant cells erode blood vessels, compounded by reduced platelet formation within the tumour. Spontaneous, profuse bleeding is extremely distressing and frightening for the patient and carers. Dressing changes may damage already delicate tissue and exacerbate bleeding (Naylor 2002). Prevention where possible is therefore important. Careful irrigation and the use of non-adherent dressings are necessary. The maintenance of humidity at the wound/dressing interface and the use of non-fibrous materials all help to prevent bleeding. Alginate dressings are absorbent and are marketed as having haemostatic properties but the fibres but may cause bleeding in fragile fungating wounds (Grocott 2000a).

Topical adrenaline 1:1000 and Sucralfate suspension can be applied in an emergency (Regnard and Tempest 1998). Gauze soaked in adrenaline 1:1000 applied with pressure for 10 minutes can be used to control haemorrhage and adrenaline can be carried by community nurses for such an emergency. Surgical haemostatic sponges can be used but are expensive.

Nutritional problems and wound healing

Cancer and cancer treatments can produce physiological changes that cause wound healing problems. The aspects of wound healing which have been altered are important when assessing a patient with a fungating wound.

In a patient with advanced cancer, cachexia may be evident, characterized by weight loss, malnutrition and anorexia. Most factors influencing wound healing are related to the patient's general health status including her nutritional status and the use of anti-cancer drug treatments. The patient needs higher levels than normal of carbohydrates, amino acids, lipids, water and minerals.

Protein metabolism is often affected in cancer patients. It may have indirect effects on wound healing. Antibody responses and certain leucocyte functions such as phagocytosis tend to be impaired if the patient is cachexic.

Glucose utilization may be increased due to altered metabolism. This results in inefficient use of energy. Carbohydrates are necessary for the cells' energy requirements, for example leucocytes and fibroblasts. Impaired healing results from an energy deficit.

Minerals and trace elements may be diminished in people with cachexia. Lack of potassium, calcium, sodium, phosphorus and magnesium will affect wound healing.

Vitamin deficiency in cancer patients is related to altered metabolism and impaired absorption. Vitamin C is the most important vitamin for wound healing. Vitamin A deficiency may influence some aspects of wound healing (Lotti et al. 1998).

The use of Miltefosine

Miltefosine (Miltex) is an unlicensed lotion used in the treatment of cutaneous lesions arising from breast cancer. It tends to be used in a clinical trials setting on a named patient only basis under close supervision by the oncologist. Miltefosine is classed as a chemotherapy agent but causes no systemic side effects. It belongs to a class of cytostatic agents. It is active at the cell membrane level, interfering with cell growth and differentiation.

Miltefosine was the first product in its family to be approved for topical application to cutaneous metasteses in skin metastatic breast cancer. It is a palliative treatment that tries to contain local recurrences and improve quality of life without systemic side effects (Cazap et al. 2001).

It is an oily lotion applied to the skin daily for a week then twice daily for as long as necessary if well tolerated. Treatment continues for eight weeks unless unacceptable side effects occur or disease progresses. It is generally well tolerated without many side effects (Cazap et al. 2001). Even if the nodules shrink the dosage should remain the same and treatment should continue for four weeks after the nodules have disappeared. Miltefosine is available in 10ml bottles. There are 40 drops in 1 ml. The dosage depends on the surface area to be treated plus a 3cm border all around the area. It will not work on a pedunculated lesion.

The area to be treated can be washed and dried gently. The required amount is then measured and applied with a gloved finger onto the lesion and the 3cm border around it. The lotion should be applied even if the wound is fungating and bleeds. The lotion will not sting and it will clean the area and encourage granulation. A period of 15–30 minutes should be allowed for it to dry, then a dressing can be applied if necessary.

Local skin reactions such as erythema, burning and pruritis may occur but aqueous cream can be applied between applications of Miltex. These reactions may be mild (Cazap et al. 2001). The number of drops can be reduced if there is still a problem until the reaction settles, then the normal dose can be reintroduced. The treatment can be undertaken by community nurses if the patient is at home as no special precautions are required. Miltefosine is an attractive treatment option as the patient can undertake the application herself if she wishes to do so. The use of Miltex is usually introduced and supervised by the research nurse attached to the unit following thorough explanation to the patient and obtaining her informed consent.

It is essential that a holistic approach be taken to caring for the patient with a fungating wound. The breasts are a symbol of femininity and the alteration of a breast by such a wound can have devastating effects on the woman's physical, psychological and social health. When breast cancer presents in this form, death is the most frequent outcome and the care of the patient should be multidisciplinary to maintain dignity and quality of life.

References

Back IN, Finlay I (1995) Analgesic effect of topical opioids on painful skin ulcers. Journal of Pain and Symptom Control 10(7): 493.

Benbow M (1999) Malodorous wounds: how to improve quality of life. Community Nurse 5(1): 43–6.

Bird C (2000) Managing malignant fungating wounds. Professional Nurse 15(4): 253–6.

Cazap E, Koliren L, Jovtis S, et al. (2001) Abstract no. 146. Phase 2 study of 6% miltefosine solution (Miltex) as local treatment in cutaneous metastatic breast cancer (MBC) patients. Preliminary results. Grupo Cooperative ASTA Medica, Mendoza 1259–1428. Buenos Aires, Argentina. www.esmo.org/reference/abstracts/bca/146.htm

Collier M (1997a) The assessment of patients with fungating malignant wounds – a holistic approach: Part 2. Nursing Times 93(46): 1–4.

Collier M (1997b) The holistic management of fungating wounds. Nursing Notes 14: 2–5.

Collier M (2000a) Management of patients with fungating wounds. Nursing Standard 15(11): 46–52.

Collier M (2000b) Wound care. In Cooper S (Ed.) Stepping into Palliative Care: A Handbook for Health Professionals. Oxford: Radcliffe Press.

Cutting KF, White R (2002) Avoidance and management of peri-wound maceration of the skin. Professional Nurse 18(1): 33–6.

Fairbairn K (1993) Towards better care for women: understanding fungating breast lesions. Professional Nurse 9(3) 204–12.

Goffman E (1963) Stigma: Notes on the Management of a Spoiled Identity. Eaglewood Cliffs, NJ: Prentice Hall.

Griffin J, Tolley EA, Tooms RE, et al. (1993) A comparison of photographic and transparency based methods for measuring wound surface area. Physical Therapy 73(2): 117–22.

Grocott P (1995) The palliative management of fungating malignant wounds. Journal of Wound Care 4(5): 240–2.

Grocott P (1998) Exudate management in fungating wounds. Journal of Wound Care 7(9): 445–8.

Grocott P (1999) The management of fungating wounds. Journal of Wound Care 8(5): 232–4.

Grocott P (2000a) The palliative management of fungating wounds. Journal of Wound Care 9(1): 4–9.

Grocott P (2000b) Palliative management of fungating malignant wounds. Journal of Community Nursing 14(3): 31-40.

Haisfield-Wolf ME, Rund C (1997) Malignant cutaneous wounds: a management protocol. Ostomy Wound Management 43(1): 56–60, 62, 64–66.

Hampson JP (1996) The use of metronidazole in the treatment of malodorous wounds. Journal of Wound Care 5(9): 421–6.

Haughton W, Young T (1995) Common problems in wound care. British Journal of Nursing 4(16): 959–63.

Ivetic O, Lyne PA (1990) Fungating and ulcerating malignant lesions: a review of the literature. Journal of Advanced Nursing 15: 83–8.

Kelly N (2002) Malodorous fungating wounds: a review of current literature. Professional Nurse 17(5): 323–6.

Lisle J (2001) Managing malignant fungating lesions. Nursing Times 97(2): 36–7.

Lotti T, Rodofili C, Benci M, et al. (1998) Wound healing problems associated with cancers. Journal of Wound Care 7(2): 81–4.

Moyle J (1998) The management of malodour. European Journal of Palliative Care 5(5): 148–51.

National Cancer Institute (2000) Skin integrity changes secondary to cutaneous metas-
tases. http://cancerweb.ncl.ac.uk/cancernet/304277.html (accessed July 2000).
Naylor W (2002) Symptom control in the management of fungating wounds.
Worldwide Wounds, www.worldwidewounds.com (accessed July 2002).
Nielsen A (1999) Management of wound exudate. Journal of Community Nursing
13(6): 27–34.
Regnard C, Tempest S (1998) A Guide to Symptom Relief in Advanced Disease.
London: Hochland and Hochland.
Schulz V (1999) Malignant wound management: The assessment and management of
patients with malignant wounds. Supplement to Hotspot Newsletter of the Rapid
Response Radiotherapy Program (RRRP) of Toronto-Sunnybrook Regional Cancer
Centre 1(3).
Thomas S (1992) Current Practices in the Management of Fungating Lesions and
Radiation Damaged Skin. Bridgend: Bridgend General Hospital Surgical Materials
Testing Laboratory.
Thomas S, Jones M, Shutler S, et al. (1996) Using larvae in modern wound manage-
ment. Journal of Wound Care 5(2) 60–9.
Thomas S, Fisher B, Fram PJ, Waring MJ, et al. (1998) Odour absorbing dressings.
Journal of Wound Care 7(5): 246–50.
Van Toller S (1994) Invisible wounds – the effect of skin ulcer malodours. Journal of
Wound Care 3(2): 103–5.
White R (2001) Managing exudate. Nursing Times Plus 97(14): 59–60.
Williams C (1998) Deodorising dressings for malodorous wounds. Nurse
Prescribing/Community Nurse May: 512.
World Health Organisation (1996) Cancer Pain Relief: With a Guide to Opioid
Availability. 2nd edn. Geneva: WHO.
Young T (1997) The challenge of managing fungating wounds. Community Nurse
(Education Series) 3(9): 41–4.

CHAPTER FIFTEEN

Recurrent breast cancer

Introduction

Potentially anyone diagnosed with breast cancer is at risk from recurrence of the disease. Recurrent breast cancer can cause a variety of symptoms and can manifest systemically and locally. A recurrent breast cancer diagnosis can have many psychological and social implications for the patient. Each patient with metastatic disease will have different needs and the care given by the multidisciplinary team must be tailored to these. The ultimate aim is to combine active treatment with symptom control and ensure that the patient has the optimum quality of life for as long as possible (Burnet 2000).

Probably more than 50 per cent of women diagnosed with operable breast cancer will develop a recurrence (Richards and Smith 1995). Cells from even a small primary, invasive breast cancer can spread locally to the breast and loco-regional nodes. It can also spread systemically to liver, lung, bones, brain and areas of soft tissue via the blood and lymphatic systems. Treatment is largely the same as for primary breast cancer – chemotherapy, radiotherapy, hormone therapy, surgery. Once a breast cancer has metastasized good symptom control is the aim of treatment as there is little chance of cure (Honig 1996).

This prospect can be devastating for patients but many women live for years with breast cancer as a chronic condition. Treatment is given when necessary and in between episodes patients are neither classed as cured nor disabled. Interventions are chosen depending on the site and extent of the metastases. Nursing care is individually tailored to the patient's needs and problems. The physical response to treatment varies between patients (Thomson 1996). (Treatments for systemic recurrence would also be used if the patient were presenting for the first time with a stage IV breast cancer and nursing care and related palliative care issues would be the same.)

Loco-regional recurrence

This is not the same as metastatic breast disease. Some residual tumour may remain at the primary site or in lymph nodes leading to a recurrence following a wide local excision. This presents as nodules on the scar or enlarged axillary or supraclavicular nodes. Residual tumour may also remain in the chest wall following a mastectomy if the tumour was large and/or adjacent to the chest wall. There are many manifestations of cutaneous involvement in patients with breast cancer including inflammatory metastatic carcinoma, carcinoma en-cuirasse, nodular metastatic carcinoma, cancer of the inframammary crease and Paget's disease (Cox and Cruz 1994).

Local recurrence can be diagnosed clinically by fine needle aspiration or biopsy, and be treated by further surgery or local radiotherapy. Radiotherapy can only be used if the patient has not already had the maximum dose. A change in hormone therapy may be ordered or chemotherapy may be introduced. If the patient has already had chemotherapy a different regimen will be used. Local cutaneous metastases can be treated by the cytostatic agent Miltefosine (Clive et al. 1999). Miltefosine is used on a named patient basis in a clinical trials setting.

The internal mammary nodes may be affected causing a mass in the mediastinum. This can cause compression on the surrounding structures resulting in dyspnoea, raised jugular venous pressure, engorged contralateral veins on the chest wall and cyanosis. This is known as superior vena cava obstruction (SVCO) and is a cancer emergency. Treatment aims to reduce the mass quickly with high dose steroids and emergency radiotherapy (Doyle 1996). The steroids help to prevent an inflammatory reaction to the radiotherapy, which would exacerbate the symptoms. The dose is reduced quickly and carefully to prevent complications. Radiotherapy is given either as a short course or possibly over four weeks (Green and Youill 2001).

Breast cancer may recur in the contralateral breast. Diagnosis and treatment would be the same as for the primary tumour using mammography, ultrasound and fine needle aspiration or core biopsy. Primary chemotherapy for a large tumour may be undertaken.

Some locally advanced breast cancers are not controlled by any treatment or are largely ignored by the patient resulting in a fungating lesion (see Chapter 14).

Very rarely breast cancer may spread across the chest wall, termed 'en-cuirasse' disease, and can be extremely debilitating. The skin of the chest is infiltrated with firm, scattered nodules overlying an erythematous or red-blue surface. These evolve into the thickening of the skin and the 'breastplate' like appearance (Cox and Cruz 1994). Treatment is generally symptom management or chemotherapy/radiotherapy can be given to reduce the mass (Lichter 1998).

Local disease can be cured locally but may also represent a systemic relapse. Tests for metastatic disease may be undertaken to restage the patient such as chest X-ray, blood profile, liver ultrasound, CT scan (computerized tomography) or MRI scan (magnetic resonance imaging) if clinically indicated (Burnet 2000). Systemic therapy (chemotherapy, hormone therapy or both) should be given and if tolerated, followed by surgery and/or radiotherapy to control local disease (National Institute for Clinical Excellence (NICE) 2002a)

Systemic recurrence

Metastatic breast cancer is cancer that has disseminated to other parts of the body from the primary site. It is the most advanced stage of breast cancer (stage IV). Some patients may present primarily with advanced disease. It may spread via the lymphatic channels and nodes supplying the breast. In some cases breast cancer may spread without involving the axillary lymph nodes. If the tumour is located near the nipple in the medial portion of the breast it may spread to the internal mammary nodes located between the ribs and beneath the sternum. Cancer cells may also directly invade the blood vessels in the breast and spread around the body in the general bloodstream without being detected in the lymphatic system. The breast cancer cells colonize forming a metastatic deposit which invades the organ supplied by that blood vessel (Burnet 2000). Lymphoedema of the arm on the affected side may be the first indication of recurrence (see Chapter 12).

Systemic metastatic breast cancer may occur following treatment for a relatively localized breast cancer. In general the more lymph nodes involved and the less differentiated the cancer cells, the greater the chance of metastatic disease. The risk of developing metastases is also related to whether the primary tumour was more than 3cm and the ER status of the patient. In 10 per cent of breast cancer diagnoses the cancer will have already spread to distant organs (Imaginis 2001). A primary diagnosis of stage IV disease may indicate either that the disease has progressed rapidly or that the breast cancer has been present for some time but not detected.

The average period of survival once metastatic disease has been diagnosed is 18–24 months but this varies depending on the site of recurrence (Leonard et al. 1995). Women with hormone sensitive tumours and a longer period between the original diagnosis and relapse are likely to do better than women who develop recurrence in soft tissue sites shortly after initial treatment. Some women will live with metastatic disease for many years.

The risk of recurrence is a question most women ask at the original diagnosis as they wish to know about the possibility of the cancer returning.

This is not an easy question to answer. The breast care nurse may have discussed it generally with the patient at diagnosis but statistics should be given with caution as there are many individual exceptions. Recurrent disease can sometimes occur many years after the initial treatment.

The patient will probably react much the same as to the original diagnosis – disbelief, horror, shock, devastation, sense of uncertainty and fear of imminent death. However, some women think about recurrence from the time of the original diagnosis and although shocked, feel that their worst fears have been confirmed and they can now positively reprioritise their lives (Mahon and Casperson 1997). Having to cope with the diagnosis and treatment, knowing that there is no cure has a profound effect on the patient and her significant others.

The breast care team need to be aware of the need to give as much care and support to the patient as at the original diagnosis. They need to ensure that they listen to her concerns and discuss the future. The consultation giving the diagnosis of recurrence must be done with sensitivity and care. Some women will wish to know everything about the prognosis and some will want only minimal information. The breast care nursing service should be available for emotional support and information (Burnet 2000). However, when it becomes clear that care will be palliative, many breast care units liaise with the palliative care service and the patient may well be taken onto the caseload of the palliative care specialist and Macmillan nurses. GPs and patients should have access to palliative care services 24 hours a day and should have continuity of contact with a named team member (NICE 2002a).

All nurses caring for the patient need to be aware of the treatments available and of their toxicities, and help the patient weigh up the treatments and quality of life. Compassion, understanding and above all, realism are required. There are various ways in which recurrent breast cancer can manifest and some treatments can be combined to provide the best possible care but the breast care team need to ensure that the side effects do not outweigh the treatment.

Bone metastases

About 9000 women with breast cancer develop bone metastases each year in the UK. Many of these will possibly survive for more than two years. The Breast Speciality Group of the British Association of Surgical Oncology (BASO) have issued guidelines for the management of metastatic bone disease in patients with breast cancer (BASO 1999). The National Institute for Clinical Excellence has updated its document *Improving Outcomes in Breast Cancer* (2002a) and also suggests guidelines for the management of metastatic disease.

The patient often presents first to the GP – in all cases where clinical suspicion is moderate or high the patient should be referred to the breast unit. BASO recommends that breast units should aim to educate GPs in the management of women with skeletal pain and a history of breast cancer.

The diagnostic process and management of women with breast cancer and metastatic bone disease should be undertaken by the multidisciplinary breast care team in the breast care unit. Additional personnel should include an orthopaedic surgeon, a pain specialist, a radiotherapist and a radiologist with an interest in metastatic breast cancer. Breast care units cope with the care and management of breast cancer from diagnosis to advanced cancer apart from delivering radiotherapy (except in Cancer Centres). Care of the patient with metastatic spread should continue to be multidisciplinary. Care is decided in multidisciplinary team meetings and each management pathway will vary from patient to patient.

Often the first site of spread is the skeleton, the spine, ribs and proximal long bones (Leonard et al. 1995). The pelvis and skull can also be affected. In a normal bone the osteoblast cells replace exactly the same amount of bone that has been resorbed by osteoclast cells. This is known as modelling and remodelling. In metastatic bone disease this cycle is unbalanced. Osteolytic bone metastases are caused by the cancer eating away at the bone and forming holes. Osteoblastic metastases increase the bone mineral density but cause bones to fracture more readily. Both types cause pain.

The primary symptom that the patient will complain of is localized, unremitting pain, unrelieved by rest and aggravated by weight bearing and movement. The presence of bone metastases should be considered in all women presenting with musculo-skeletal pain who have had breast cancer (BASO 1999). An X-ray and bone scan will demonstrate a bony lesion and the bone may be weakened by tumour resulting in a pathological fracture. This may be the first presentation; a common site is the proximal femur. As the management is different to standard fracture management the diagnosis is vital. All patients with a long bone fracture should initially be managed with rest and splintage and discussed fully with the orthopaedic team.

Further investigations to exclude other likely primary tumours are carried out such as chest X-rays, ultrasound of the liver and kidneys, MRI scans and bone biopsies (BASO 1999). Routine skeletal surveys and routine bone scans are not recommended for women with a history of breast cancer who are asymptomatic (Roselli del Turco et al. 1994).

If a bone scan is ordered, a small amount of mildly radioactive material is injected into a vein, generally in the arm, and travels round the body in the bloodstream. It is then taken up by the bones, which absorb more radioactivity if affected. A scanner then shows the bone and abnormal areas will show – these are known as 'hot spots'.

Bone scans may not always accurately show the response to treatment so tumour markers may be tested for. These are substances often detected in higher than normal amounts in the tissues of patients with certain cancers. Tumour marker tests (blood tests) measure non-specific markers that can be followed over time. CA15-3 is a serum cancer antigen that measures the amount of a specific protein produced by breast cancer cells after cell division and growth have occurred. Minor changes in levels are common and do not necessarily indicate activity of the tumour but high levels indicate an increase in cell activity when the cancer has metastasized (Genentech online 2002). This has limited use in detecting the response of metastatic disease as the tumour has to express one of these markers (Chapman and Goodman 1997).

However, if a patient presents with an apparently solitary bone metastasis it is important to ensure that it does come from the breast cancer. Tumour markers can be useful in this case as over 30 per cent of patients with one or two lesions will show elevation of the CA15-3 (Crippa et al. 1992). This may be regarded as confirmation of metastatic disease in this group of patients.

CEA (carcinoembryonic antigen) is a marker for cancer recurrence; it is a special protein that is produced in embryonic cells and regenerating cells as well as in cancer cells. It is found on the cell surface and measured in blood tests as the cells shed these proteins. It can also, however, be elevated in a number of benign conditions including cigarette smoking and stomach ulcers. Some oncologists do not use these markers as they can cause unnecessary anxiety (Imaginis 2001).

All patients with confirmed solitary or multiple metastases are clinically assessed and restaged prior to treatment to evaluate the extent of the disease. Blood is taken for full blood count, creatinine, electrolytes, liver function, serum calcium, alkaline phosphatase, tumour markers CEA, CA15-3 and erythrocyte sedimentation rate (ESR). ER and PR levels are repeated as ER status may change at the time of recurrence. The tumour may also be tested for HER2/neu positivity (see later). In addition to a chest X-ray, X-rays are taken of the pelvis and an ultrasound of the liver is carried out. Previous imaging and staging should always be reviewed (BASO 1999). If ER and PR status are still unknown then the site or sites of recurrence, length of disease free interval, menopausal status and response to previous therapy are all useful for selecting treatment.

Treatment aims to strengthen the bone, prevent pathological fractures and relieve pain. Surgery may be carried out – internal fixation to stabilize the bone or replacement of the femoral head. Patients who may benefit from orthopaedic surgery are those who have spinal instability or some degree of vertebral collapse, which can be treated by decompression of the spinal cord and nerve roots, followed by stabilization of the affected vertebrae. Prophylactic fixation of metastatic deposits is carried out where there is a risk of fracture. A pathological fracture is stabilized or reconstructed. These procedures are different to normal surgery for trauma and the patient may need to be transferred to a centre for orthopaedic oncology. If the patient's life expectancy is very short the team must consider the benefit of carrying out major surgery but a patient immobilized by a fracture will have a very poor quality of life, which will not improve without surgery (BASO 1999). The multidisciplinary team must discuss and plan treatment regimes for each patient individually.

Radiotherapy can be given for localized bone pain in a single or several fractions. Patients may get immediate pain relief after the first fraction of radiotherapy but usually there is an improvement two weeks after treatment or improvement may take up to six weeks. Approximately 70–80 per cent of patients will respond. A single fraction is given as a fraction of 8–10 Gy using megavoltage radiotherapy; 20 Gy may be given in five fractions following surgical stabilization.

If the patient has pain occurring at several sites systemic treatment of hormone therapy or chemotherapy may be undertaken. All patients with metastatic breast cancer should be considered for systemic therapy determined by their overall condition, ER status, site and extent of metastases and any previous adjuvant therapy. Systemic therapy will be discussed later in the chapter.

The patient is assessed for appropriate analgesia, which will include mild analgesics such as paracetamol and non-steroidal anti-inflammatory drugs (NSAIDs), which are very effective for pain relief. Progress is then made up the 'analgesic ladder' (WHO 1996) of drugs of increasing strength to potent drugs such as DF118 and morphine.

Bisphosphonates can reduce the incidence of new bony and visceral metastases in women at high risk of developing them (Diel et al. 1998). For women already diagnosed with bony metastases oral bisphosphonates such as disodium pamidronate and sodium clodronate given regularly can stabilize bone mineral. Bisphosphonates naturally inhibit bone demineralization by interrupting the osteoclast cell cycle. They are difficult to take orally so monthly intravenous infusions of disodium pamidronate 60–90mg are administered as an alternative (Burnet 2000). If the patient does wish to take the medication orally they must be informed that calcium and other minerals bind to it, rendering it inactive. The patient needs to take it with plain tap water only, and should not take it within one hour of eating, having a milky drink or taking other medication.

Pamidronate provides effective relief of bone pain, therefore improving quality of life. High dose bisphosphonates can also be useful for patients with severe bone pain that is unresponsive to analgesics and too widespread for radiotherapy. Pamidronate can cause renal damage if the infusion rate is too high, possibly due to accumulation in the renal tubules

(Houston and Rubens 1998). Newer bisphosphonates are under investigation such as zoledronic acid and ibandronate. These have a higher potency, a more pronounced effect and will simplify treatment.

Treatment of bone disease should be continued indefinitely as osteoclastic bone resorption does not appear to become resistant to bisphosphonates (BASO 1999). The financial and logistical implications of long-term bisphosphonate therapy may be balanced by the reduced need for radiotherapy and orthopaedic services as the risk of fractures is reduced. Studies have shown that pamidronate and clodronate can reduce pathological fractures by 28 per cent and reduce the need for radiotherapy for bone pain by 39 per cent. Serious side effects are uncommon. Bisphosphonates should be given for as long as bone disease remains an important clinical problem (NICE 2002a).

Hypercalcaemia

Hypercalcaemia is frequently associated with widespread, active bone metastases increasing osteoclastic activity and bone resorption, releasing calcium into the bloodstream. Urinary output is increased, loss of fluid leads to dehydration and then to a decrease in urine output as the kidneys try to excrete the excess calcium. Calcium levels rise leading to slowing of muscles. Hypercalcaemia is seen in about 20 per cent of patients with bone metastases. It can affect every organ system and may be confused with end-stage disease. Hypercalcaemia is also associated with the production of a parathyroid hormone-related protein by the tumour, a process unrelated to bone metastases (Regnard and Tempest 1998).

Hypercalcaemia is classed as a cancer emergency. Signs and symptoms are anorexia, nausea and vomiting, constipation, dehydration, polyuria, polydipsia, lethargy, confusion and coma. These are variable and symptoms can be mild, although it depends on the degree of hypercalcaemia, rapidity of onset, the patient's general condition and the ability of the kidneys to maintain homeostasis. The patient may be asymptomatic and diagnosis made by a routine blood calcium. Prognosis and survival are poor if treatment is not initiated rapidly. If the patient receives the appropriate treatment she may recover to live for a long period of time. It is necessary to be alert to the possibility of hypercalcaemia as it is reversible if treated promptly. It is important that the symptoms are not dismissed as being part of the progress of the cancer in a patient whose cancer is advanced. Blood calcium levels need to be monitored regularly in vulnerable patients (Thomson 1996).

Treatment involves rehydration with intravenous fluids designed to lower the calcium level. Saline rehydration (3–4 litres a day) replaces lost sodium and increases urinary output by restoring glomerular function.

Calcitonin and steroids may be used. Calcitonin is a natural hormone, which rapidly produces an inhibitory effect on bone resorption and enhances the excretion of calcium in the urine (Barnett 1999). However its effect is not long lasting. BASO (1999) recommend that high-dose bisphosphonates are administered by intravenous infusion as well as saline rehydration. These are regarded as first-line therapies in patients with hypercalcaemia. Pamidronate produces marked and rapid reduction of serum calcium levels and is the drug of choice. Bone pain, nausea and vomiting, hypercalcaemic episodes and pathological fractures are reduced. Quality of life is improved and the need for palliative radiotherapy reduced. Clodronate is also used but does not appear to be quite as effective. Both are well tolerated, although the patient may experience mild flu-like symptoms at the start of treatment.

The patient's fluid intake and output are closely monitored. General nursing care to maintain hygiene and comfort is necessary as the patient may be quite ill. A diet low in vitamin D and calcium is also recommended.

Following recovery explanation of the signs and symptoms can be given along with what action to take if symptoms recur. It may be advisable to further investigate the progress of the breast cancer to ascertain whether a change of treatment is necessary (Thomson 1996).

Spinal cord compression

Whilst the use of bisphosphonates can reduce the risk of fractures and spinal cord compression, they cannot always prevent them. Therefore, each breast care team should ensure that the patient is assessed as quickly and efficiently as possible by professionals who have expertise in dealing with problems caused by bone metastases (NICE 2002a). These personnel should include radiotherapists, radiologists, neurosurgeons and specialist orthopaedic surgeons.

Spinal cord compression is a cancer emergency and warrants immediate surgical, radiological and oncological assessment. It is caused by metastatic deposits of breast cancer within the dura or vertebrae. Density is lost from the bones supporting the spinal cord with compression of the nerves and possibly sudden, dense paralysis of the lower body below the area of collapse. Around 3–7.4 per cent of women with breast cancer will develop it (Jacobs 1999). Most will occur in the thorax and there is compression at more than one level in some patients. Below the level of L2 vertebra the compression is of the peripheral nerves (cauda equina) rather than the spinal cord (Twycross 1999).

Signs and symptoms include weakness of legs and arms, sphincter disturbance and sensory changes. The patient may not be aware of sensory loss until examined especially if the only loss is in the sacral or perineal area (Twycross 1999). Pain of several preceding weeks or months is generally a feature. This is caused by root compression, compression of the tracts of the spinal cord or vertebral metastases. Pain can be exacerbated by neck flexion, straight leg raising, coughing or straining.

If plain X-rays are negative the investigation of choice is an MRI scan, preferably carried out and assessed by a spinal surgeon within 2–4 hours. A bone scan can also be ordered to assess the condition of other bones.

The patient is given dexamethasone 16–32mg orally for a week, which is then reduced (Twycross 1999). Emergency radiotherapy is commenced. Surgical decompression for isolated metastases followed by surgical stabilization may be carried out if the patient is relatively fit, followed by post-operative radiotherapy (BASO 1999). Surgery and radiotherapy need to be carried out within 12 hours.

This situation is extremely frightening and distressing for the patient as she faces the risk of paralysis. Also metastatic disease compromises the healing process and post-operative complications such as slow wound healing, bleeding and deep vein thrombosis may occur (Burnet 2000). Nerve damage must be minimized and further injury to the spinal cord prevented.

The patient is nursed flat, catheterized and given intravenous fluids for rehydration. The patient may be still for a short while following surgery and/or radiotherapy but care must be taken to prevent pressure sores and deep vein thrombosis. The degree of recovery depends on the condition of the spine and nerve damage but patients can make an almost complete recovery with early recognition and treatment (Thomson 1996). Patients with any residual disabilities or functional difficulties should be referred for rehabilitation including physiotherapy and occupational therapy (NICE 2002a). Counselling services for patients and carers should also be available. The patient may also be referred to the community services on discharge.

The most important aspect of spinal cord compression is early recognition and there is great potential for professional education to ensure that all those in contact with the patient can recognize the early symptoms (BASO 1999).

Lung metastases

Some patients will develop lung involvement. A cough, pain and dyspnoea may be symptomatic of a pleural effusion or infiltrating lung disease. The patient may also complain of fatigue and loss of appetite. A chest X-ray, CT or MRI scan will be undertaken to diagnose lung metastases and a biopsy may be ordered. Treatment consists of steroids, salbutamol, diazepam, morphine (to reduce dyspnoea and anxiety) and oxygen therapy, carefully monitored. Oxygen does not always help and should be used only if the patient is clearly benefiting (Twycross 1999). The patient will be assessed for systemic therapies of chemotherapy, radiotherapy and hormonal treatments.

Approximately 50 per cent of women with metastatic breast disease develop a malignant pleural effusion. They may not all be symptomatic, depending on the location and amount of fluid (Leonard et al. 1995). Diagnosis is usually by X-ray but a CT scan can be used. If this is unclear a MRI scan can be carried out. Prolonged tube drainage is the most effective treatment, with bleomycin or tetracycline instilled into the pleural space following drainage. These cause pleuradhesis (the pleural lining sticks to itself) therefore preventing fluid reaccumulating (Leonard et al. 1995). Thoroscopy or partial thoracotomy may be used to drain fluid and insert the adhesive substance.

The patient may be taught behavioural changes by the physiotherapist such as breathing control, relaxation exercises and activity pacing. Psychosocial support can help (Bredin et al. 1999). It is important to acknowledge the feelings of fear and panic associated with exacerbations of breathlessness. General measures that can be taken include plenty of rest between activities, space and fresh air in the room, loose clothing and help with tasks. Complementary therapies may be useful for some patients.

Liver metastases

Two-thirds of women with metastatic breast cancer will eventually have it spread to the liver. Symptoms are subtle at first but increase in intensity over time (Imaginis 2001). Liver metastases occur mainly in younger women and often presents with nausea and pain in the hypochondrium, which is worse on turning or inspiration. Pain is caused by the liver enlarging causing pressure by stretching the capsule. The patient may experience referred pain in the right shoulder. Weight loss, fatigue, anorexia and fever is also indicative of liver disease. The liver may be palpably enlarged. The patient may be anaemic with blood clotting problems and jaundiced as the bile duct becomes blocked causing itching. A stent may need to be inserted into the bile duct to keep it patent. The presence of ascites may necessitate paracentesis and diuretics to relieve bloating, nausea and dyspnoea (Breast Cancer Care online 2002). Spironolactone is the diuretic of choice, 300mg once daily or less (Twycross 1999).

A blood test for liver function and an ultrasound scan of the liver confirms how much function is impaired. A CT or MRI scan may be requested. Endoscopic retrograde cholangiopancreatography (ERCP) confirms whether or not the bile duct is blocked (Breast Cancer Care online

2002). A liver biopsy is necessary to confirm the diagnosis of metastases. Liver metastases carry a very poor prognosis and their presence needs to be explained very gently with great sensitivity and compassion.

Radiotherapy, systemic chemotherapy or monoclonal antibodies if appropriate can be given to shrink the tumour but care is taken with the drug dosages if liver impairment is significant. Hormone therapy may be changed if the woman cannot tolerate chemotherapy (Burnet 2000). Steroids to reduce swelling around the liver, anti-inflammatory and morphine-based drugs can be given for pain. Nausea caused by the enlarged liver pressing on the stomach or toxins from liver damage can be controlled by anti-emetics.

Brain metastases

Brain metastases are especially distressing as the effect they will have on the patient's life is very uncertain. Symptoms depend on the part of the brain affected and the degree of raised intra-cranial pressure, and include a wide range – headache, nausea, vomiting, fatigue, dizziness, loss of balance, general weakness or weakness of one side, fits, double vision, behavioural changes and difficulty with speech.

A MRI or CT scan will confirm the diagnosis. Treatment consists of steroids and possibly whole brain irradiation with steroid cover to reduce cerebral oedema. If the lesion is single surgery may possibly be carried out. The patient also has the side effects of the steroids to deal with including fluid retention, weight gain, susceptibility to infection, steroid-induced diabetes and hair loss at the radiotherapy site (Burnet 2000). Survival rates are very poor.

Pain

The subject of pain is vast and pain relief in palliative care is a specialist area. Details of the mechanisms of pain and descriptions of drugs used and their actions can be found in palliative care texts. A very brief overview has been included here as, of all advanced cancer symptoms, pain is probably the most prominent and the most feared by patients.

Pain is difficult to evaluate as it is a subjective experience. The pain threshold is the intensity at which pain is first perceived and is relatively constant in individuals. However, pain tolerance varies greatly, from person to person and within the same individual under differing circumstances. Pain tolerance can be lowered by many factors including fear, depression, anxiety, exhaustion, anger and social problems (Bycroft and Brown 1996). Patients may also have low expectations that their pain can be controlled and may fear becoming addicted to the drugs. Pain associated with a life-threatening illness has spiritual and emotional components and will limit the social function of the patient and her carers (Farrer 2001).

Assessment of pain is an essential part of nursing care and a prerequisite of effective pain control. The aim is to ensure the optimum quality of life – this aim is multidisciplinary. Holistic pain management will achieve pain control in most cases but in patients where pain control is difficult to achieve the palliative care services can be consulted.

The nurse can gather a wide scope of information about the patient's experience of pain and how it is affecting her life. Assessment is ongoing as pain can change frequently and cancer pain can often be multi-focal. A patient may also experience pain from other medical conditions unrelated to the cancer, and from problems such as pressure sores and constipation. Recent studies show that approximately one-third to a half of cancer patients needlessly experience pain (McCaffrey and Ferrell 1997). According to NICE (2002a) there is evidence that cancer pain is undertreated and this is due to failure to assess pain properly. Other reasons could be that staff have a poor knowledge of cancer pain management, have inappropriate attitudes such as fear of addiction and tolerance to opioids, have poor clinical skills or have a lack of understanding how emotional issues can affect pain (McCaffrey and Ferrell 1997). Health care professionals need to recognize the severity of the patient's pain and become familiar with the use of appropriate drugs. Active listening to the patient and empathy are vital.

A history is taken and clinical examination and investigations are undertaken to define the pathology. A formalized approach is required to manage pain effectively.

The use of pain charts can help the assessment process and aid communication between staff and patient (Bycroft and Brown 1996). This should include a body chart to illustrate multiple pains and rate the severity. The patient's description should be included, for example if the pain is worse on movement or at night. A pain diary may be useful in the community where the patient is not under observation day and night (de Wit et al. 1999). The pain management or palliative care specialist may be consulted as there may not be a pain assessment tool available in every setting (Farrer 2001).

Realistic goals should be set, ideally the patient should be pain-free at night, on moving and at rest. Careful discussion with the patient and family and the setting of realistic, achievable goals and treatment option can help to alleviate fear and anxiety. The use of the analgesic ladder (WHO 1996) is recommended, commencing with paracetamol or aspirin and progressing to a strong opioid such as morphine. An adequate dose is prescribed to be taken at regular intervals to anticipate the pain.

The WHO analgesic ladder

The WHO (1996) recommend that analgesia is given orally as far as possible and given regularly by the clock and by the ladder. If oral analgesia is not appropriate transdermal fentanyl patches or continuous subcutaneous infusion can be used. Radiotherapy may be used in conjunction with analgesia.

- Mild pain: Non-opioid +/- adjuvant analgesia.
- Mild–moderate pain: Weak opioid + non-opioid +/- adjuvant analgesia.
- Moderate–severe pain: Strong opioid + non-opioid +/- adjuvant analgesia.
- Uncontrolled pain with opiate side effects: Consider alternative opioid if previously responsive to an opioid, if still uncontrolled review adjuvant analgesia and consider anaesthetic block.
- Adjuvant analgesia includes:
NSAIDs, for example Naproxen, Diclofenac.
Steroids, for example Dexamethasone.
Amitriptyline.
Carbamazepine

Other pain relief measures can be employed in conjunction such as positioning, complementary therapies, for example relaxation, massage, acupuncture where appropriate or the use of a TENS machine. Nerve blocks may be ordered for intractable pain.

Side effects from analgesics especially opioids include constipation for which a laxative is given alongside the pain relief, nausea and vomiting for which an anti-emetic is given, and transient drowsiness which settles quite quickly. Addiction and tolerance are almost never an issue in clinical practice (WHO 1996).

It is very important to explain and provide relevant information for the patient and family. Explaining the common myths and including the patient in the decision over which drugs to employ will maximize compliance with the drug regimens. Non-physical distress needs to be recognized along with the physical management of the pain. This can be addressed much of the time by good communication and supporting the patient and family during the illness. Palliative care nurses need to keep patients informed and involved in the decision-making process. Health care professionals need to remain flexible when involving patients and families and ensure that they have correct and accurate information at all times so that an informed decision can be made (Farrer 2001). This can become vitally important if the patient and family wish to take a decision that the multidisciplinary team would not always choose such as only alternative therapies or an alternative diet for example.

Constant modifications to the regime will probably be required. A patient with advanced cancer will present with various symptoms, all of which can be addressed using the same principles of assessment and diagnosis of underlying pathology. If pain and other symptoms are controlled the patient can begin the process of grieving and adjusting to dying (Bycroft and Brown 1996).

Systemic therapies for recurrent breast cancer

Metastatic breast cancer is incurable and therefore any treatment is aimed at producing the optimum survival time and quality of life. The breast care team and palliative care specialists need to ensure that side effects from systemic therapies do not cause more problems than benefits. The choice of hormone therapy or chemotherapy as first-line treatment for metastatic breast cancer is based on various clinical factors. The choice of drugs will depend on which drugs were given as an adjuvant treatment, side effects and the patient's tolerance to the drug. A disease-free interval of less than one year between surgery for early breast cancer and the development of metastases suggests that the recurrence is very likely to be resistant to the drug used originally for adjuvant treatment.

Hormone therapy

(Hormone therapies have been discussed in some detail in Chapter 9.)

Treatments for advanced disease need to be low toxicity wherever possible. Hormone therapy is the first-line therapy for women with metastatic disease who are oestrogen receptor or progesterone receptor positive. The oestrogen receptor (ER) status is sometimes unknown when the patient presents for the first time with metastatic disease and then a trial of hormone treatment is commenced without knowing this information. Positive responses are seen in about 60 per cent of patients with metastatic disease who are ER positive and less than 10 per cent in patients who are ER negative (BASO 1999). Simultaneous measurements of ER and PR status appear to give a better indication of the likelihood of response to hormone therapy. If the breast cancer is hormone sensitive the prognosis is better – endocrine treatment will give longer survival. Hormone insensitive disease generally means a shorter disease-free interval and shorter survival.

Hormone therapy would also be given to a patient who has newly diagnosed metastatic disease and/or who has not received any adjuvant treatment. Hormone therapy can also be used in women who have a non-aggressive relapse in the lymph nodes or bones, or have a long interval free of disease. Menopausal status is also taken into account – it would be the first treatment of choice for the post-menopausal woman.

Tamoxifen is the first-line therapy of choice. Even some ER negative patients may benefit which suggests that part of the activity of Tamoxifen may be independent of its hormonal action. Bone disease often responds to Tamoxifen, anastrazole (a highly specific aromatase inhibitor) or Zoladex (a luteinizing hormone-releasing hormone inhibitor).

Hormone therapy largely depends on menstrual status. Zoladex may be given to pre-menopausal women to achieve ovarian ablation instead of oopherectomy or radiotherapy. Tamoxifen or an aromatase inhibitor would be given in addition if the tumour was ER positive (NICE 2002a).

The introduction of aromatase inhibitors such as anastrazole, lestrozole and exemestane has been a leap forward as these inhibit oestrogen synthesis by 97–99 per cent (Geisler et al. 1998). (Aromatase inhibitors block the way oestrogen is produced in post-menopausal women by interfering with the adrenal glands.) Some studies have shown these to be superior to Tamoxifen. These would be used as second-line treatment if the patient was unresponsive to Tamoxifen. If the patient is unresponsive to aromatase inhibitors, megestrol or medroxyprogesterone acetate can be tried or can be used for women who cannot tolerate aromatase inhibitors.

Failure of hormone therapy necessitates further endocrine therapy if there has been an objective response or static disease for at least six months. Careful assessment of response to treatment is necessary (BASO 1999).

Chemotherapy

Chemotherapy can give effective palliation of symptoms, especially in patients whose disease is progressing rapidly, who do not respond to hormone treatment or who are oestrogen receptor negative. It is usually the first treatment of choice for patients with advanced visceral metastases. It may also be given initially to a patient presenting for the first time with a large tumour to shrink it. A variety of chemotherapy agents should be available. The regimen chosen will depend on previous chemotherapy given, the extent of the disease and the patient's general health. The wishes of the patient should also be taken into consideration. Advantages and disadvantages of embarking on the treatment should be clearly explained and expectations should be discussed. Patients should be given clear written and verbal information about the treatment and side effects. A contact number is always given to ring day or night if there is a chemotherapy-related problem. (Treatments and side effects of chemotherapy are discussed in Chapter 7.)

Some of the cytotoxic drugs used in early breast cancer as an adjuvant treatment are also used in metastatic disease. These include the cytotoxic antibiotics such as the anthracyclines, the taxanes, vinca alkaloids, antimetabolites and alkylating drugs for example. These can be given singly or can be combined in a number of different ways depending on the previous treatment given. The taxanes, paclitaxel and docetaxel (Taxol and Taxotere) appear to be more effective than other forms of chemotherapy for progressive or metastatic breast cancer, offering longer remission, better response rates and an increase in survival time of about 20–25 per cent (NICE 2002a).

Capecitabine is an anti-metabolite that interferes with the growth of cancer cells, eventually destroying them. It is activated by several enzymatic steps. It is converted to 5FU by an enzyme that is found at high levels in tumour tissues. The metabolism of 5FU is thought to interfere with the synthesis of DNA. The 5FU also leads to inhibition of RNA and protein synthesis. The effect of 5FU is thought to cause unbalanced growth and cell death (NICE 2002b).

Capecitabine is used in metastatic breast cancer for patients who are resistant to paclitaxel and an anthracycline-containing chemotherapy regime, and for those for whom further anthracycline therapy is not indicated. As it is converted in the body to 5FU it should not be given to any patient who has had problems with 5 fluorouracil in the past.

A recent study (O'Shaughnessy et al. 2002) showed that patients with advanced breast cancer who received a combination of capecitabine and docetaxel survived for three months longer. As taxanes are being used earlier in the course of the disease it is more likely that patients with recurrence will have already had these drugs. Combining docetaxel and capecitabine is thought to boost effectiveness and is an important option for women who have also had anthracyclines as a previous treatment. It works differently to anthracyclines or taxanes therefore offering a new approach unlikely to suppress bone marrow (National Cancer Institute 2002b). It is not recommended for patients who are pregnant or breastfeeding.

Possible side effects of capecitabine include diarrhoea, pain, blistering or swelling of the palms of the hands or soles of the feet, pain and swelling in the mouth or mouth ulcers. Nausea and vomiting are less common. Rare side effects include abdominal pain, chest pain, tarry stools, fever, severe constipation, painful urination, breathing problems. Any patient with any worrying symptoms when on chemotherapy should report immediately to the chemotherapy unit.

Capecitabine is given at the moment on a named patient basis in a clinical trials setting. The dosage is 2500mg per metre squared per day, orally, in two divided doses 12 hours apart, after meals for two weeks followed by a one-week rest period. It is still awaiting approval by NICE for widespread use within the NHS.

Another chemotherapy drug, vinorelbine, is also awaiting approval by NICE for use in metastatic breast cancer. This can be used in addition to 5FU either as a bolus dose or in a pump for continuous infusion. This is useful as the patient is less likely to lose her hair.

Administration of intravenous chemotherapy may be problematic especially if the patient has undergone previous chemotherapy treatments. It may be necessary to insert a PICC line (peripherally inserted central catheter) or a central venous line. Side effects can be a considerable cause of distress in the patient with advanced cancer. The patient may be unable to deal with them due to her depleted health status resulting from recurrent disease and emotional and psychological distress. Psychological and emotional support is vitally important (Burnet 2000).

Herceptin (trastuzumab)

Increased knowledge of the biology of tumours and the anti-tumour properties of antibodies have resulted in the development of monoclonal antibody therapies such as trastuzumab (Herceptin), recently approved for widespread use on the NHS. Monoclonal antibodies can be made in the laboratory in large quantities and are an innovative cancer therapy that utilizes the body's immune system. Trastuzumab is now licensed in the UK and approved for use in certain circumstances by NICE.

Trastuzumab is a humanized monoclonal antibody, which binds to HER2 (also known as HER2/neu or c-erb-2), an epidermal growth factor receptor found on a breast cancer cell surface. Epidermal growth factor is a protein produced naturally by the body. When this protein attaches itself to the HER2 protein the cancer cells are stimulated to divide and grow. The HER2 gene is associated with cell growth and normal cells usually contain two copies. The receptor is a proto-oncogene situated in the cell membrane (Sanders 2002). A study by Slamon et al. (1989) first demonstrated that HER2/neu is over-expressed in as many as 30 per cent of all breast cancers as well as other cancers. This results in the uncontrolled cell proliferation, which is linked to the development of cancer (Cooke 2000)

Herceptin blocks this action, attaching itself to the HER2 protein so that epidermal growth factor does not reach the cancer cells so that they are prevented from replicating. Herceptin also attracts the body's immune cells to help destroy the cancer cells.

Positive HER2 status is generally associated with a poor prognosis and the identification of HER2 can have implications on decision making and treatment planning. HER2 positive tumours can be associated with chemo resistance to certain cytotoxic agents such as CMF, commonly used in adjuvant treatment although breast tumours are not routinely tested for HER2. Only patients with HER2 positive disease are eligible for treatment with trastuzumab, therefore it is important to identify HER2 patients (Sanders 2002). A variety of methods are used to measure HER2 status including:

- immunohistochemistry (IHC)
- fluorescence in-situ hybridization (FISH)
- polymerase chain reaction (PCR)
- enzyme linked immunosorbent assay (ELISA)
- blot analysis (Rovelon 2000).

Testing can be undertaken years after the initial breast surgery if necessary, depending on which test is used as testing requires fresh, frozen or archival tumour samples. Only women who have high levels of HER2 are offered treatment, not all HER2 positive patients will be suitable as there are various levels of HER2 positivity. Herceptin will only be used in patients whose tumour over-expresses HER2 at a 3+ level as determined by an immunohistochemistry (IHC)-based assessment of fixed tumour blocks. The testing must be undertaken in a specialized laboratory to ensure accurate results and validation of the testing procedures. The recommended scoring system to evaluate the IHC staining patterns is:

0 no staining observed or membrane staining is observed in less than 10 per cent of tumour cells – HER over-expression negative.

1+ a faint or barely perceptible membrane staining is detected in more than 10 per cent of tumour cells. Only part of the cells' membrane is stained – HER over-expression negative.

2+ a weak – moderate complete membrane staining is detected in more than 10 per cent of tumour cells – HER over-expression weak to moderate.

3+ moderate – strong complete membrane staining is detected in more than 10 per cent of tumour cells – HER over-expression moderate to strong (Roche Pharmaceuticals 2000).

Herceptin can be given as a single agent or in combination with chemotherapy. It may be used as a single agent in women who are unresponsive to chemotherapy and hormone therapy. As it targets the cancer only it has few side effects. It is given as a short intravenous infusion while the woman is an out-patient. Some patients report chills, fever and pain experienced with the initial infusion. The patient must be closely monitored during and after the treatment for a specified time. About 40 per cent of patients experience this (Cobleigh et al. 1999).

Herceptin is associated with cardiac toxicity when combined with doxorubicin. Consequently patients with metastatic breast cancer with over-expression of HER2/neu are candidates for treatment with the combination of Herceptin and paclitaxel. This is provided that the tumour expresses HER2 levels at 3+, the patient has not had chemotherapy for metastatic breast cancer and has not been a candidate for anthracyclines (NICE 2002c). Taxanes have a lower risk of associated cardiotoxicity than anthracyclines and when given with Herceptin may be more effective and increase survival (Cancer Bacup 2001). Patients undergo left ventricular ejection fraction measurement before and during treatment. They may also be asked to participate in clinical trials of Herceptin combined with taxanes and other chemotherapeutic agents (Burstein et al. 2001).

Patients who are HER2 negative may be psychologically devastated as they are excluded from a potentially helpful new treatment. It is important to stress that the determination of HER2 status will facilitate a more individualized approach to their treatment (Sanders 2002). Information, support and counselling are very important.

Further developments in systemic therapies

Research carried out at the Royal Marsden has recently resulted in the discovery of a new form of therapy called Zarnestra, which blocks signals in cancer cells. A series of key proteins that transmit signals from the surface of cells toward the nucleus have been identified. Some of these proteins function abnormally and play a part in the growth and behaviour of cancer cells. Zarnestra is a famesyl transferase inhibitor, a new generation of signal transduction inhibitors (STIs).

It appears to inhibit the function of these proteins and stops tumours from growing. In the clinical trials it was given in tablet form for three weeks in every month to patients with advanced breast cancer who had already received several hormone and chemotherapy treatments. Up to a quarter had shrinkage or prolonged control of their tumour. Most experienced few side effects. It may be most effective given in combination with hormone treatment. More of these new inhibitor drugs will be the subject of clinical trials over the next few years (Royal Marsden Hospital 2002).

Other drugs currently being researched include anti-angiogenesis drugs, which inhibit the rapid, tumour-induced formation of the new blood vessels that are required to nourish malignancies. A sub-class of these drugs is Marimastat, an inhibitor of tumour growth, which works by inhibiting enzymes responsible for the breakdown of the external cell matrix that occurs during the growth of a tumour (Healthlink 1999). Clinical trials of new drugs will continue over the next few years.

Psychosocial issues

Women who have apparently similar tumours at the time of presenting with breast cancer differ considerably in their disease-free and overall survival. Differences in outcome may be explained by host and environmental factors, including psychological and social variables. A recent study examined the relation between severely stressful life experiences and the recurrence of breast cancer. No increased risk of recurrence was found in women who had one or more severely stressful life experiences in the year before diagnosis compared with women who had not. Stressful life experiences would be divorce for example and severe life difficulties could be caring for a severely handicapped child. The study concluded women who had had one or more severely stressful life events in the five years after the breast cancer diagnosis had a lower risk of recurrence. Therefore, women with breast cancer need not fear that stressful events and experiences will cause their disease to return (Graham et al. 2002). (The study allowed for lymph node infiltration and histology.)

When breast cancer recurs the nature and course of the illness is not as clearly defined as the course at initial diagnosis. The focus has shifted from cure to promoting quality of life, controlling symptoms and extending life expectancy. The condition becomes chronic, causing the individual to change their perspective and probably their lifestyle. Recurrent cancer brings about many changes to the patient's and family's lives.

The experience of being told of a recurrence is similar to the original diagnosis. Shock, disbelief, surprise and devastation are characteristic. The news may be more traumatic than the original diagnosis as the future becomes uncertain. Whatever the patient's expectations are, the news is still painful and a shock. However, some patients may feel a sense of relief that now their worst fear has been confirmed, they can reprioritize their life. Relationships become more significant and the support and information needs of the patient and carers are paramount (Burnet and Robinson 2000). Having to cope with the diagnosis and treatment and live with it, knowing that there is no cure, has a profound effect on patients and families.

Patients will have already had experience of cancer treatments and their side effects. A recurrence will reinforce feelings of unattractiveness and altered body image as the patient contemplates further therapies. However, oncologists tend to offer treatments with the attitude that there is always something to offer the patient so she may feel reassured that new interventions are available. It would be emphasized to the patient presenting primarily with advanced disease that there are a whole range of therapies to offer.

Health care professionals must ascertain what is distressing for the patient on an individual basis with careful assessment to ascertain the patient's needs and concerns. The breast care team cannot assume that the patient with cancer recurrence has adequate information and that information needs are similar to those at the time of the original diagnosis. They may assume that patients are aware of the symptoms of cancer recurrence. Women who have had breast cancer may want information on signs and symptoms as they will be quicker to seek advice and gain referral back into the breast care system (Burnet and Robinson 2000).

Patients need the correct information regarding their condition and life expectancy. There may be hope for a cure at diagnosis but hope changes when it becomes clear that there is a time limit, and the patient may give up hope. Patients who are deteriorating and developing symptoms are generally aware of the truth.

The multidisciplinary team need to assess each patient individually and where appropriate discuss the realistic outcomes of the illness. This then gives the patient chance to discuss fears and anxieties openly (Faulkner 1995).

The patient may have new fears about treatments such as chemotherapy and radiotherapy, so the multidisciplinary team needs to reappraise her perception of past treatments. She may also fear becoming a burden to family and friends as she experiences increased pain and fatigue. Reduced independence and inability to carry out activities of daily living will be another concern. Patients may be more fearful of a life prolonged by disability and altered mental state than of actually dying (Faulkner 1995).

However, some women may be determined to live with a recurrence and lead a normal life. Whatever the patient's attitude to her illness, the prospect of dying can bring life into sharp focus and encourage self-appraisal (Colyer 1996). Life becomes precious and some patients may wish to make their lives more meaningful. Families also reappraise their situation to adapt to the patient's disease. Patients and carers may set goals to achieve, and things that seemed important before may seem less so now. The whole family is affected and relationships may change. Families go through a period of change in order to adapt to the demands of the disease on the patient. Younger women experience great distress as they try to come to terms with not being able to see their children grow up. Worry about how the family will cope adds to their anxiety.

Friends and family may feel an increasing sense of loss as the illness progresses (Langford 1995). Support and information is of prime importance for the family so that they can support the patient (Burnet and Robinson 2000). Breast care and palliative care nurses need to be supportive, facilitate adjustment and promote well-being.

Health care professionals should also be alert for symptoms of depression. Great sadness can be detected between couples coping with a recurrent cancer diagnosis and depression would seem a predictable reaction. Symptom distress and hopelessness may cause marital dysfunction along with difficulty in communication. This is where the palliative care approach is so vital as it addresses the psychological, social and spiritual well-being of the patient and family as well as symptom control.

Children may be protected from the reality of the illness by not being given information in case of distress. Alternatively, more responsibility may be given to older children who may have difficulty coping with high expectations. Feelings of isolation may result (Langford 1995).

Women with recurrent breast cancer (and patients with a primary diagnosis of advanced cancer who will also experience feelings of shock and devastation) should have access to services based in hospitals, the community and hospices to ensure effective delivery of palliative care (NICE 2002a). Palliative care should be integrated between services provided by the palliative care team, the breast care team and the primary health care team. Palliative care teams should consist of the palliative care consultant, palliative care nurse specialist, social worker, occupational therapist, physiotherapist and counsellor. A pain relief team and access to spiritual support whatever the patient's beliefs should also be available. If the patient has a strong religious faith she may derive great comfort from this. Religion may provide support and guidance for some people. Health care professionals should respect religious beliefs and be aware of the rituals and beliefs of patients of differing religions.

The patient should be assisted to remain in the place she wishes, whether this is her home, nursing home or hospice and should be able to choose where to die (NICE 2002a). Attendance at a day care facility, often at a hospice, can provide respite for carers. Complementary therapies, bathing, outings and creative therapies are usually on offer and may enable the patient to remain at home for longer.

Community nurses need to offer time, support and reliability to patients with advanced cancer. A contact number is given in case of problems arising outside the scheduled visit. Community nurses often offer a 24-hour service, which is accessed frequently as symptoms and anxieties tend to be exacerbated at night.

The patient should be assessed at home, needs identified, goals set and care planned. The patient's understanding of her disease is noted. The community nursing team may have very little input initially but can act as an advocate for the GP and can get to know the patient and family when more care is required (Langford 1995). The patient's condition may deteriorate rapidly with the progression of the disease. The care plan needs to be adaptable and change on a regular basis. All care is discussed with the patient and family. The Macmillan nurse is often accessed for advice on symptom control and both health professionals build up a close relationship with the family. The local hospice can be accessed by the patient and family via the Macmillan nurse for periods of short-term care to provide respite and symptom control. Ideally the patient should be helped by all the multidisciplinary team to remain at home to die wherever possible.

However, if the patient is unable to manage any longer at home or the symptoms cannot be managed in the community, the community or Macmillan nurse may need to facilitate the final transfer from home to hospice. Communication between the patient, family and professional carers is very important. Relatives are often reluctant to relinquish the patient, feeling perhaps that they have failed to care for her. Guilt, anger and fear may be displayed. Relatives can be encouraged that they will still be involved in the patient's care if they wish and be involved at all stages of decision making.

The patient in turn may feel fear, loneliness, anxiety and abandonment, which can lead to depression and fatigue. Anxiety will be felt over dying and how the family will cope. There is often a social worker attached to the palliative care team who can give advice and practical assistance on matters such as benefits, making a will, assistance with child care and practical help in the home. The social worker is usually attached to a hospice and will visit the family at home. Referral is usually through the breast care or palliative care nurse and the social worker can also provide counselling and bereavement care (Clark and McDermott 1995).

The issue of finances can cause anxiety and restlessness, the patient will probably want to conclude unfinished business and put her affairs in order. Once this is done and a will is made she may gain peace of mind that the family will be cared for.

(Hospice care and end of life issues are discussed in many excellent and more specialized texts.)

Conclusion

The wide variety of treatments can be confusing and the nurse needs to explain and support throughout. Each woman will have different needs. Treatment should be realistic and discussed at all stages. It is vital that quality of life issues are considered and the team needs to ensure that the patient has all the information necessary about treatments available in order to make an informed decision. The multidisciplinary team also need to ensure that she understands that time is limited.

It is difficult to ascertain where treatment ceases to be active and becomes palliative with symptom management necessary. Nurses and carers in the community need to be involved in care especially when it becomes palliative. District and community nurses can provide invaluable professional support to patients with recurrent breast cancer. However, many have not received any post-registration training in the principles. One of the commitments of the NHS Cancer Plan was to fund additional education for community nurses in the principles and practices of palliative care. Programmes are clinically focused and delivered locally. Cancer Networks nationwide are running the programme for their network, developing workshops on all aspects of palliative care and also on portfolios and clinical supervision/reflective practice (Department of Health 2002).

References

Barnett ML (1999) Hypercalcaemia. Seminars in Oncology Nursing 15: 190–201.

Breast Cancer Care online (2002) www.breastcancercare.org.uk/Breastcancer/Secondarybreastcancer/Secondarylivercancer (accessed August 2002).

Bredin M, Corner J, Krishnasamy, et al. (1999) Multicentre randomised controlled trial of nursing intervention for breathlessness in patients with lung cancer. British Medical Journal 3(318): 901–4.

British Association of Surgical Oncology (BASO) (1999) The management of metastatic bone disease in the United Kingdom. The Breast Speciality Group of the British Association of Surgical Oncology 25(1): 3–23.

Burnet K (2000) An overview of the management of recurrent breast cancer. International Journal of Palliative Nursing 6(7) 318–30.

Burnet K, Robinson L (2000) Psychosocial impact of recurrent cancer. European Journal of Oncology Nursing 4(1): 29–38.

Burstein HJ, Kuter I, Campas SM, et al. (2001) Clinical activity of trastuzamab and vinorelbine in women with HER2 over-expressing metastatic breast cancer. Journal of Clinical Oncology 19(10): 2722–30.

Bycroft L, Brown JG (1996) Care of the dying. In Tschudin V (Ed.) Nursing the Patient with Cancer. 2nd edn. Hemel Hempstead: Prentice Hall.

Cancer Bacup (2001) Trastuzumab (Herceptin). The Cancer Bacup Factsheet. London: Cancer Bacup.

Chapman DD, Goodman M (1997) Breast Cancer. In Groenwald SL, Goodman M, Frogge MH, et al. (eds) Cancer Nursing Principles and Practice, 4th edn. Sudbury, MA: Jones & Bartlett.

Clark J, McDermott M (1995) Nursing assessment. In Robbins J, Moscrop J (eds) Caring For the Dying Patient and the Family. London: Chapman & Hall.

Clive S, Gardiner J, Leonard RC (1999) Miltefosine as a topical treatment for cutaneous metastases in breast carcinoma. Cancer Chemotherapy & Pharmacology 44 (suppl): 529–30.

Cobleigh M, Charles LV, Tripathy D, et al. (1999) Multi-national study of the efficacy and safety of humanised anti-HER2 monoclonal antibody in women who have HER2 over-expressing metastatic breast cancer that has progressed after chemotherapy for metastatic disease. Journal of Clinical Oncology 17(9): 2639–48.

Colyer H (1996) Women's experiences of living with cancer. Journal of Advanced Nursing 23: 496–501.

Cooke T (2000) What is HER-2? European Journal of Oncology Nursing 4 (Suppl 1): 2–9.

Cox SE, Cruz PD Jr (1994) A spectrum of inflammatory metastases to skin via lymphatics: three cases of carcinoma erysipeloides. Journal of American Academy of Dermatology 30: 304–7.

Crippa F, Bombardieri E, Seregni E, et al. (1992) Single determination of CA15-3 bone scintigraphy in the diagnosis of skeletal metastases of breast cancer. Journal of Nuclear Biological Medicine 36: 52–5.

Department of Health (2002) Education and support for district nurses in principles and practice of palliative care – Sharing our practice. The NHS Cancer Plan. London: Department of Health.

De Wit R, Van Dam F, Hanneman M, et al. (1999) Evaluation of the use of a pain diary in chronic cancer pain patients at home. Pain 79(1): 89–99.

Diel IJ, Solomeyer EF, Costa SD, et al. (1998) Reduction in the new metastases in breast cancer with adjuvant clodronate treatment. New England Journal of Medicine 339: 357–62.

Doyle D (1996) Domiciliary Palliative Care: A Handbook for Family Doctors and Community Nurses. Oxford General Practice series. Oxford: Oxford University Press.

Farrer K (2001) Pain control. In Kinghorn S, Gamlin R (eds) Palliative Nursing: Bringing Comfort and Hope. London: Harcourt Publishers.

Faulkner E (1995) Importance of communications with the patient, family and professional carers. In Robbins J, Moscrop J (eds) Caring for the Dying Patient and the Family. London: Chapman & Hall.

Geisler J, King N, Anker G, et al. (1998) In vivo inhibition of aromatisation by exemestane, a novel irreversible aromatase inhibitor, in post-menopausal breast cancer patients. Clinical Cancer Research 4: 2089–93.

Genentech online (2002) Genentech: Products – Product Information – Breast Cancer Tumor Marker Testing. www.gene.com/gene/products/education/oncology/factsheet-tumormarkertest.jsp (accessed August 2002).

Graham J, Ramirez A, Love S, et al. (2002) Stressful life experiences and risk of relapse of breast cancer: observational cohort study. British Medical Journal 324: 1420–2.

Green P, Youill J (2001) Promoting comfort through surgery, chemotherapy and radiotherapy. In Kinghorn S, Gamlin R (eds) Palliative Nursing – Bringing Comfort and Hope. London: Harcourt Publishers.

Healthlink (1999) New Drug Tested Against Advanced Breast Cancer. www.healthlink.mcw.edu/article/943940081.html (accessed August 2002).

Honig SF (1996) Treatment of metastatic disease. In Harris JR, Lippman M, Morrow M, et al. (eds) Diseases of the Breast. 2nd edn. Philadelphia,PA: Lippincott Rowen.

Houston SJ, Rubens RD (1998) The tolerability and adverse event profile of pamidronate disodium. Reviews in Contemporary Pharmacotherapy 9: 213–24.

Imaginis (2001) www.imaginis.com/breasthealth/metastatic.asp (accessed August 2002).

Jacobs P (1999) Malignant spinal cord compression. Palliative Care Today 8(2): 20–2.

Langford L (1995) Care in the home. In Robbins J, Moscrop J (eds) Caring for the Dying Patient and the Family. London: Chapman & Hall.

Leonard RC, Rodger C, Dixon JM (1995) Metastatic breast cancer. In Dixon JM (Ed.) ABC of Breast Diseases. London: BMJ Publishing Group.

Lichter AS (1998) Breast cancer. In Lieber SA, Philips TL (eds) Textbook of Radiation Oncology. Philadelphia, PA: WB Saunders.

McCaffrey M, Ferrell BR (1997) Nurses' knowledge of pain assessment and management: how much progress have we made? Journal of Pain and Symptom Management 14(3): 175–88.

Mahon S, Casperson D (1997) Exploring the psychosocial meaning of recurrent cancer: a descriptive study. Cancer Nursing 20(3): 178–86.

National Cancer Institute online (2002a) Stage IV recurrent and metastatic breast cancer. www.nci.nih.gov/cancerinfo/pdq/treatment/breast/healthprofessional/#Section211

National Cancer Institute online (2002b) Capecitabine-Docetaxel combo improves survival in advanced breast cancer. www.cancer.gov/ClinicalTrials/results/capecitabine-combo0602

National Institute for Clinical Excellence (2002a) Guidance on Cancer Services. Improving Outcomes in Breast Cancer: Manual update August 2002. www.nice.org.uk/pdf/Improving_outcomes_breastcancer_manual.pdf (accessed September 2002).

National Institute for Clinical Excellence (2002b) A rapid and systematic review of the clinical effectiveness and cost-effectiveness of capecitabine (Xeloda) for metastatic breast cancer. www.nice.org.uk (accessed September 2002).

National Institute for Clinical Excellence (2002c) Press Release. NICE approves Trastumuzab (Herceptin) for advanced breast cancer. www.nice.org.uk/article.asp?a=29316

O'Shaughnessy J, Miles D, Vukelia S, et al. (2002) Superior survival with capecitabine plus docetaxel combination therapy in anthracycline pre-treated patients with advanced breast cancer: Phase III. Journal of Clinical Oncology 20(12): 2812–23.

Regnard CFB, Tempest S (1998) A Guide to Symptom Relief in Advanced Disease. 4th edn. Hale: Hochland and Hochland Ltd.

Richards MA, Smith IE (1995) Role of systemic treatment for primary operable breast cancer. In Dixon JM (Ed.) ABC of Breast Diseases. London: BMJ Publishing Group.

Roche Pharmaceuticals (2000) Summary of Product Characteristics. Herceptin. Welwyn Garden City: Roche Registration Ltd.

Roselli del Turco M, Palli D, Carridi A, et al. (1994) Intensive diagnostic follow-up after treatment of primary breast cancer: a randomised trial. National Research Council on breast cancer follow-up. Journal of the American Medical Association 271: 1593–7.

Rovelon P (2000) A practical guide to HER2 testing. European Journal of Oncology Nursing 4(Suppl 1): 18–23.

Royal Marsden Hospital (2002) New Breast Cancer Drug Shows Early Promise. www.royalmarsden.org/news/pressrelease/137.asp (accessed July 2002).

Sanders A (2002) Developments in breast cancer care. Cancer Nursing Practice. 1(1): 22–5.

Slamon D, Godolphin W, Jones LA, et al. (1989) Studies of the HER-2/neu proto-oncogene in human and ovarian breast cancer. Science 244: 707–12.

Thomson L (1996) Breast cancer. In Tschudin V (Ed.) Nursing the Patient with Cancer. 2nd edn. Hemel Hempstead: Prentice Hall.

Twycross R (1999) Introducing Palliative Care. 3rd edn. Oxford: Radcliffe Medical Press Ltd.

World Health Organisation (1996) Cancer Pain Relief: With A Guide To Opioid Availability. 2nd edn. Geneva: WHO.

CHAPTER SIXTEEN

Rare breast cancers

Breast cancer in men

Causes

Men can develop breast cancer in the small amount of breast tissue behind the nipple. The pathology is similar to female breast cancer with infiltrating ductal carcinoma being the most common type of tumour (Harris et al. 1997). Men can also develop Paget's disease and inflammatory carcinoma. Breast cancer in men is rare with about 200–250 per year diagnosed; there were 73 male breast cancer deaths in the UK in 1999 (Cancer Research Campaign 2001). It is more common in men over 60 years, with increasing age being the most important risk factor (Breast Cancer Care 2001a). Men who have had close members of their family affected by breast cancer, cancer of the colon or ovarian cancer can also be affected (Cancer Bacup 2001). The genetic link appears to be more common in men, with the BRCA2 gene most commonly associated with male breast cancer (Breast Cancer Care 2001a). Whereas the risk in women is five per cent, the risk of a man with the BRCA2 gene contracting breast cancer is 10–20 per cent.

Men who have been exposed to repeated radiation doses at a young age may be at increased risk. A genetic condition called Klinefelter's Syndrome where a man is born with an extra female chromosome will also result in an increased risk of breast cancer although the condition is rare (Breast Cancer Care 2001a). Men with Klinefelter's are 20 times more likely to develop breast cancer, possibly in both breasts.

The growth of breast tissue in older men can be stimulated by some diseases – usually those with a hormonal component such as chronic liver conditions and obesity which raises oestrogen levels – and some drugs, for example oestrogen preparations that are administered for cancer of the prostate (Donegan 1979). However, the effect of oestrogen for prostate cancer is small. Men having treatment for this may develop breast cancer as a secondary rather than a primary (Everson and Lippman 1979). Men with breast cancer tend to display abnormal patterns of hormone excretion and metabolism.

A study found that men employed in motor vehicle manufacturing, in blast furnaces, steel works and rolling mills appeared to have an increased risk of breast cancer and that the role of these workplace exposures should be further investigated (Cocco et al. 1998).

Ethnic factors may play a part. Eight white men per million are affected as opposed to 14 black men per million. The incidence may also be higher among Jewish men who have European ancestors (Fentiman 1998).

Signs and symptoms

Signs and symptoms are the same as in the female – a lump, a change in the size or shape of the breast, skin ulceration, inversion of the nipple or nipple discharge. There may also be fixation to the underlying tissues or skin. Often there is local spread before diagnosis due to the smallness of the breast – the nearby structures are readily invaded. Most are centrally located around the areola and may have access to the internal mammary lymph pathways, therefore spreading easily. A fine needle aspiration, biopsy, mammogram and ultrasound are used as in women. Tests such as chest X-ray, bone scan and liver ultrasound may be carried out to rule out metastases.

Treatment

Male breast cancer is treated in much the same way as in females. Surgery usually consists of a mastectomy as the amount of breast tissue is small. Axillary lymph nodes are likely to be removed.

Men have a small amount of oestrogen in their bloodstream. As the majority of breast cancers need oestrogen to grow, hormone therapy is very effective in reducing the amount in the body and is used to try to prevent recurrence. Tamoxifen is most commonly used and men may experience hot flushes, loss of libido and decreases in erections (Cancer Bacup 2001). Chemotherapy and radiotherapy are used in the same way as for female breast cancer. Orchidectomy may be considered as some patients respond but this may not be acceptable to many men (Peate 2001).

Support

Men may find difficulty accessing support and information when diagnosed with breast cancer as the condition is so rare. Men may feel angry, embarrassed, guilty, resentful, anxious and fearful. Many men are unaware that they can develop breast cancer and tend not to examine their breasts. Some may develop gynaecomastia (over-development of the breasts) and may think that this is a tumour (Peate 2001). Some may perceive it as a flaw in their masculinity and do not acknowledge it. Men in general are not comfortable discussing their health and may delay seeking help (Beare and Priddy 1999).

Loss of arm strength following a mastectomy can be incapacitating for a man whose work involves physical activity. Lymphoedema may develop, which will further impede activities of living.

The treatments can also be seen as a threat to their masculinity especially if taking feminizing hormones. As breast cancer is very much a female disease, a man may feel isolated as much of the information and support available is aimed at women (Peate 2001). Breast care nurses play a very important role in supporting these patients. The same physical and psychological support is required as for a woman but the nurse must be aware that the man's needs are different. Help with coping strategies is required for the patient and his family so that they can come to terms with his cancer and the treatments. The charity Breast Cancer Care has male volunteers staffing the telephone helpline if the patient does not wish to talk to a woman.

Nurses are also in the ideal position to address their patients' sexual problems. Limited information can probably be given but it is important to know when to refer on to a sexual therapist or other clinical nurse specialist when the problem is outside the scope of the breast care nurse (Peate 2001).

Pregnancy and breast cancer

Breast cancer is the most common cancer in pregnancy and in post-partum women, occurring in around 1 in 3000 pregnancies. The average age is between 32 and 38 years (Cancerweb – National Cancer Institute online 2002). Pregnant women with breast cancer are a small but significant group. Clinicians will probably see few cases.

Discrete masses may not be noticed due to the natural engorgement and tenderness of the breasts in pregnancy. The patient may assume that any changes are due to the pregnancy. Delays in diagnosis are common, averaging 5–15 months from the onset of symptoms (Gwyn and Theriault 2001). A pregnant woman has a 2.5-fold higher risk of being diagnosed with metastatic breast cancer and a decreased chance of being diagnosed with stage 1 (Zemlickis et al. 1992). Axillary lymph node metastases are more likely to be present. The prognosis by grade does not differ from that of non-pregnant women with the same grade.

Diagnostic procedures are very important to reduce the delay in diagnosis. Mammography can be used, with proper shielding it poses little threat of radiation exposure to the foetus (Barnavon and Wallack 1990). However, due to the changes in the breasts in pregnancy it is not always helpful. Therefore mammograms may not be carried out. Breast ultrasound is safe and accurate in differentiating solid tumours from cysts (Liberman et al. 1994). Fine needle aspiration could result in a false positive result due to the hyperproliferative state of the breast tissue in pregnancy.

Biopsy is essential as 25 per cent of mammograms in pregnancy may be negative. The pathologist should be advised of the patient's pregnancy (Novotny et al. 1991). Breast biopsy can be performed without risk to mother or baby although local problems such as infection, milk fistula and haematoma may occur due to hypervascularity and oedema of the breasts (Motherisk 2002).

About 60 per cent will be stages 1 and 2 so surgical treatment is usually a mastectomy to avoid radiotherapy. A lumpectomy with radiotherapy may provide radiation to the foetus but if the patient is near to term this can be delayed and carried out after delivery (Motherisk 2002). Stages 3 and 4 breast cancer will require chemotherapy following surgery and possibly radiotherapy for local control after delivery.

Chemotherapy can be given after the first trimester. The risk of malformations when chemotherapy is administered during the first trimester is estimated to be approximately 10 per cent for single agent chemotherapy and 25 per cent for combined (Berry et al. 1999). There is no evidence of increased risk of foetal malformation during the 2nd and 3rd trimesters. However, the long-term effects remain largely unknown. There have been reports of low birth weight and increased risk of stillbirth (Zemlickis et al. 1996). Delivery of the child should be timed to avoid the chemotherapy low points and associated problems (Motherisk 2002). Tamoxifen is not recommended until after the baby is born as its safety during pregnancy is still being questioned.

Lactation should be suppressed to decrease the vascularity and size of the breasts. Women receiving chemotherapy should not breastfeed (Cancerweb – National Cancer Institute online 2002). Any radiotherapy to the breast prior to pregnancy would mean that the treated breast would be unlikely to produce much milk. After a mastectomy the remaining breast would still produce milk, possibly more to compensate (Breast Cancer Care 2001b).

Pregnancy has a dual effect on the risk of breast cancer. The risk after childbirth is transiently increased but the risk is reduced in later years. This could be because pregnancy increases the short-term risk by stimulating the growth of cells that have undergone the early stages of malignant transformation but differentiates normal mammary stem cells that are potentially likely to change, thereby conferring long-term protection (Lambe et al. 1994).

Many specialists advise women to wait two years after a diagnosis of breast cancer before becoming pregnant as this is the most likely time that it will recur. There does not appear to be any extra risk of breast cancer recurring if pregnancy occurs (Breast Cancer Care 2001b). Breast cancer is not thought to affect the baby's development and cancer cannot be passed on. There is also no evidence that the child would develop cancer in later life due to the mother's breast cancer.

Termination is not thought to have any effect on breast cancer and is not a therapeutic option. However, the patient may consider this if chemotherapy and radiotherapy options are severely limited by continuing the pregnancy (Giacalone et al. 1999). Termination may only be recommended if it is necessary to administer chemotherapy during the first trimester. Also, a termination may be considered if the breast cancer is progressing rapidly and has spread to other body parts. The decision is very difficult and the patient needs to discuss it fully with the specialist breast care team and the obstetrician.

It is devastating for patients who discover that they have breast cancer at a time when they should be happy and hopeful for the future. A cancer diagnosis will have a major impact on the experience of giving birth. It may be difficult to cope with caring for a new baby and recovering from breast surgery and the treatment's side effects. Also the decision to terminate can give rise to feelings of helplessness and grief as well as the fear, shock and anxiety of a cancer diagnosis.

The team of surgeon, oncologist, breast care nurse, obstetrician and midwife should all work together to ensure that the patient receives the best support and treatment. The patient with pregnancy-associated breast cancer is undergoing two life-changing events simultaneously. The multidisciplinary team are facing a unique set of problems – cancer care, maternity care and possible psychological morbidity. The breast cancer diagnosis will impact on the family and on child care issues. It may be helpful to put the patient in touch with another who has been in a similar situation, either one to one or in a support group (Breast Cancer Care 2001b).

At the moment, women who have undergone IVF treatment do not appear to be at any greater risk than the general population.

References

Barnavon Y, Wallack MK (1990) Management of pregnant patients with carcinoma of the breast. Surgery, Gynaecology and Obstetrics 171(4): 347–52.

Beare H, Priddy N (1999) The Cancer Guide for Men. Guildford: Sheldon Press.

Berry DL, Teriault RL, Holmes FA, et al. (1999) Management of breast cancer during pregnancy using a standardised protocol. Journal of Clinical Oncology 17: 855–61.

Breast Cancer Care (2001a) Male Breast Cancer. Factsheet 2. www.breastcancercare. org.uk/breastcancer/diagnosis/malebreastcancer (accessed May 2002).

Breast Cancer Care (2001b) Breast Cancer and Pregnancy. Factsheet 13. London: Breast Cancer Care.

Cancer Bacup (2001) Male Breast Cancer. www.cancerbacup.org.uk (accessed May 2002).

Cancer Research Campaign (2001) Cancerstats: Mortality – UK. London: Cancer Research Campaign.

Cancerweb – National Cancer Institute online (2002) Breast Cancer and Pregnancy. cancerweb.ncl.ac.uk/cancernet/105380.html

Cocco P, Figgs L, Dosemeci M, et al. (1998) Case control study of occupational exposures and male breast cancer. Occupational and Environmental Medicine 55(9): 599–604.

Donegan WL (1979) Cancer of the male breast. In Donegan WL, Spratt JS (eds) Cancer of the Breast. Philadelphia, PA: WB Saunders Co.

Everson RB, Lippman ME (1979) Male breast cancer. In Williams L. Maguire (Ed.) Breast Cancer, vol. 3. New York: Plenum.

Fentiman IS (1998) Detection and Treatment of Breast Cancer. 2nd edn. London: Martin Dunitz.

Florica JV (1994) Breast cancer and pregnancy. Obstet. & Gynae. Clinic of N. America 2: 721–32.

Giacalone PL, Laffargine F, Benos P (1999) Chemotherapy for breast carcinoma during pregnancy. A French national survey. Cancer 86(11): 2266–72.

Gwyn K, Theriault R (2001) Breast cancer during pregnancy. Oncology. (Huntingdon NY) 15(1): 39–46.

Harris J, Morrow M, Norton L (1997) Malignant tumors of the breast. In DeVita VTJ, Hellman S, Rosenberg SA (eds) Cancer: Principles and Practice of Oncology. 5th edn. Philadelphia, PA: Lippincott-Raven Pub.

Lambe M, Hsieh C, Trichopoulios D, et al. (1994) Transient increase in the risk of breast cancer after giving birth. New England Journal of Medicine 331(1): 5–9.

Liberman L, Giess CA, Dershaw DD, et al. (1994) Imaging of pregnancy associated breast cancer. Radiology 191(1): 245–8.

Motherisk (2002) Breast Cancer and Pregnancy. www.motherisk.org/cancer/ index.php?content_id=200&name=Breast%20Cancer%20in%20Pregnancy (accessed May 2002).

Novotny DB, Maygarden SJ, Shermer RW, et al. (1991) Fine needle aspiration of benign and malignant breast masses associated with pregnancy. Acta Cytologica 35(6): 676–86.

Peate I (2001) Caring for men with breast cancer: causes, symptoms and treatment. British Journal of Nursing 10(15): 975–81.

Zemlickis D, Lishner M, Degendorfer P, et al. (1992) Maternal and fetal outcome after breast cancer in pregnancy. American Journal of Obstetrics and Gynaecology 166: 781–7.

Zemlickis D, Lishner M, Koren G (1996) Review of fetal effects of cancer chemotherapeutic agents. In Koren G, Lishner M, Farine D (eds) Cancer in Pregnancy. Cambridge: Cambridge University Press.

Useful websites

Breakthrough Breast Cancer: www.breakthrough.org.uk
An organization which researches breast cancer and raises awareness.

Breast Cancer Care: www.breastcancercare.org.uk
Information on every aspect of breast cancer for patients and health care professionals.

Breast Care Campaign: www.breastcare.co.uk
Information on all aspects of benign breast disease.

Breast Doctor: www.breastdoctor.com
A US website offering clear information about breast disease for patients.

British Lymphology Society: www.lymphoedema.org/bls
Information for patients, carers and health care professionals about lymphoedema.

CancerBACUP: www.cancerbacup.org.uk
The leading cancer information service in the UK.

Cancer Research UK: www.cancerresearchuk.org or www.cancerhelp.org.uk
Formed by the amalgamation of the Imperial Cancer Research Fund and the Cancer Research Campaign. Information on all aspects of cancer and research into the disease.

Imaginis. The Breast Health Specialists: www.imaginis.com
A US website specializing in breast cancer.

Lymphoedema Support Network: www.lymphoedema.org/lsn
Information and support for patients with lymphoedema. The network
aims to encourage uniform and high standards of care and treatment for
lymphoedema.

Macmillan Cancer Relief: www.macmillan.org.uk
A charity which supports patients and carers and also assists in funding specialist cancer nursing posts.

National Cancer Institute: www.nci.nih.gov
A US Government website covering cancer nursing and research.

Oncolink – Abramson Cancer Center of the University of Pennsylvania:
www.oncolink.com
A US website covering all aspects of cancer.

UK National Electronic Library for Health: www.nelh.nhs.uk
The NHS UK information site.

Index